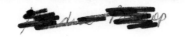

Clinical Management of Voice Disorders

Clinical Management
of Voice Disorders

SECOND EDITION

JAMES L. CASE

pro·ed

8700 Shoal Creek Boulevard
Austin, Texas 78758

Printed in the United States of America

Library of Congress Cataloging-in-Publication Data

Case, James L.
    Clinical management of voice disorders / James L. Case. — 2nd ed.
        p.   cm.
    Includes bibliographical references and index.
    ISBN 0-89079-425-1
    1. Voice disorders—Treatment. 2. Speech therapy. I. Title.
    [DNLM: 1. Voice Disorders—therapy.   WV 500 C337c]
    RF510.C37   1990
    616.85'5—dc20
    DNLM/DLC
    for Library of Congress   90-14313
                                                                          CIP

pro·ed
8700 Shoal Creek Boulevard
Austin, Texas 78758

1 2 3 4 5 6 7 8 9 10   96 95 94 93 92 91

Dedication

T his book is dedicated to many individuals: the many voice-disordered persons with whom I have worked and from whom I learned so much about clinical management, the many graduate students personally taught, and the special mentors who taught me while I was learning as a graduate student.

The book is especially dedicated to my wife, Diane; my children, Jeff, Brian, Darren, and Christy; my beautiful daughters-in-law, Rebecca and Leigh; my son-in-law, Damon; and my granddaughters, Tamra and Erica, whose voices are an inspiration to me.

James L. Case

Contents

Preface / xi

1   Anatomy and Physiology of Phonation / 1
VOCAL TRACT ANATOMY AND PHYSIOLOGY / 2
ANATOMY AND PHYSIOLOGY OF THE LARYNX / 10
MEMBRANES OF THE LARYNX / 18
THE VOCAL FOLDS / 18
PHONATION THEORY / 22
THE PHASES OF PHONATION / 23
SPECIFIC CHARACTERISTICS OF VOICE / 24
AGE AND SEX DIFFERENCES IN THE VOICE / 32
THE AGING VOICE / 33
ELECTROMYOGRAPHIC DATA ON VOICE PHYSIOLOGY / 35
SUMMARY / 37

2   Medical Aspects of Voice Disorders / 39
MEDICAL SPECIALTIES IN VOICE DISORDER / 40
MEDICAL PROCEDURES IN VOICE DISORDER / 43
DRUG TREATMENT IN VOICE DISORDER / 50
SURGERY AND THE VOICE PATIENT / 51
SUMMARY / 54

3 Evaluation Procedures in Voice Management / 55
MEDICAL REFERRAL / 56
SCREENING AND IDENTIFICATION / 58
THE CASE HISTORY / 60
EVALUATION OF SPECIFIC VOICE PARAMETERS / 63
VOCAL QUALITY / 71
COMBINATION OF FACTORS IN DYSPHONIA / 74
INSTRUMENTATION IN VOICE QUALITY EVALUATION / 77
INSTRUMENTATION FOR LOUDNESS MEASUREMENT / 79
INSTRUMENTATION FOR RESONANCE EVALUATION / 80
INSTRUMENTATION FOR RESPIRATION MEASUREMENT / 80
MAXIMUM PHONATION DURATION / 83
PERCEPTUAL RATING SCALES / 85
CASE EXAMPLE OF VOICE EVALUATION / 90
SUMMARY / 92

4 Voice Disorder from Vocal Abuse / 93
VOCAL NODULES / 94
VOICE CHARACTERISTICS WITH NODULES / 96
ETIOLOGY OF VOCAL NODULES / 98
EVALUATION AND THERAPY PROCEDURES IN VOCAL NODULES / 116
PHONOSURGERY FOR VOCAL NODULES / 131
CASE EXAMPLE OF POOR SURGICAL MANAGEMENT / 133
CASE EXAMPLE OF VOCAL NODULES MANAGEMENT / 135
SUMMARY: VOCAL NODULES / 137
CONTACT ULCERS / 138
VOICE CHARACTERISTICS / 138
SPECIFIC ETIOLOGIES / 140
EVALUATION PROCEDURES / 141
THERAPY FOR CONTACT ULCERS / 143
CASE EXAMPLE OF CONTACT ULCERS / 145
SUMMARY: CONTACT ULCERS / 148

5 Neurogenic Voice Disorders / 149
INNERVATION OF LARYNGEAL STRUCTURES / 150
DISORDERS IN CHILDREN AND ADULTS / 152
VAGUS NERVE LESIONS / 153
CASE EXAMPLE OF LARYNGEAL NERVE PARALYSIS / 155
LESION OF SUPERIOR LARYNGEAL NERVE / 156
ETIOLOGIES OF VAGUS NERVE LESIONS / 157
MEDICAL TREATMENT OF LARYNGEAL PARALYSIS / 158
CNS/PNS LESIONS AND DYSARTHRIA / 163

DYSTONIA / 164
PARKINSONISM / 165
AMYOTROPHIC LATERAL SCLEROSIS / 166
MULTIPLE SCLEROSIS / 168
MYASTHENIA GRAVIS / 169
MISCELLANEOUS CENTRAL DYSARTHRIAS / 170
SPASTIC (SPASMODIC) DYSPHONIA / 173
ABDUCTOR SPASTIC (SPASMODIC) DYSPHONIA / 177
TREATMENT FOR NEUROGENIC VOICE DISORDER / 179
CASE EXAMPLE OF HYPERFUNCTIONAL DISORDER / 183
SUMMARY / 185

6 Psychogenic (Nonorganic) Voice Disorders / 187
VOCAL SYMPTOMS OF PSYCHOGENIC DISORDER / 189
PHYSIOLOGICAL SPEECH CHANGES UNDER STRESS / 190
CASE EXAMPLES OF PSYCHOGENIC VOICE DISORDER / 192
APHONIA (CONVERSION) / 194
EVALUATION PROCEDURES / 199
THERAPY PROCEDURES / 201
CASE EXAMPLE OF APHONIA TREATMENT / 203
THERAPY FOR CONVERSION DYSPHONIA / 204
VOCAL ABUSE AS A PSYCHOGENIC DISORDER / 207
PUBERPHONIA (MUTATIONAL FALSETTO) / 207
MANAGEMENT PROCEDURES IN PUBERPHONIA / 213
A CASE EXAMPLE OF PUBERPHONIA / 214
SPECIAL CONSIDERATIONS IN PUBERPHONIA / 216
LITERATURE REVIEW IN PUBERPHONIA / 217
ORGANIC MUTATIONAL FALSETTO / 218
TRANSSEXUAL VOICE DISORDER / 219
STAGE FRIGHT / 222
THE SPEECH–LANGUAGE PATHOLOGIST AND THE PSYCHOLOGY
OF VOICE / 222
SUMMARY / 224

7 Alaryngeal Phonation Therapy / 225
THE NATURE OF CANCER IN THE LARYNX / 226
TREATMENT OF LARYNGEAL CANCER / 230
EXTRINSIC METHODS OF ALARYNGEAL PHONATION / 232
INTRINSIC METHODS OF ALARYNGEAL PHONATION / 235
ESOPHAGEAL SOUND MECHANISMS / 238
METHODS OF AIR INTAKE / 238
AIR RESERVOIR (NEOLUNG) / 241

NATURE OF THE VIBRATOR / 241
PERCEPTUAL AND ACOUSTIC CHARACTERISTICS / 242
REHABILITATION OF LARYNGECTOMIZED PERSONS / 247
GOAL OF FUNCTIONAL ESOPHAGEAL SPEECH / 258
CASE EXAMPLE OF ALARYNGEAL PHONATION / 259
ADDITIONAL METHODS OF REHABILITATION / 260
CHALLENGES IN LARYNGECTOMEE REHABILITATION / 267
SUMMARY / 268

8 *Resonance and Miscellaneous Disorders* / 269
DISORDERS OF RESONANCE / 270
HYPERNASALITY / 270
TREATMENT OF HYPERNASALITY DISORDERS / 277
VOICE THERAPY FOR HYPERNASALITY / 284
HYPONASALITY / 289
VELOPHARYNGEAL EXAMINATION / 294
VOICES OF THE HEARING IMPAIRED AND DEAF / 295
MISCELLANEOUS DISORDERS OF VOICE / 298
AIDS AND THE SPEECH–LANGUAGE PATHOLOGIST / 305
SUMMARY / 305

References / 307

Author Index / 331

Subject Index / 341

Preface

Professionals who daily manage persons with voice disorders are challenged by the many aspects of this area of communication dysfunction. Persons with voice disorder range from a simple case of laryngitis that usually is resolved spontaneously by time and body healing, to a life-threatening condition such as laryngeal cancer. Between these extremes the speech–language pathologist is challenged by numerous organic, psychogenic, and functional voice disorders. To manage these clients successfully requires great skill on the speech–language pathologist's part, along with the cooperation of many other professionals, primarily from the medical field.

Although this book is intended primarily for speech–language pathologists, other professionals will find it helpful as a reference as to their role in voice management. It is designed to provide comprehensive coverage of the many clinical aspects of voice disorder.

I recognize that several less common voice disorders are not discussed. References are provided, however, to guide the reader to obtain information on the clinical management of such disorders.

Chapter 1 deals with normal aspects of laryngeal and voice function, including the anatomy and physiology of laryngeal and vocal tract structures. Specific characteristics of voice, such as pitch, loudness, voice quality, and resonance, are described, as are age and sex characteristics. The instrumentation that has helped clarify the inner workings of the larynx, particularly electromyography, is discussed.

Chapter 2 is directed specifically toward medical aspects of voice treatment. Medical specialties, medical procedures of evaluation and treatment, information regarding common drug usage, and some common surgical techniques are covered.

Chapter 3 presents the general procedures involved in the evaluation of persons with voice disorder without respect to etiology. Principles of taking a good case history, and of evaluating laryngeal parameters of pitch, loudness, and voice quality, are covered. Both instrumental and perceptual evaluation procedures are discussed, along with a case example of a voice evaluation.

Chapter 4 studies the broad aspect of vocal abuse that is so common in society. The disorders of vocal nodules and contact ulcers, including details of significant etiological, symptomatic, evaluative, and treatment aspects, are provided. This chapter contains a checklist that provides a practical guide to identification of most specific forms of vocal abuse, as well as a description of each abuse form. A case example discusses management of both vocal nodules and contact ulcers.

In Chapter 5 on neurogenic disorders, I had trouble determining what to include and what to omit. Entire books could have been written on many of the topics in this book, particularly neurogenic disorders. A review of general aspects of this problem lays the foundation for understanding the many neurogenic voice disorders. Several specific disorders of the nervous system that have laryngeal and voice sequelae are analyzed. Many forms of dysarthria are omitted, but the more common ones are discussed. There is considerable detail on the controversial disorder of adductor spastic dysphonia, which I believe to be essentially neurogenic in etiology.

Chapter 6 covers the varied aspects of psychogenic or nonorganic voice disorder. One unique aspect of this chapter is the section of physiological changes in the speech system that occur under stress and emotional states. The American Psychiatric Association's list of all mental disorders is accompanied by a discussion of those that affect the voice. Conversion aphonia, dysphonia, puberphonia (mutational falsetto), and transsexual voice change are covered.

Chapter 7 includes a description of medical aspects of laryngeal cancer, with special emphasis on the speech–language pathologist's role in the rehabilitation of persons who have been laryngectomized. Details of the usage of intrinsic and extrinsic forms of alaryngeal phonation are supplemented by a case example on alaryngeal management. Considerable detail on prosthetic devices for alaryngeal phonation is provided.

Chapter 8 serves two main functions: (1) it provides background for the management of persons with the resonance disorders of hypernasality and hyponasality, and (2) it provides a forum for discussion of miscellaneous disorders of voice that do not fit in previous chapters. These miscellaneous disorders include the vocal quality of hearing-impaired persons, papillomatosis, ventricular dysphonia, laryngeal webs, and other less commonly observed disorders.

Although significant and recent references are included, information processing is sufficiently rapid that readers will need to augment it from even more current literature. However, the references will help readers fill gaps of information not provided directly in the text.

1

Anatomy and Physiology of Phonation

Any chapter titled "Anatomy and Physiology of Phonation" is likely to generate as much enthusiasm as is experienced by the prisoner on death row about to "enjoy" a last meal. It is simply something that must be endured before the real excitement begins. It might be asked whether it is necessary to know "that stuff" in such pedantic detail. Of course, some individuals actually become excited about the details of muscle origin, insertion, course, and function, or the manner in which anatomical processes are related to each other (notwithstanding that such a person is likely to be the anatomy professor in the university training program). Others might think, "Who cares?"

Every book on voice disorder contains the ominous anatomy and physiology chapter, and it usually is the first one. Is this necessary? Can the author instead simply refer readers to other references on the subject and proceed to the essence of the book without the burden of all that anatomy and physiology? After all, how much can the body change from year to year to justify such duplication? Although I contemplated referring readers to other sources, I quickly rejected the idea. Why?

Anatomy and physiology do not change significantly by evolutionary processes from year to year or even from decade to decade. George Washington's laryngeal functions probably were the same as those of the current president of the United States—and everyone else as well. What is changing from decade to decade, year to year, and even month to month, however, is the understanding of the details involved.

Anatomy and physiology do not constitute a static science. This is evidenced by the fact that the physiology book used as the primary reference for this chapter in the first edition (Stevens & Hirano, 1981) has been supplanted by others published a few years later (Baken, 1987; Bless & Abbs, 1983). Both contain contributions from many of the same investigators, but data and information appear in the latter references that are not contained in the former. This is also true of additional references used for this second edition.

Science moves forward, but the presses must roll. Such a dilemma is faced by every author of a reference book. When does one stop reading and begin writing? No book can remain a current source. Readers must try to remain informed of the recent advances in knowledge about vocal anatomy and physiology, as well as review factors that appear constant or at least have not been changed by contemporary investigation.

Because most readers probably are familiar with the information presented in Chapter 1 from their basic anatomy and physiology courses, this chapter is intended as a review of the highlights.

The birth of a human infant usually is signaled by a loud cry. That cry constitutes the infant's first attempt to signal its presence in the world and, in a basic sense, to establish communication, as if to say, "I am here. Please take note of my existence." Although the birth cry is reflexive and unlearned, the anatomical and physiological functions of the structures involved are extremely complex. The birth cry could be considered the first stage of speech and language development since it is the first time the infant uses biological structures in the nonbiological function of voice in communication.

The technical term for voice production is phonation. It is a process of sound generation that occurs when air exhaled from the lungs is interrupted by the closed vocal folds. As exhaled air is forced through the trachea, pressure is increased below the closed vocal folds, setting them into vibration and producing a sound wave. The sound produced by the vibrating vocal folds is resonated in the chambers above and shaped into the sounds of the particular language being spoken.

Vocal Tract Anatomy and Physiology

The vocal folds are housed in a complex valving structure called the larynx, which is situated immediately above the trachea. The larynx as a sound generator of voice constitutes the inferior or lowest structure in the human vocal tract. Figure 1–1 shows a sagittal section through the human head and neck

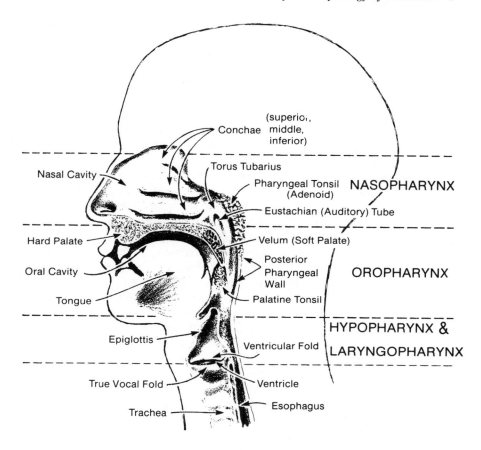

Figure 1–1 The Human Vocal Tract.

regions demonstrating the structures that comprise the vocal tract. In a biological sense, the vocal tract also could be labeled the upper respiratory tract or part of the upper digestive tract, depending on which function is being studied: respiration (breathing) or deglutition (mastication and swallowing). The vocal tract is composed of regions called the nasal cavity, oral cavity, and pharyngeal cavities (nasopharynx, oropharynx, and laryngopharynx).

The Nasal Cavity

The most superior aspect of the vocal tract is the nasal cavity. Its superior borders are formed by the bones that form the cranial floor, the lateral margins by the nasal turbinates (conchae), the anterior aspect by nasal bones and alar cartilage of the external nose, the floor by the bony hard and muscular soft palates, and the posterior border by the posterior pharyngeal wall.

The pharyngeal orifice for each auditory (eustachian) tube is located on each lateral and somewhat posterior wall of the nasal cavity. This auditory tube connects the nasopharynx with the middle ear to maintain pressure equilibrium between the middle ear space and the external atmosphere. The auditory tube orifice is bounded by a cartilage called the torus tubarius. Also in the posterior nasopharynx is the mass of lymphoid tissue called the pharyngeal tonsils or adenoids.

Biologically, the nasal cavity contains the sensory end organs from the bulbs of the olfactory nerve (cranial nerve I) for the sense of smell. Also, during inhalation, the nasal cavity warms, moistens, and filters air. The nasal turbinates (conchae) provide an extensive surface in the nasal cavity for the accomplishment of these biological tasks.

In speech, the nasal cavity functions as a resonator when coupled to the oral and pharyngeal cavities. This coupling process occurs at the velopharyngeal port, which is located at the posterior entrance to the nasal cavity. (This process is discussed in detail later in this chapter.) Essentially, the nasal cavity is completely separated from other cavities during the production of all speech sounds in English except the nasal consonants /m/, /n/, and /ŋ/.

The Oral Cavity

The oral cavity is bounded anteriorly by the lips, anteriorly and laterally by the maxillary and mandibular dental arches, superiorly by the hard and soft palates, posteriorly by the faucial pillars and the posterior pharyngeal wall, and inferiorly by the muscular structures of the mandibular cavity and the tongue. The oral cavity is variable in its dimensions because of the movement potential of the tongue, lips, and oropharyngeal structures. In speech, the oral cavity functions as a resonator of sound produced by the larynx, and the structures contained in it serve as articulators to shape sounds into specific vowels and consonants. Biologically, the oral cavity functions in the mastication and swallowing of food and liquid.

The Pharyngeal Cavity

The pharyngeal cavity extends from the base of the skull to the lower aspect of the larynx at approximately the level of cervical vertebra number six. It is formed in a major sense by the three constrictor muscles (superior, middle, and inferior) that constitute a muscular tube or passageway from the nasal and oral cavities down to the opening to the larynx and esophagus. This passageway connects the oral and nasal cavities with the larynx, trachea, and lungs during respiration, as well as the esophagus during deglutition. In speech, the pharyngeal cavity acts as a resonating cavity and forms the posterior and lateral borders of the vocal tract. The pharyngeal cavity is divided anatomically into the nasopharynx, oropharynx, and laryngopharynx as it connects these three cavities.

Velopharyngeal Mechanisms. From a voice production standpoint, one of the most important mechanisms for resonance management in the vocal tract occurs at the velopharyngeal port. The soft palate or velum is a musculature extension from the bony hard palate that either separates or couples the oral and nasal cavities. During breathing, the velopharyngeal port is open, allowing air to be drawn into and forced out through the nasal cavity. This port also is open during the articulation of the nasal consonants /m/, /n/, and /ŋ/. During deglutition and the production of all other English consonants, the velopharyngeal port essentially is closed.

The mechanisms involved in velopharyngeal closure are complex, involving different patterns and muscle groupings for deglutition and speech. The muscles include the superior constrictor, levator veli palatini, palatoglossus, palatopharyngeus, and uvulus. Three additional muscles have origin and insertion in the area but are not directly involved in regulating the velopharynx: tensor veli palatini, stylopharyngeus, and salpingopharyngeus. Of these three, the tensor veli palatini has received the most attention in the literature.

Superior Constrictor. The paired superior constrictor (Figure 1–2) originates from the general area of the pterygoid hamulus of the sphenoid bone and a raphe (tendon) that connects the pterygoid hamulus with the mandible (pterygomandibular raphe). The course of the muscle is on a horizontal plane in a posterior and then medial direction to insert into the midline pharyngeal raphe. At this raphe, the fibers from the left constrictor connect to those from the right side. Upon contraction, the superior constrictor decreases the cross-sectional space of the upper pharynx. Below the superior constrictor are the middle and inferior constrictors that complete the ring of muscles forming the bulk of the pharynx.

Levator Veli Palatini. The levator veli palatini is a paired muscle that forms the bulk of the musculature of the velum (Figure 1–3). From a complex origin on the petrous portion of the temporal bone and lateral and posterior to the torus tubarius (the cartilage of the auditory tube), this muscle courses downward, medialward, and slightly anteriorly to enter the velum. As the muscle enters and forms the bulk of the velum, the fibers fan out as they approach the midline. At midline, the fibers from the right side join with those from the left. This muscle forms a sling, lifting the velum upward and posteriorly

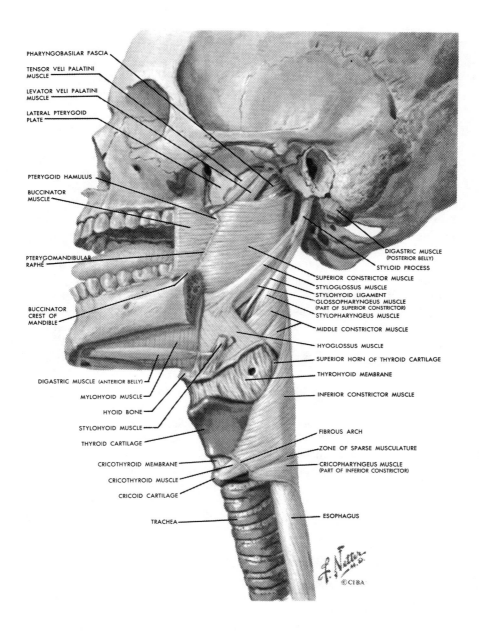

Figure 1–2 Pharynx Musculature. Copyright 1959 CIBA-GEIGY Corporation. Reproduced with permission from *The CIBA Collection of Medical Illustrations* (p. 22) by Frank H. Netter, MD. All rights reserved.

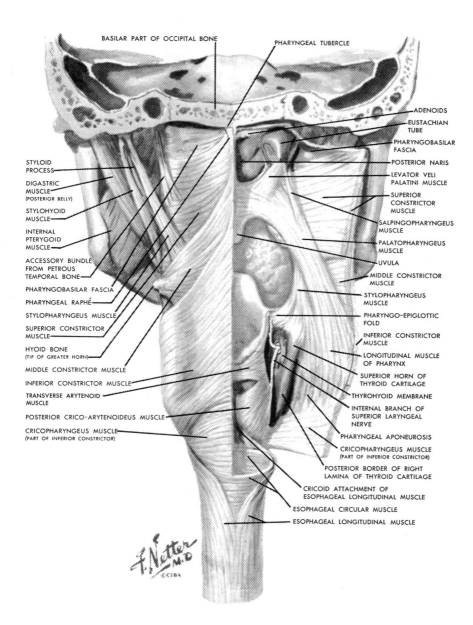

Figure 1–3 Velopharyngeal Musculature. Copyright 1959 CIBA-GEIGY Corporation. Reproduced with permission from *The CIBA Collection of Medical Illustrations* (p. 23) by Frank H. Netter, MD. All rights reserved.

toward the cranial base and against the superior constrictor area of the posterior pharyngeal wall.

Palatoglossus.   The palatoglossus is a paired muscle that influences the velum in a downward direction. It also can be considered a muscle that lifts the posterior and lateral margins of the tongue. It extends from the lateral margins of the velum in a downward and slightly anterior direction to insert into the tongue. The muscular basis of the anterior faucial pillar is formed by this muscle. During velopharyngeal closure, the palatoglossus is passive.

Palatopharyngeus.   The palatopharyngeus is a paired muscle that can be considered a muscle of either the pharynx or the velum. It originates in the velum and courses in an inferior direction to form the muscular basis of the posterior faucial pillar. Some fibers of this muscle integrate with muscle fibers of the superior constrictor. Although not active in velopharyngeal closure, the palatopharyngeus can function to depress the velum, constrict the pharynx, or even elevate the pharynx during swallowing.

Uvulus.   The uvulus muscle also is paired and forms the longitudinal midline of the velum. It originates on the posterior nasal spine, a bony projection from the horizontal plates of the palatine bone that form the posterior portion of the hard palate. The uvulus courses posteriorly and then inferiorly along the superior aspect of the velum to terminate and form the bulk of the uvula. The uvulus muscle has been found to be more important in velopharyngeal closure than previously described (Zemlin, 1988) by adding bulk to the portion of the velum that is most directly involved in closure (D. R. Dickson & W. M. Dickson, 1982). The uvulus also can shorten the velum upon contraction.

Tensor Veli Palatini.   The tensor veli palatini is a paired muscle of the velum that originates from the base of the skull generally at the medial pterygoid plate and surrounding structures. The muscle courses vertically in an inferior direction, ending as a tendinous connection around the hamulus of the medial pterygoid plate. From this hamulus, the tensor becomes a fibrous sheet of connective tissue entering the velum. Some of the fibers attach to the posterior border of the bony palate, whereas others become continuous with fibers from the opposite side of the velum.

The tensor muscle functions more to open the normally collapsed auditory tube for middle ear ventilation than any activity during velopharyngeal closure.

Patterns of Velopharyngeal Closure

Examination of velopharyngeal closure processes from several angles (lateral, anterior, superior, and multiview projection), as well as by several different methods (lateral radiography, tomography, baseview projection, endoscopy, and ultrasound), seems to indicate clearly that velopharyngeal closure is accomplished by the synergistic involvement of several muscles when swallowing and speech are considered. The bulk of velar lifting is accomplished by the levator veli palatini. The mass of velar muscle is lifted upward and slightly posteriorly by action of this muscle.

Evidence seems to be contradictory regarding the involvement of the superior constrictor in velopharyngeal closure. Skolnick, McCall, and Barnes (1973) described velopharyngeal closure as a sphincteric process in which the velar musculature and the superior constrictor progressively narrow the velopharyngeal port until it is obliterated. D. R. Dickson and Dickson (1972) contended that the mesial movement of the lateral pharyngeal walls in closure is a passive result of the movement of the tori tubari and the salpingopharyngeal folds medially and posteriorly against the velum, and not a function of superior constrictor contraction. This statement was not repeated in their 1982 book (D. R. Dickson & Dickson, 1982), in which they asserted that velopharyngeal closure mechanisms for swallowing involve the levator veli palatini and superior constrictor contraction and speech velopharyngeal closure resulting from levator and uvulus contraction only.

There is little disagreement that lateral wall movement is an important part of the velopharyngeal valving process (Zagzebski, 1975), and that the process appears as essentially sphincterical in nature (Figure 1–4). It is merely the anatomical mechanisms of closure that appear controversial. Electromyographic (EMG) measurement of direct muscle activity provides important information regarding the muscular processes of velopharyngeal closure. Bell-Berti

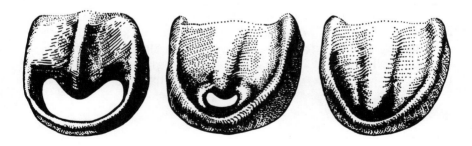

Sphincteric closure of velopharyngeal portal in a normal subject seen from base view. Left: portal at rest. Middle: portal during partial closure (note that a coronal pattern is developing as velum moves posteriorly and pharyngeal walls contract centrally. Right: full closure has occurred, producing coronally oriented slit.

Figure 1–4 Velopharyngeal Closure. Reprinted with permission from *"The Sphincteric Mechanisms of Velopharyngeal Closure"* by M. L. Skolnick, G. N. McCall, & M. Barnes, 1973, *The Cleft Palate Journal, 10*, p. 288.

(1976) obtained EMG recordings from the levator veli palatini, superior constrictor, middle constrictor, palatoglossus, and palatopharyngeus muscles of three normal speakers of American English. The levator palatini was found to be the primary muscle of velopharyngeal closure for each of the subjects. Other findings regarding the role of the palatopharyngeus and constrictors were less consistent.

Obtaining clear patterns of velopharyngeal closure has been difficult when only small numbers of subjects have been studied by electromyography. The hook-wired technique of inserting an electrode into the muscle tissue remains highly experimental and has been done on only small numbers of subjects, often members of the research team. Given the state of knowledge of variation in patterns of closure in males and females (McKerns & Bzoch, 1970), as well as other variables, caution must be used in interpreting the results of research not involving large samples and control of independent variables that traditionally have been shown to influence velopharyngeal closure.

The normal function of velopharyngeal closure is very complex. For example, when a person with normal closure says, "I'll paint it," the soft palate or velum is closed for all sounds until the /n/ in "paint." The brain sends messages via the nerves innervating closure directing the closure muscles to relax. This allows rapid opening of the velopharyngeal port and nasal resonation to occur on the /n/ sound. A reversal of this process is needed instantaneously, however, because the nasal sound /n/ is followed immediately by a nonnasal /t/. For the pressure for the /t/ sound to be released orally, complete velopharyngeal closure must occur. These rapid and precise movements are necessary to articulate accurately one word containing a nasal consonant (e.g., "paint"), and the complexity of the process is magnified in an ongoing stream of verbal behavior in which the nasal consonants /m/, /n/, and /ŋ/ are liberally disbursed. Dalston and Keefe (1988) described the reaction time of velopharyngeal closure using a photodetector system and determined an average reaction time of 206 msec among normal speakers. More information is provided on this complex process in Chapter 8.

Anatomy and Physiology of the Larynx

The larynx is composed of five major cartilages, four minor cartilages, one bone, and several intrinsic and extrinsic muscles, all bound together by complex ligaments and membranes into a functional unit (Exhibit 1–1). The adult larynx is situated at the superior aspect of the trachea, just anterior to the third through sixth cervical vertebrae.

Exhibit 1–1 Components of the Larynx

Major Cartilages	*Minor Cartilages*
Cricoid (unpaired)	Corniculate (paired)
Thyroid (unpaired)	Cuneiform (paired)
Arytenoids (paired)	*Bone*
Epiglottis (unpaired)	Hyoid
Intrinsics	*Extrinsics*
Posterior cricoarytenoids	Stylohyoids
Lateral cricoarytenoids	Diagrastics
Transverse arytenoids	Geniohyoids
Oblique arytenoids	Thyrohyoids
Thyroarytenoids	Sternohyoids
Cricothyroids	Sternothyroids
	Omohyoids

The Hyoid Bone

The single bone involved is the hyoid, which can be considered a bone of the tongue and pharynx since muscles of the tongue and pharynx attach to it from above, or of the larynx since structures of the larynx (muscles and cartilages) attach to it from below.

Figure 1–1 shows the relationship between the larynx (vocal folds) at the top of the respiratory tract and the esophagus leading to the stomach. The laryngopharynx and hypopharynx are also shown. During swallowing, the larynx is tilted and sphincterically closes so that food or liquid is channeled into the esophagus, avoiding the respiratory tract. This valving process during swallowing occurs on three levels: inferior, the true vocal folds; middle, the ventricular folds; superior, the epiglottis and aryepiglottal folds.

The larynx can be seen and detected externally by palpating the laryngeal prominence in the middle of the neck. This prominence, also called the Adam's apple, is more prominent in adult males. During swallowing, the marked tilting of the larynx can be observed easily. The hyoid bone (body) can be palpated just superior to the laryngeal prominence; just inferior to the prominence, the anterior ring of the cricoid cartilage can be detected. Other than these significant landmarks, the intricate structures that compose the larynx are hidden from view except through peroral inspection using a mirror, laryngoscope, or endoscope.

The Five Major Cartilages

The five major cartilages that comprise the larynx are the unpaired cricoid, the unpaired thyroid, the two paired arytenoid cartilages, and the unpaired epiglottis. Figures 1–5 and 1–6 show the functional relationships of these cartilages.

The Cricoid Cartilage. The cricoid cartilage constitutes a superior extension of the top tracheal cartilage and is shaped similarly to a signet ring. Its major landmarks include an anteriorly directed arch or ring and a large posterior quadrate (four-sided) lamina. Four articular facets (surfaces for articulation) are located on the cricoid: two on the lateral aspect of the quadrate lamina to which the thyroid cartilage attaches and two on the superior aspect of the lamina for arytenoid articulation.

The Unpaired Thyroid. The largest of the laryngeal cartilages is the unpaired thyroid, which consists of two rather large flat plates called the thyroid lamina. These lamina are joined anteriorly to form the thyroid angle. Whereas A. E.

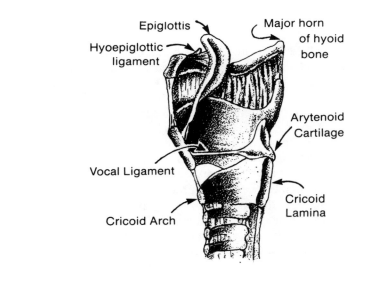

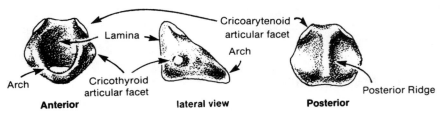

Figure 1–5 Laryngeal Cartilages.

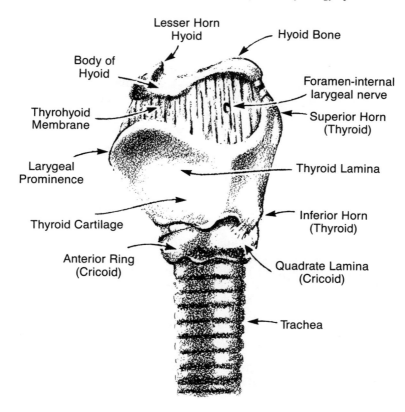

Figure 1–6 Laryngeal Cartilages: Lateral View.

Aronson (1985) stated that the angle of the thyroid is significantly different between postpubescent males (90°) and females (120°), and that this angle difference is an important factor in pitch differences between the sexes, Kahane (1982) found the angle difference to be much less (84.2° for males and 92.5° for females, mean values). Kahane's findings are compatible with several studies of thyroid angles in males and females (Zemlin, 1988). Regardless of the angle, the superior aspect just below the thyroid notch forms the laryngeal prominence, or the Adam's apple, which is the most anterior aspect of the larynx.

Arising from the superior surface of each thyroid lamina is the superior horn, which indirectly attaches to the major horn of the hyoid bone. The remaining space between the superior aspect of the thyroid and the hyoid bone is filled with the thyrohyoid membrane. The superior aspect of each thyroid lamina depresses downward in front to form the thyroid notch just above the angle. This notch is easily palpated and helps in the identification of these laryngeal landmarks.

The essential landmarks of the thyroid cartilage are completed by the paired inferior horns that extend from the posterior and inferior aspects of each thyroid lamina to articulate on the lateral aspects of the posterior quadrate lamina of the cricoid. This joint between the thyroid and the cricoid is the most significant factor in voice pitch adjustments. (The functional aspects of this joint relationship are discussed in detail later in this chapter.)

The Paired Arytenoid Cartilages. The tiny and complex paired arytenoid cartilages are responsible for most of the laryngeal valving processes involved in biological and phonation functions of the larynx. Each arytenoid is comprised of three significant processes. Posteriorly, the apex and muscular processes are well defined.

A lateral view of a sagittal section through the laryngeal cartilages reveals the vocal process directed anteriorly (see Figure 1–5). The joint relationship between the arytenoid cartilages and the superior aspect of the cricoid is such that arytenoid rocking and sliding along a longitudinal axis is possible. The rocking and sliding of the arytenoids are responsible for most laryngeal valving functions for the true vocal folds (D. R. Dickson & W. M. Dickson, 1982).

The Unpaired Epiglottis. The final significant cartilage is the unpaired epiglottis. This is a thin, leaflike structure comprised of yellow elastic cartilage. It is attached to the posterior surface of the thyroid cartilage at the angle just inferior to the notch. From this attachment, the epiglottis rises to overhang the entrance to the larynx. It is held in position over the entrance by a series of ligaments. Arising from each arytenoid cartilage is a muscle structure called the aryepiglottal fold that attaches to the lateral aspects of the epiglottis. This combination of tissue formed by the epiglottis posteriorly and the aryepiglottal folds laterally circles the entrance to the larynx like a collar. During deglutition, this laryngeal collar sphincterically closes the laryngeal opening to protect the respiratory tract from aspiration.

The Four Minor Cartilages

The four minor laryngeal cartilages are the paired corniculates, which are tiny extensions of the apex of each arytenoid, and the paired cuneiforms, which are small bits of cartilage imbedded in each aryepiglottal fold. The function of these cartilages in biological and phonation valving processes appears unclear and perhaps is vestigial in humans.

Extrinsic Laryngeal Muscles

The extrinsic laryngeal muscles listed in Exhibit 1-1 have been discussed thoroughly in general books of anatomy and physiology for speech (D. R. Dickson & W. M. Dickson, 1982; Zemlin, 1988). These muscles are important for laryngeal function in deglutition to lift and tilt the larynx as part of biological valving (Shin, Hirano, Maeyama, Nozoe, & Ohkubo, 1981), but their phonation function is less well defined. Functions of the extrinsic muscles have been found to be important in laryngeal adjustments in singing (Mason & Zemlin, 1969; Shin et al., 1981). The function of these muscles in speech appears much less clearly defined and is not detailed here since they play a secondary role to the intrinsic muscles.

Intrinsic Laryngeal Muscles

The cartilages mentioned above are bound together by ligaments and membranes to form a valving structure for respiratory protection during swallowing and phonation. The joints between these cartilages determine the limits of potential movement in the valving processes. Several intrinsic muscles (having both origin and insertion within the larynx) are responsible for the intricate and well-coordinated movements involved in valving (see Figure 1-7). The origin, course, insertion, function, and research evidence of each such laryngeal muscle are discussed later, with a special section on laryngeal innervation in Chapter 5 on neurogenic disorders.

Thyroarytenoid.   The paired thyroarytenoid (TA) is the most important mass of muscle tissue in the larynx for phonation because it forms the muscular mass for each vocal fold. It starts on the deep and posterior surface of the thyroid cartilage at the angle, and courses posteriorly in a horizontal plane to insert onto the arytenoid cartilage at the vocal process. The medial fibers in this muscle often are identified separately as the vocalis muscle. The vocalis muscle runs parallel and lateral to the vocal ligament or lamina propria, which are discussed in detail later.

The lateral fibers of the thyroarytenoid course more directly to the anterior surface of the muscular process of the arytenoid. Whether the medial (vocalis) and lateral portions of the thyroarytenoid are separate muscles is unclear and controversial. However, the threefold function of this muscle in phonation is well understood: (a) it constitutes the main vibrating mass, (b) it shortens the distance between the thyroid and arytenoid cartilages, and (c) it thereby increases the longitudinal tension of the vocal folds for pitch modification. These processes occur as the thyroarytenoid muscle acts in synergistic harmony with other laryngeal muscles. The vocalis muscle also has been associated

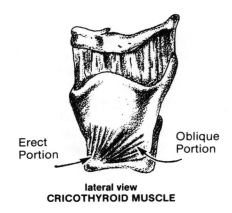

Erect Portion

Oblique Portion

lateral view
CRICOTHYROID MUSCLE

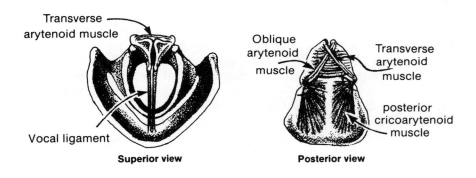

Transverse arytenoid muscle

Vocal ligament

Superior view

Oblique arytenoid muscle

Transverse arytenoid muscle

posterior cricoarytenoid muscle

Posterior view

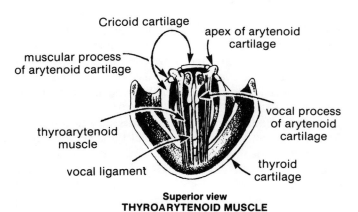

Cricoid cartilage

apex of arytenoid cartilage

muscular process of arytenoid cartilage

vocal process of arytenoid cartilage

thyroarytenoid muscle

thyroid cartilage

vocal ligament

Superior view
THYROARYTENOID MUSCLE

Figure 1–7 Intrinsic Laryngeal Muscles.

with rapid decreases in fundamental frequency through isotonic contraction (Harvey & Howell, 1980).

Titze, Luschei, and Hirano (1989), using EMG measurements, reported increased thyroarytenoid activity for both positive and negative changes in the fundamental frequency of the voice. Similar findings on the role of the thyroarytenoid and the cricothyroid muscles in fundamental frequency changes have been reported by Larson, Kempster, and Kistler (1987).

Posterior Cricoarytenoid. The posterior cricoarytenoid is a fan-shaped paired muscle that originates on the posterior surface of the quadrate lamina of the cricoid. It courses and converges in a lateral direction to insert on the posterior surface of the muscular process of the arytenoid by means of extensive ligaments. Contraction of the posterior cricoarytenoid functions to rock and slide each arytenoid along a longitudinal axis on the cricoid. The effect of such contraction is to part the arytenoid cartilages and open or abduct the glottis. The converging nature of this muscle generates force at excellent mechanical advantage in abduction of the vocal folds. Laryngeal dilation or abduction occurs entirely by the function of the posterior cricoarytenoid (Figure 1–7).

Lateral Cricoarytenoid. The lateral cricoarytenoid muscle is paired and originates on the superior and lateral surface of the cricoid arch. It courses posteriorly and slightly superiorly to inset on the lateral aspect of the muscular process of the arytenoid in a plane rather directly antagonistic to the posterior cricoarytenoid. It functions to facilitate glottal closure (adduction) (Figure 1–7).

Transverse Arytenoid. The unpaired transverse arytenoid muscle extends across the posterior surface of each arytenoid cartilage, entirely covering the surface. Upon contraction, the transverse arytenoid, or interarytenoid, functions to slide the arytenoid cartilages medially to adduct the glottis (Figure 1–7).

Oblique Arytenoid. The oblique arytenoid is a paired muscle that crosses superficial to the interarytenoid from the base of one arytenoid cartilage to the apex of the other. In harmony with the interarytenoid, the oblique arytenoid functions to adduct the arytenoid and the glottis. Some of the fibers of this muscle extend beyond each apex and become the aryepiglottal muscle forming the aryepiglottal fold (Figure 1–7).

Cricothyroid. The cricothyroid is a paired muscle that is divided into erect and oblique portions (pars recta and pars oblique). The cricothyroid muscle directly influences the cricothyroid joint in such a manner that the cricoid arch is adducted in relation to the thyroid cartilage. The limit of this joint movement is determined by restricting influence of the ligaments that connect the inferior horn of the thyroid to the cricoid on each side. Upon contraction of the cricothyroid muscle, either the cricoid is moved relative to the thyroid (A. E. Aronson, 1985) or vice versa (D. R. Dickson & W. M. Dickson, 1982). In either case, the relative distance between the arytenoid cartilages positioned on the cricoid and the thyroid cartilage is increased when this muscle contracts. Thus the paired cricothyroid muscle is responsible for increasing the length of the vocal folds. This increase produces stretching of the vocal folds, which in turn causes an increase in longitudinal tension and a decrease in cross-sectional mass. Under these conditions, the fundamental frequency of vocal fold vibration rises, which is heard as increased pitch. The cricothyroid muscle also adducts the vocal folds by generating longitudinal tension (Figure 1–7).

The cricothyroid muscle is also a likely significant factor in producing the changes in the vocal fold tension which result in normal jitter measurements (Larson et al., 1987).

Membranes of the Larynx

Several connective tissue membranes bind and integrate the cartilages and muscles of the larynx into a functional valving mechanism. The thyrohyoid membrane fills the space from the superior margin of the thyroid cartilage to the hyoid bone. The conus elasticus is composed mainly of yellow elastic tissue and is divided into an anterior and two lateral portions. The anterior portion fills the space between the inferior thyroid margin and the anterior arch of the cricoid. The lateral portions are thinner and fill the lateral portions of the larynx close to the mucous membrane that lines the larynx.

The superior border of the conus elasticus becomes the fibrous tissue that covers the vocalis muscle and acts as a cushion to protect the folds from mechanical damage that may be caused by the constant vibration of the vocal folds. This fibrous cushion is called the lamina propria (vocal ligament) and is divided into superficial, intermediate, and deep layers (Figure 1–8) (Hirano, Kurita, & Nakashima, 1981). Another mass of connective tissue is the quadrangular membrane that binds the aryepiglottal folds superiorly and the ventricular folds inferiorly.

The Vocal Folds

The vocal folds constitute one of the valving mechanisms in the larynx that protect the respiratory tract. They also are the source of air impedance in phonation. They are comprised of muscle, connective tissue, and epithelium. A coronal section through the larynx reveals these combination layers of tissue (Figure 1–8).

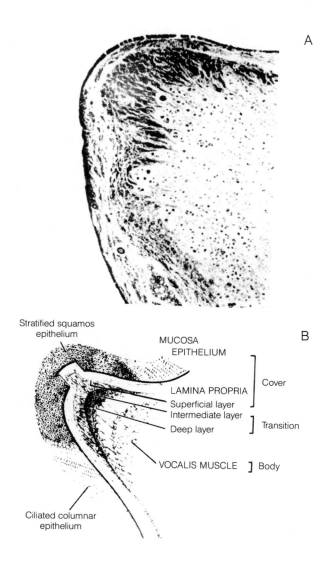

Figure 1–8 Larynx: Coronal View Through Vocal Folds. Reprinted with permission from "The Structure of the Vocal Chords" by M. Hirano, S. Kurita, and T. Nakashima in *Vocal Fold Physiology* (p. 34) by K. N. Stevens and M. Hirano (Eds.), 1981, Tokyo: Tokyo University Press. Copyright 1981.

The bulk of the vocal fold is composed of the vocalis muscle, which, as discussed previously, constitutes the medial portion of the thyroarytenoid. Surrounding the muscular portion of the vocal fold are the lamina propria (superficial, intermediate, and deep layers). Their layer structure, which varies along the length of the vocal fold, is thickest at the midportion of the vocal fold and becomes thinner toward the anterior and posterior aspects. Variance in the relative contribution of the superficial, intermediate, and deep layers also occurs along the anterior and posterior dimensions of the vocal fold.

The vocalis muscle and lamina propria are covered by stratified squamous epithelium, which also varies in thickness along the length of the vocal fold, with the greatest thickness in the middle region. The squamous epithelial layer differs from the mucosa of most surrounding tissues in the larynx that are involved in biological valving (e.g., the ventricular folds). These tissues are lined with columnar epithelium.

Although the structural layers of the vocal folds seem to vary between children and adults, little variance is seen between adult sexes. Stevens and Hirano (1981) wrote that the vibrating tissue that constitutes the vocal folds is composed of the cover (epithelium and superficial layer of the lamina propria), the transitional tissue (intermediate and deep layers of the lamina propria), and the body (vocalis muscle).

The blood supply to the vocal fold is an important consideration for understanding normal and pathological larynges. The larynx is supplied by (a) the superior laryngeal artery, (b) the cricothyroid branch of the superior thyroid artery, and (c) the inferior laryngeal artery. These arteries are branches of the superior thyroid artery from the external carotid artery. Angiography of the vocal folds in fresh cadavers has revealed the following:

- Vessels of the free edge run parallel to the longitudinal axis of the vocal fold.

- The blood stream on the free edge flows posteriorly from the anterior end and anteriorly from the posterior end of the fold.

- The blood vessels in the mucosal free edge are clearly differentiated from upper and lower mucosal surfaces of the vocal fold as well as from the vocalis muscle portion.

- A reticulated vascular network in the midportion of the vocal fold provides for blood distribution.

- The distribution and direction of blood flow is highly suitable for a structure undergoing constant mechanical vibration.

- The blood volume of the vocal fold decreases markedly during vibration. If this did not occur, the distribution and circulation of blood would be markedly disturbed during vibration. This blood reduction constitutes a fail-safe system to prevent abnormal hemorrhaging as a result of normal vibration (Mihashi et al., 1981).

- A slight rise in temperature of the vibrating vocal folds occurs during pho- nation as a result of viscous friction, which complements what would ordi- narily be a drop in temperature with reduced blood flow during phonation (Cooper & Titze, 1985).

From a superior view (Figure 1-9), the vocal folds appear as the most medial projection from the lateral walls of the larynx. Between the vocal folds is the variable fissure or chink called the glottis. The glottis is the space between the vocal folds formed by the rima glottidis, which is the margin of the vocal folds medially. The anterior-to-posterior dimensions of the glottis are divided into the intermembranous and intercartilaginous portions. The intermembranous portion includes the glottal length from the most anterior point to the junc- tion of the vocal processes and the muscular folds. The point where the vocal folds converge anteriorly is called the anterior commissure. The intercar- tilaginous portion is the remaining area formed by the vocal processes of the arytenoid.

The color of the vocal folds appears whitish compared with the pinkish tone of the surrounding tissues. This whitish appearance is a result of reduced blood supply compared with that of the surrounding tissues. The white color is one indicator of a healthy larynx.

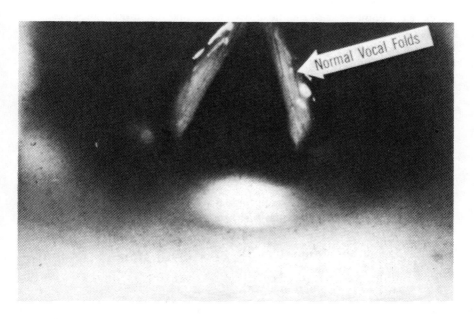

Figure 1-9 Superior View of the Vocal Folds. Reproduced with permission from *Voice Disorders: A Programmed Approach to Voice Therapy* by F. B. Wilson and M. Rice, 1977, Hingham, MA: Teaching Resources Corp. Copyright 1977 by F. B. Wilson.

Phonation Theory

Two theories of phonation have prevailed in the voice science literature: neurochronaxic and myoelastic–aerodynamic. The neurochronaxic theory explains the vibration process of the vocal folds in phonation as occurring in response to individual neural impulses causing the abduction–adduction necessary to produce glottal pulsing. In direct conflict is the myoelastic–aerodynamic theory, which explains phonation as a phenomenon of passive vibration of the vocal folds in response to subglottal airflow and pressure.

Phonation is undoubtedly a myoelastic–aerodynamic phenomenon (Titze, 1980). The process of using airflow and pressure through a constriction to produce vibration of tissue can be demonstrated through an analogy. Lips vibrate if they are relaxed in light approximation and air is forcedly blown from the lungs through the mouth. Horses do it all the time to generate the sound that, in addition to the "whinny," can almost always be identified as coming from a horse. The lips vibrate in rhythmic response to airflow and oral pressure. In phonation, this same process occurs as the adducted vocal folds are blown apart in rhythmic sequence in response to airflow from the lungs and subglottal pressure.

It is important to understand the concept of normal variability in the anatomy and physiology of the normal larynx. We all notice variation in human faces, each comprised of one nose, two eyes, and one mouth with lips, and each combination forming a unique but normal and recognizably unique pattern. Similar normal variation occurs in the form and function of the human larynx. Casper, Brewer, and Colton (1987) documented variations in configuration and movement patterns in selected laryngeal structures during a phonation protocol among men and women. These variations were observed fiber optically. The authors concluded that, when no clear tissue changes or lesions are observed, distinction between normal and abnormal variation is indeed difficult and at times impossible.

Although the process of phonation, as described, seems simple, it is actually very complex when studied in detail. Information on vibration patterns has been obtained by research methods including fiber optic endoscopy, highspeed cinematography, X-ray, stroboscopy, ultrasonic analysis, electromyography, aeromechanical analysis, and electroglottography (Baken, 1987; Stevens & Hirano, 1981).

Moore and von Leden (1962) pioneered high-speed cinematography and provided extensive new information regarding phonation. Hirano, Kakita, Kawasaki, Gould, and Lambiase (1981) elaborated on the basic technique and used computer enhancement to store and measure x-y coordinates of selected points in the vibratory cycle. The detail provided in this form of analysis allows millisecond-by-millisecond description of a typical cycle of vibration, which would be so pedantic that it would put the most alert reader into a deep sleep. However, a generalization of the highlights provided by such careful investigation of phonation is helpful to speech pathologists. The following is an attempt to provide such a generalization.

The Phases of Phonation

Phonation can be described by detailing three phases of vibration: opening, closing, and closed. When a person initiates phonation, the vocal folds are set at the paramedian position. In this position, the mucous membrane of the vocal fold begins to move as a rippling wave. Several vibrations of this ripple effect occur before the glottis completely closes.

Complete closure of the glottis is effected by the adductive musculature moving the arytenoid cartilages into medial compression. As this is happening, air from the lungs through the trachea is forced through an increasingly narrowed glottis. According to Bernoulli's principle, as the glottis narrows, air is forced through the constriction with increased velocity, causing a drop in pressure at the point of constriction. The final effect of these pressure-flow dynamics involved in Bernoulli's principle is complete medial compression of the vocal fold along its entire medial surface.

It often is difficult to imagine how airflow can generate such negative pressure. This can be demonstrated, however, by holding two pieces of typing paper close together and blowing air between them. The papers will vibrate and will be sucked together during portions of the vibration cycle. This same effect occurs in the larynx between the vocal folds.

With the vocal folds in a closed state, one cycle can be analyzed further. The glottal closure causes an increase in subglottal pressure until it is sufficient to overcome glottal resistance. When this happens, the opening phase of vibration begins. In this phase, the vocal folds are blown upward in a traveling wave that undulates from the lower lip of each vocal fold to the upper lip.

After the pressure has forced the vocal folds apart completely, the closing phase begins as the lower lips protrude from each vocal fold. This closure process also undulates from this lower lip contact upward until the entire medial surface of the vocal fold is closed once again. This closed phase remains complete for a time that depends on the intensity of the sound being produced. After the duration of the closed phase, the cycle repeats itself in the same fashion. Each cycle involves this undulating traveling wave from the lower lip to the upper in both the opening and closing phases.

These rhythmic pulses produced by the vibrating vocal folds constitute the glottal tone. The frequency of the tone depends on the number of cycles occurring each second. The glottal tone represents a sound wave of compressed and rarefied air. These sound wave vibrations then are resonated by the chambers of the vocal tract.

The sound that is present in the vocal tract under conditions of phonation is composed of the fundamental frequency of vibration and harmonics of the fundamental. The harmonics are multiples of the fundamental, so if the fundamental were a 100 Hz tone, the multiples would be 200, 300, 400, 500 Hz, and so on. Thus a complex tone is present in the vocal tract, where it is resonated and shaped into the vowels and consonants of the language being spoken. Underlying these sounds of the language is the voice of the speaker.

Specific Characteristics of Voice

The basic sound produced by the vibrating vocal folds is characterized by parameters of frequency, intensity, and quality. Frequency and intensity are dependent on factors at the level of the vocal folds or below in the respiratory system. Vocal quality is a function of characteristics in the vibrating vocal folds coupled with factors of resonance.

Frequency

Voice frequency is determined by the rate of vibration or cycles that occur each second. This value is expressed in hertz. If a person's vocal folds were vibrating 100 times each second, that individual's fundamental frequency (F_0) equals 100 Hz. Frequency is a physical measurement expressed in hertz; its psychological correlate is pitch.

Frequency and pitch are roughly equivalent. The frequency is the specific hertz of the tone, and the pitch is what the listener hears or perceives. Frequency also can be expressed as a musical scale value. For example, the 100 Hz tone essentially corresponds to the note G_2, meaning two Gs below middle C on the musical scale.

Several factors determine the specific F_0 of vibration: (a) the length of the vocal folds, (b) the cross-sectional mass of the vocal folds, and (c) the longitudinal tension of the vocal folds. Subglottal pressure also influences frequency in a less significant manner.

Length, cross-sectional mass, and tension interact to account for intersubject and intrasubject differences in frequency or pitch. Longer and thicker vocal folds vibrate slower, producing a lower frequency. Adult males typically have longer and thicker vocal folds than females and thus have lower pitches. These sex differences in pitch do not occur until puberty.

In a recent study on voice frequency, Kempster, Larson, and Kistler (1988) found that stimulation of both the cricothyroid and the thyroarytenoid muscles produces elevation of vocal pitch. They reported that the thyroarytenoid muscle has a faster contraction speed than the cricothyroid, but both synergistically function to raise the pitch.

Factors in Frequency Fundamental Change

Changes in longitudinal tension of the vocal folds account for intrasubject increases or decreases in pitch. The anatomical and physiological mechanisms involved in altering longitudinal tension are found in the cricothyroid and thyroarytenoid musculature. Contraction of the cricothyroid muscle moves the cricoid in relation to the thyroid cartilages, increasing the thyroarytenoid distance. The vocal folds are stretched by this effort, which increases the longitudinal tension. Under this stretching condition, the vocal fold frequency of vibration increases and the pitch rises. A similar phenomenon occurs when the tension is increased on a guitar or piano string: the frequency or pitch rises as tension is increased.

The increased longitudinal tension produced by cricothyroid contraction can be complemented by simultaneous contraction of the vocalis muscle. Vocalis contraction generates an isometric tension in the vocal fold when it occurs with cricothyroid contraction. Increased vocal fold tension results from this synergistic effect.

It can be confusing when trying to understand the relationship between greater length as being associated with lower frequency vibration in inter-subject comparisons and greater lengthening as producing higher frequency vibrations in intrasubject changes. It is helpful to remember that greater lengthening within a subject is associated with a corresponding reduction of cross-sectional mass of the vocal fold and an increase in longitudinal tension that accounts for the higher pitch.

As expected, vocal folds producing a low-frequency sound are thicker than vocal folds producing higher pitches. For example, in falsetto, the vocal folds are sufficiently tense to decrease the vertical layer of the vibrating vocal fold, eradicating the influence of the upper and lower lips.

One significant factor involving frequency and pitch is pitch variability. Cycle-by-cycle frequency variation in a speech signal is called jitter or pitch perturbation. Horii (1982a) defined jitter as the average period difference between consecutive cycles divided by the average period. This value can be expressed as a percentage of jitter by multiplying that value by 100. He found an average jitter value of .75% among eight English vowels produced by 20 adult males with no laryngeal pathology.

Increased jitter is one vocal characteristic noted in the voice spectrum of persons with laryngeal pathology. W. S. Brown, Morris, and Michel (1989) reported data that indicate mean jitter ratio values (mean jitter in milliseconds divided by the period in milliseconds times 100) to range between .50 to .90%. Perhaps the most significant finding of their study relates to the stability of jitter as a measure of normal phonation. Comparing jitter ratio (and other values not reported here) among healthy young and aged female speakers, no significant change in jitter ratio was found as a function of aging. This finding is in contrast to earlier research, which indicated that jitter values increase as part of the aging process (Wilcox & Horii, 1980).

Another important concern for jitter analysis is the method of capturing the vocal signal for analysis. Doherty and Shipp (1988) found that jitter analysis is best obtained from live samples since recorded samples introduce abnormal jitter to the signal. In descending order of adequacy, they reported that direct sampling is superior, FM (frequency modulation) recorders are slightly less accurate, audio reel-to-reel recorders are marginally adequate, and audio-cassette recordings should be avoided.

Intensity

The intensity of a sound produced by the vocal mechanism is the physical measurement of sound pressure and is expressed in decibels. The psychological correlate of intensity is loudness. Intensity and loudness are roughly equivalent: The intensity of a sound is a specific decibel level and the loudness is the sound level perceived by the listener. Several factors are responsible for increases in the intensity or loudness of a vocal sound: (a) increased airflow from the lungs and (b) increased resistance to flow by the vocal folds that causes (c) increased subglottal pressure.

Increased resistance to airflow is equivalent to greater medial compression by the vocal folds. If the vocal folds do not resist this increased airflow, the resulting sound merely sounds breathier. When resistance occurs, however, greater pressure builds below the closure for each vibration. The result is greater compression of air molecules in the trachea below the glottis.

When this compressed air finally overcomes the laryngeal resistance and displaces the vocal folds, the compression wave collides with the column of air in the vocal tract with greater energy, sending a more intense shock wave into the vocal tract. The result is a sound with greater intensity that is perceived as louder. To sustain this intense sound, the greater airflow and glottal resistance must be maintained.

The intensity of the human voice must vary to sustain the prosodic factors of stress and intonation. A normal adult larynx is capable of generating a tone of 108 dB at a distance of about 1 meter from the mouth (Daniloff, Schuckers, & Feth, 1980). This represents a remarkable amount of sound pressure. For very soft speech, as little as 2 to 3 cm H_2O pressure are sufficient to cause the vocal folds to vibrate and produce a soft tone. For loud speech, 15 to 20 cm H_2O pressure are needed, and 40 to 60 cm H_2O pressure are needed for a loud shout. The normal human respiratory system is capable of providing the needed laryngeal driving force to accommodate those extreme needs (Daniloff et al., 1980).

As increased subglottal pressure occurs during louder phonation efforts, it must be met with increased laryngeal airway resistance. This resistance cannot be measured directly, but can be calculated when pressure-drop factors from the trachea to the pharynx across the laryngeal valve are known and compared with translaryngeal airflow.

Smitheran and Hixon (1981) demonstrated that laryngeal airway resistance can be calculated without physically invading the trachea to determine tracheal pressure. The peak oral pressure during the production of a voiceless stop-plosive can be taken as an estimate of the tracheal pressure existing at the corresponding moment. This value had been difficult to obtain in previous studies and required puncturing the trachea or having the client swallow a pressure transducer to locate it on a horizontal level to measure tracheal pressure.

On 15 normal adult males, Smitheran and Hixon calculated mean laryngeal airway resistance values of 35.7 cm H_2O/LPS (liters per second). This method provides a reliable and valid method of analyzing laryngeal potential for airway resistance for producing voice in normal and dysphonic persons. The norms in limited form for laryngeal airway resistance provide speech–language pathologists or voice scientists opportunities for subject comparison. Intra-subject comparisons also can be made with this method to document improvement in laryngeal efficiency as a result of vocal management.

The three phases of vocal fold vibration (opening, closing, and closed) are modified in duration under conditions of increased intensity. The increased laryngeal airway resistance to increased flow and pressure is manifested by a lengthened duration of the closed phase in a vibration cycle.

One significant factor related to intensity and loudness is variability. Cycle-by-cycle variation in intensity is called shimmer, which Horii (1982a) defined as the average decibel difference between peak amplitudes of consecutive cycles. He reported a value of .17 dB shimmer across eight vowels produced by 20 adult males with no laryngeal pathology. Abnormal shimmer and jitter values often are present in dysphonic patients. The concerns expressed about jitter analysis reported above also pertain to shimmer analysis (see Doherty & Shipp, 1988).

It should also be kept in mind that vocal pitch (frequency) and loudness (intensity) are interactive and it is difficult to modify one without changing the other. This is fundamental to understanding good vocal hygiene. Gramming, Sundberg, Ternstrom, Leanderson, and Perkins (1988) reported that trained singers increase the frequency of their voices by about one-half semitone per decibel of increased intensity.

Vocal Quality

Vocal quality is much more difficult to describe than vocal frequency and intensity. Several terms are used in the literature to describe vocal quality. Most of the following terms have limited communicative potential:

mellow, rich, clear, bright, ringing, hollow, hooty, smooth, harmonious, pleasing, velvety, sharp, heady, clangy, chesty, throaty, covered, open, breathy, balanced, coarse, crude, heavy, golden, warm, brilliant, cool, flat, round, dull, pointed, pingy, pectoral, shallow, deep, buzzy, reedy, whiney, orotund, light, toothy, white, dark, metallic, dead, cutting, constricted, strident, shrill, blatant, poor, faulty, whispery, thin, whining, piercing, raspy, guttural, pinched, tight, twangy, hard. (Murphy, 1964)

Such terms, although not commonly used, would not contribute to understanding important parameters of voice quality. Even more common terms, such as harsh, hoarse, tense, spastic, and breathy, have limited communicative potential. Most people can distinguish vocal quality in the extreme sense when it is either excellent or significantly defective but are less adept at analyzing the subtle voice quality factors heard in most persons. Speech–language pathologists must be competent in distinguishing vocal parameters of quality.

Several factors contribute to voice quality. Some occur at the level of the larynx and depend on the status of the vocal folds that generate the sound. Others are resonance phenomena that occur in the supralaryngeal structures of the vocal tract. Voice quality is a composite phenomenon of sound source and sound resonance.

The sound spectrum present in the vocal tract includes frequencies from the fundamental and its harmonics. A fundamental of 100 Hz could have multiple harmonics reaching as high as 3000 Hz in the typical male speaker (Lieberman, 1977). Although the intensity of each multiple harmonic decreases up the spectrum from the fundamental, the energy nevertheless is present in the vocal tract and available for resonance and articulation.

The vocal tract functions as an acoustic filter that suppresses sound energy at certain frequencies, allows maximum sound energy to be maintained at other frequencies, and considerably amplifies the energy of other bands of frequency energy. The frequencies at which maximum sound energy is fostered and amplified are called formant frequencies. The terms resonance or vocal tract resonance apply to these regions of sound amplification.

Acoustic filtering and resonance, as it applies to the sounds of human speech, are described in detail by Baken (1987) and Lieberman (1977). However, the speech–language pathologist working with a voice-disordered client is not interested in the process of shaping the vocal tract to modify the acoustics of the glottal tone into a speech signal, but rather in the process of shaping the sound produced by the vocal folds into a quality voice.

Because voice quality is a composite of sound source and sound resonance, several characteristics must be present in the spectrum to ensure good quality. The sound source factors include vocal folds capable of vibrating in phase with each other (i.e., the left and right vocal folds are vibrating at all times at the same point in the vibratory cycle). For this to happen, the mass, length, tension, and approximation characteristics of each vocal fold must be equal. Under such conditions, the waveform generated is periodic.

When pathology is present in the larynx, a high probability exists that one vocal fold will have mass, shape, tension, and approximation characteristics that differ from the other vocal fold. In such a case, the glottal waveform generated is aperiodic. When the glottal waveform is aperiodic and abnormal, it does not matter how well the tone is resonated—it always sounds abnormal. On the other hand, if the waveform is periodic and normal but the resonance is abnormal in some sense, the vocal quality sounds abnormal. (Several other chapters discuss abnormal voice qualities resulting from abnormal glottal wave generation, poor resonance factors, or combinations.)

Periodic glottal waves and certain aspects of normal resonance can be demonstrated objectively by means of spectrographic analysis. A spectrographic pattern of normal phonation and resonance for a steady-state vowel is shown in Figure 1–10. The periodicity of the waveform and the formant frequencies are clearly defined. The spectrographic pattern for a dysphonic patient, in Figure 1–11, shows the contrasting aperiodicity of the waveform and indistinct formant frequencies.

An additional factor related to vocal quality relates to the supraglottal structures of the vocal tract, the structures above the vocal folds which provide vocal resonance. Trained singers appear able to produce voice with a vocal tract setting that includes a low laryngeal height, as well as moderately dilated, rounded, yet tense pharyngeal walls about the glottis. This supraglottal configuration appears related to the improved vocal quality heard in the trained singer. Pershall and Boone (1987) confirmed this vocal tract configuration by direct observation of supraglottal structures of the vocal tract by means of videoendoscopy. In an attempt to somewhat quantify the notion of vocal quality, researchers have proposed the use of the phonetogram. Phonetography is the registration of the dynamic range of a voice as a function of fundamental frequency. For example, F_0 and sound pressure are measured simultaneously and plotted on an x-y diagram. From these measurements, three additional acoustical voice quality parameters can be measured with the F_0 and sound pressure: The jitter value in the F_0 can be used as a measure of vocal roughness, the sound pressure difference among frequency bands (0 to 1.5 kHz vs. 1.5 to 5 kHz) can be used as a measure of vocal sharpness, and the vocal noise level above 5 kHz can be used as an index of breathiness (Pabon & Plomp, 1988).

Vocal Registers

One of the most confusing aspects of vocal quality from a resonance perspective is that of vocal registers. The terms head voice, chest voice, midvoice, and falsetto are only a few of the terms used by voice (musical performance) teachers, voice scientists, and speech–language pathologists to describe the resonance focus in voice production. As persons sing a tone from the lowest

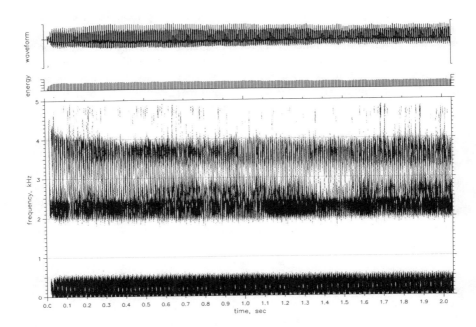

Figure 1-10 Normal Spectrographic Pattern.

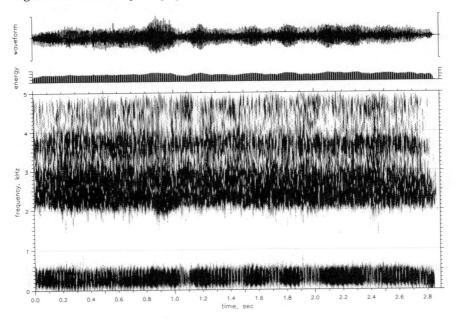

Figure 1-11 Abnormal Spectrographic Pattern.

to the highest of their range, several shifts of resonance focus can be heard independent of the pitch. These shifts are labeled as vocal register and occur in speaking as well as singing. Although several registers are described in the literature of musical pedagogy and voice science, Daniloff et al. (1980) maintained that three definite vocal registers exist: pulse, modal, and loft.

Pulse Register.   The pulse register, also called the low-frequency register, corresponds to the vocal quality described in the literature as vocal fry (Boone & McFarlane, 1988). It represents a pattern of vibration so slow that individual vibrations can be heard, from a low of 3 Hz to 50 Hz tone. Pulse register tone can be produced under conditions of extreme glottal resistance (tension) or when the vocal folds are relaxed and floppy. There also is an increase in the closed phase of a vibrating cycle in pulse register.

Modal Register.   In modal register, the entire vocal fold is involved in the vibration and the thickness of the folds produces an upper and lower lip to the vibrating margins. This layered nature of the vocal folds is evident in vibration until the upper ends of the modal register are reached. Most speaking and trained singing and most of the tones in the vocal pitch range are in the modal register. Within this register, the larynx functions most efficiently so tremendous potential for loudness increases exists (110 dB) (Daniloff et al., 1980).

Loft Register.   The highest register is the loft or falsetto. As the upper end of the pitch range is reached, the shift into loft register involves a laryngeal adjustment in which only the margins of the vocal folds are involved in vibration. The upper and lower lips of the vocal folds are obliterated by the tension, and only tight phonating edges remain. The tension involved in this loft register also tends to stabilize the anterior and posterior aspects of the intermembranous glottis so that only the midregion of the folds is vibrating. This reduced length factor also increases the frequency of vibration (Daniloff et al., 1980).

Many popular singers have learned to produce voice almost entirely in the loft register, and others can shift from modal to loft with little obvious transition. One goal of vocal performance training is to teach students to make smooth transitions from low to high tones without obvious breaks so as to utilize the voice's entire frequency range; however, significant intensity increase is possible only in the modal register.

Titze (1988) proposed that the human voice has only two types of register transition: periodicity and timbre. The periodicity transition involves a specific F_0, below which the human ear seems able to detect individual pulses in the speech waveform. These perceptions would correspond to the pulse register or vocal fry. Above that specific F_0, the human ear perceives a continuous tone. The timbre transition is characterized by an abrupt quality change resulting from a loss or gain of high-frequency sound energy corresponding to the voice heard in the primo passaggio and secondo passaggio (the primary and secondary passages or transitions) in the male and female singers' voices. Titze also stated that subglottal resonance in the trachea plays in important role in vocal resonance, voice quality, and vocal register.

Vibrato

One interesting and rather complex aspect of voice, particularly of the singing voice, is vocal vibrato. The perception of vibrato is that of periodic or regular fluctuations in pitch or frequency and loudness or intensity above and below modal levels. The typical level of frequency fluctuation is from 5 to 7 Hz, but may range from 3 to 10 Hz. The loudness or intensity variations can be from a near nonmeasurable increase to several decibels. When intensity or amplitude modulations are identifiable, they are usually synchronous with the frequency modulations (Horii, 1989). Most singers consider vibrato to be a desirable aspect of the singing voice. If a vibrato-type sound is heard in the speaking voice, it is called vocal tremor and usually reflects an undesirable aspect, often reflecting neurological disorder. An issue of the *Journal of Voice* was devoted entirely to the study of vibrato in singing, and the interested reader is referred to this issue for further study (Sataloff, 1987).

Age and Sex Differences in the Voice

The first use of the larynx as a sound generator usually is the infant's cry at birth. Regardless of the sex, the frequency of the cry is essentially equal, around 400 Hz (Lieberman, Harris, Woolff, & Russell, 1971). Some researchers have claimed that different physical and psychological states can be discriminated in infant cries (Wasz-Hockert, Lind, Vuorenkoski, Partenen, & Valanne, 1968). However, the basic differences between cries do not seem to categorize into discrete segments, and little acoustic or perceptual information is imparted to the listener regarding the stimulation behind the cry (Hollien & Muller, 1973).

At birth, the intermembranous length of the vocal folds is approximately 3 mm. The vocal folds of both sexes increase steadily and equally until around puberty, when the male larynx undergoes more dramatic enlargement than the female. The distinguishing growth changes after puberty are well documented by Kahane (1982):

• A high level of morphologic congruence appears in the male and female prepubertal larynx.

- Clear sexual dimorphism is manifested in laryngeal structures at puberty.

- Prepubertal female laryngeal dimensions are closer to adult size and weight than male counterparts, suggesting that the female larynx requires less growth per time unit to reach maturity.

- Laryngeal cartilage growth occurs through oppositional (external expansion) and interstitial (internal expansion) processes so the basic shape is not changed in cartilage growth.

- Extensive regional growth characterizes the enhancement of the anterior aspect of the male thyroid cartilage. This growth, rather than the thyroid angles, produces the typical male Adam's apple. This growth produces a thicker thyroid lamina at the angle, and the prominence cannot be interpreted as indicating greater length of the male vocal folds.

- Male growth changes are two to three times those of females in almost every aspect, particularly in the thyroid cartilage, in which the mean increase from anterior to posterior is 15.04 mm for males and 4.47 mm for females.

- Growth of the vocal folds likewise is greater in males than females (mean: 11.57 mm [63%] in males and 4.16 mm [34%] in females).

- Vocal fold length and thickness grow independently, with data supporting the possibility that thickness continues to increase after length has reached adult dimensions.

Table 1–1 presents information on fundamental voice frequencies for various ages of males and females.

The Aging Voice

Much information is now available regarding the changes that occur in voice during the aging process. Because aging often is accompanied by disease processes, the effect on voice must be analyzed. What is known about the healthy male and female voice during the Golden Years?

Fundamental Frequency

Whereas a clear vocal divergence of vocal fundamental frequency occurs at puberty between males and females, it appears that a slight vocal convergence occurs in the menopause stage, and men's and women's voices become closer in pitch. This convergence occurs as the older male voice rises in pitch and the older female voice remains more stable until extreme old age (Hollien, 1987).

TABLE 1–1
Fundamental Frequency of Voice

Males				Females			
Age	Hz	Note[a]	Investigator/Date	Age	Hz	Note[a]	Investigator/Date
7	294[b]	D	Fairbanks, Wiley, & Lassman, 1949	7	273[b]	C#	Fairbanks, Herbert, & Hammond, 1949
10	226	A_1	Holcik, 1967	11	266	C	Duffy, 1970
14	185	$F\#_2$	Hollien, Malcik, & Hollien, 1965	15	237	$A\#_1$	Ibid.
18	115	$A\#_2$	Ibid.	17	211	$G\#_1$	Hollien & Paul, 1969
30–39	112	A_2	Hollien & Shipp, 1972	30–39	196	G_1	Saxman & Burk, 1967
60–69	112	A_2	Ibid.	40–49	189	$F\#_2$	Ibid.
80–89	146	D_1	Ibid.	72	196	G_1	McGlone & Hollien, 1963
				85	199	G_1	Ibid.

[a] Approximate
[b] Mean values

Note. Adapted with permission from "A Study of the Reading Fundamental Vocal Frequency of Young Black Adults" by A. I. Hudson and A. Holbrook, 1981, *Journal of Speech and Hearing Research, 24,* p. 201. Copyright 1981 by American Speech–Language–Hearing Association, Rockville, MD.

Vocal Intensity

The effect of aging on vocal intensity is not clearly understood. The stereotype of the older voice is that intensity is increased perhaps due to hearing loss in the aged. However, the compensation for hearing loss must be understood in the context of reduced respiratory support and vital capacity for speaking. It is more likely that older speakers have at least reduced capacity to significantly increase the intensity of their voices (Hollien, 1987).

Vocal Tremor

One commonly perceived aspect of the older voice is vocal tremor, a rather rhythmical fluctuation of pitch and intensity much like the quality of vocal vibrato in singing. Hollien (1987) stated that although vocal tremor accompanies the aging process, it can signal the neurological changes of clinical dysarthria.

Voice Quality

Voice quality abnormalities such as vocal roughness, aperiodicity, and breathiness are found more prevalently in the aged. For example, Linville, Skarin, and Fornatto (1989) studied 20 women ranging from 67 to 89 years of age. One significant finding they reported is frequently inadequate glottal closure during voice production. This would be correlated with increased breathiness in the voice, as well as reduced loudness potential.

Many of these aging acoustic changes are reflected in changes in the tissues of the larynx. Hirano, Kurita, and Sakaguchi (1989) reported many of the changes that occur in the vocal folds during the aging process. For example, they noted the following tendencies in 70- to 104-year-olds:

- The membranous vocal fold shortens in males in aging.
- The mucosa thickens in females.
- The cover of the vocal fold thickens in females.
- Edema develops in the superficial layer of the lamina propria of both sexes.
- The intermediate layer of the lamina propria thins and its contours become deteriorated in males.
- Elastic fibers in the intermediate layer become less dense and atrophy in males.
- The deep layer of the lamina propria thickens in males.
- Collagenous fibers in the deep layer become denser and fibrotic in males.

Kahane (1987) also reported on the connective tissue changes that occur in the larynx as a result of aging, and related those changes primarily to changes in vocal pitch.

One of the most complete studies of phonational frequency range for adult males and females was reported by Hollien, Dew, and Philips (1971). It covered the total range from lowest to highest pitch of 332 male and 202 female subjects (ages 18 to 36). The mean frequency range is in excess of three octaves, specifically 38 semitones (halftones) for the males and 37 semitones for the females. The mean values for the lowest fundamental are 78 Hz for males and 139 Hz for females. The mean values for the highest fundamental are 698 Hz for males and 1108 Hz for females.

Electromyographic Data on Voice Physiology

Several electromyographic analysis studies of muscle activity have been completed on the intrinsic laryngeal muscles. Every such muscle has been studied by hooked-wire electrodes placed in the muscle either percutaneously or perorally. The percutaneous approach generally is selected to reach the thyroarytenoid (vocalis) (TA), lateral cricoarytenoid (LCA), and cricothyroid (CT). The peroral approach is used to reach the posterior cricoarytenoid (PCA) and interarytenoid (IA). Although the number of subjects generally is small in these studies, several consistent patterns of electromyographic activity seem apparent:

- Increases in pitch are accompanied by progressive increases in the activity of the CT and TA (Gay & Hirose, 1972).

- Glottal abduction during inhalation is generated by sustained activity of the PCA with an accompanied reduction of activity of the IA, LCA, CT, and TA.

- Increased activity occurs in CT, TA, LCA, and IA during adduction for phonation.

- Voiceless consonants are produced during running speech by quick bursts of PCA activity producing milliseconds of nonphonation. This is complemented by simultaneous suppression of the adductor muscles. Figure 1–12 demonstrates this reciprocity.

An additional EMG study on laryngeal control in singing (Stevens & Hirano, 1981) has contributed to professionals' understanding of the delicate adjustments involved in laryngeal adduction, abduction, and quality control for human phonation. It is marvelous how well these adjustments are controlled to produce, for example, the voice of a great singer or actor. Even nonprofessionals can communicate rather well with subtle nuances of pitch, intensity, and quality control that enhance and add meaning to the messages being communicated.

It is intriguing to contemplate the sensitivity of instant adjustment a singer must be capable of accomplishing in the larynx to match a note perfectly without

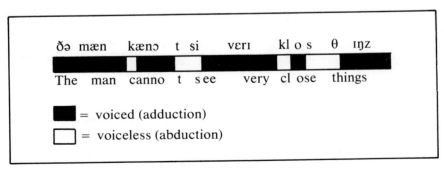

Figure 1–12 Phonation Reciprocity.

trial-and-error feedback. These adjustments are produced as the singer is hearing the note to be sung while establishing in the larynx the longitudinal tension and medial compression adjustments necessary to match the tone. This must happen instantaneously as exhaled air hits the adducting vocal folds. If the adjustments are not right, the singer is out of the show. Even in speech, these same adjustments are made but with less serious consequences when errors occur. Fortunately, the adjustments are highly programmed in people's brains, and for the most part require little conscious control. Otherwise, people would find themselves as confused as the proverbial centipede trying to control the action of leg number 39.

These fine-tuning mechanisms within the structure of the vocal folds are now clearly understood. Wyke (1983) described this neuromuscular control system of voice production as intralaryngeal mechanoreceptors which act reflexively in response to aerodynamic forces from the lungs. Three types of mechanoreceptors are described: subglottal mucosal, laryngeal myotatic, and laryngeal articular mechanoreceptors. These mechanoreceptors found in the mucosa, muscle spindles, and connective tissue joints of the larynx provide sensory feedback to the brain regarding aerodynamic forces acting on the larynx. As a function of this feedback and the motor adjustments to it, vocal fold stability is maintained in a constantly changing aerodynamic system. This feedback also allows the speaker or singer to preset the vocal folds in a specific state of tension to allow a specific pitch to be produced. This occurs almost instantaneously in the case of great singing, and the perfect note is sung with little adjustment.

Summary

This chapter has introduced many of the basic principles of voice science. Recent evidence on the anatomy and physiology of voice science has been presented to provide a basis for understanding principles of normal phonation. Details of intrinsic laryngeal structures, basic phonation theory, aspects of frequency, intensity, and quality control have been emphasized. These normal aspects provide a basis for understanding the deviations found in the various dysphonias presented in the remaining chapters.

2

Medical Aspects of Voice Disorders

The speech–language pathologist working with voice-disordered clients must be comfortable with medical relationships, terms, and procedures. The following sample of a physician's report on a patient referred for voice management is typical of the language used in such communications:

I am referring Mr. J. _____ for voice therapy. He recently underwent Jako laryngoscopic surgery under general endotracheal intubation for removal of suspected bilateral vocal nodules. Under surgery, the larynx, epiglottis, true and false cords, ventricles, pyriform sinuses, and valleculae were all carefully examined and found to be normal, with the exception of the true and false cords which appeared to be chronically infected and had a peculiar nodular hypertrophy. These were examined bilaterally for pathological diagnosis. The pathology report is as follows:

The specimen is stated to be the right and left vocal cord strippings. The right portion consists of approximately a 2 × 1 mm portion of somewhat translucent epithelially surfaced soft tissue. The left portion consists of a 5 mm aggregate of tissue similar to the right portion. Under microscopic analysis, multiple sections reveal a fragment of tissue surfaced by benign squamous epithelium which focally contains mucus-producing cells. No hyperkeratosis or dyskeratosis is noted. The underlying stroma contains a few scattered collections of mononuclear cells. Sections also reveal the presence of focal hyalinization with congested vascular structures present in the underlying stroma as well as a few small focal strands of skeletal muscle fibers.

This patient also has probable neuromuscular deformity involving the lower extremities which could be a form of Charcot–Marie–Tooth syndrome. There is no evidence of upper motor neuron signs, although lateral sclerosis is a possible cause.

Please evaluate and advise on speech pathology findings. Thank you for seeing this patient.

No matter how well the speech–language pathologist is trained, the physician typically will use language with which the speech–language pathologist may not be familiar, causing a frantic search through a medical dictionary for definitions and clarification. The speech–language pathologist cannot hope to acquire, in the course of training in communication disorders, the necessary background in medical management to communicate equally with the physician and should not be expected to do so, just as the typical physician is somewhat unfamiliar and perhaps uncomfortable with the language used by speech–language pathologists to describe communication disorder. However, for competent management of voice-disordered patients, a common understanding of terms and procedures involved in medical management can be helpful to the clinician whose job it is to provide behavior modification of abnormal voice habits.

This chapter introduces basic information regarding medical procedures in the treatment of voice disorder, including the background, training, and certification procedures of medical specialties commonly involved. General procedures of medical evaluation, drug therapy, and surgery for voice-disordered patients also are explained.

Medical Specialties in Voice Disorder

Although many medical specialists can be involved in the treatment of patients with voice disorders, the bulk of evaluation and treatment is done by specialists in otolaryngology, neurology, psychiatry (psychology), radiology, plastic surgery, and pathology. The reference for the following medical specialty training procedures is the *Directory of Residency Training Programs* (1989).

Otolaryngology: Head and Neck Surgery

Otolaryngology is the medical specialty for the ears, nose, throat, and head–neck surgery. Physicians in this field are trained in general medicine and have fulfilled a specialization residency, usually of 5 years, in both general surgery and the surgical and medical treatment of diseases of the ears, nose, and throat. This is the discipline that works most closely with speech–language pathologists in the treatment of most voice disorders. Otolaryngologists manage most disorders involving the larynx and many involving the general vocal tract. Their certification of specialization is by the American Board of Otolaryngology: Head and Neck Surgery, of the American Medical Association (AMA).

Neurology

A neurologist is a physician who specializes in the clinical evaluation and treatment of diseases and disorders of the nervous system. The clinical neurologist is certified by the American Board of Psychiatry and Neurology, and therefore has considerable background in the psychiatric condition of patients. The methodology used by the clinical neurologist includes general reflex assessment, administration, and interpretation of diagnostic procedures including roentgenologic studies, electroencephalography, electromyography, psychological testing, biochemical testing, and ophthalmological and otological procedures pertaining to the nervous system. The neurologist is most helpful in the evaluation and treatment of voice-disordered patients in terms of assessment of the integrity of the innervation of the larynx, pharynx, and general vocal tract anatomy and physiology. Several central nervous system disorders also can affect the voice and speech functions, making the clinical neurologist a valuable member of the treatment team.

Psychiatry

The specialty of psychiatry includes training in a 3-year residency preparing the physicians for competence in the diagnosis, treatment, and prevention of all psychiatric disorders. Certification of training is from the American Board of Psychiatry and Neurology (AMA) so that, in addition to the training in psychiatry, some experience is obtained in general neurology. Most medical procedures in psychiatry involve individual psychotherapy, family and individual counseling, crisis and stress management, pharmacological assessment and treatment as it pertains to mental illness, hypnosis, biofeedback of biological processes as they relate to mental states, and general behavioral management training. Psychiatrists are particularly helpful in management of patients with psychogenic (nonorganic) voice disorders.

Psychology

The nonmedical discipline of psychology is highly correlated with psychiatry. The differences are centered on the fact that the psychiatrist is a physician and can treat patients with prescribed medicines, whereas the psychologist usually has a doctoral degree in clinical psychology. The psychologist cannot directly prescribe medicines and treats mental illness and general psychological disturbance or maladjustment through counseling, group or individual psychotherapy, hypnosis, biofeedback, and so forth, without pharmacological support other than that prescribed by a physician.

Radiology

The specialty of radiology requires 4 years of residency in diagnostic oncology and 3 years in radiation oncology. Certification is through the American Board of Radiology (AMA). Radiologists also receive some training in nuclear medicine. They use various methods to examine the human body to diagnose and sometimes treat disease. The therapeutic portion of training includes extensive experience in the treatment of malignant tumor disease by means of radiotherapy. Several of the specific radiological techniques used in the evaluation and treatment of voice-disordered patients are described in this chapter.

Plastic Surgery

The plastic surgeon is certified by the American Board of Plastic Surgery (AMA) as having completed a minimum of 3 years of general surgery followed by at least 2 years of plastic surgery. Specific training supports medical competency in the treatment of traumatic defects requiring reconstructive surgery of the maxillofacial region, general body and extremities, burns, aesthetic operations, plastic surgery of the hands, treatment of congenital anomalies such as absence of external ear structures, cleft lip and palate, and other orofacial defects. The plastic surgeon works most closely with the speech–language pathologist in the management of cleft lip and palate patients who have velopharyngeal insufficiency. Some plastic surgeons have specialized training for surgical management of the cranium and have the additional title of Craniofacial Surgeon.

Pathology

The medical pathologist is a physician certified by the American Board of Pathology (AMA) as having completed a residency in microscopic analysis of normal and clinical tissues of the body. Several certification procedures can be followed to become board certified, including an emphasis on normal or clinical tissues. Each takes a minimum of 2 years of residency training.

Medical pathologists analyze tissue removed in biopsies and in tonsillectomy, adenoidectomy, and tumor surgery. This pathological diagnosis confirms whether a tissue removed is benign or malignant and identifies the nature of the tissue. Pathologists generally work directly with other physicians rather than with speech–language pathologists; however, the latter often receive medical reports containing pathology reports and therefore must have some familiarity with this specialty.

Medical Procedures in Voice Disorder

The thorough examination and treatment of a person with voice disorder can involve several of the disciplines identified above in order to clarify the etiological and treatment procedures necessary for competent management. The specific procedures covered here are those directly involved in the examination and treatment of laryngeal pathology, including the vocal tract.

Indirect (Mirror) Laryngoscopy

Perhaps the most common evaluation procedure in examining the status of the laryngeal structures is indirect laryngoscopy. The procedure usually is done by the laryngologist and involves directing a light into the oral cavity to reflect off a laryngeal mirror to inspect the larynx and hypopharynx.

To maximize the probability of success, the patient's position is of great importance. The client should be seated in an erect manner with the jaw protruded forward a little. As the patient protrudes the tongue, it is wrapped with gauze and held firmly by the examiner. The patient then is asked to breathe gently through the mouth or pant like a dog. After warming the surface of a laryngeal mirror, the examiner inserts it into the oropharynx region over the tongue. Often the back of the mirror touches and elevates the velum. Light is directed against the mirror by a headlight system. When the mirror is positioned properly, the light is reflected off the mirror into the regions of the larynx for examination. Once the examiner can see the structures of the larynx, including the vocal folds, the patient is asked to phonate and "think" of saying an "ee" sound to help elevate the epiglottis so the anterior commissure can be observed more readily.

This indirect inspection method permits general examination of the larynx. Mass changes, movement disorders, growths, infections, and phonation abnormalities generally can be discerned by indirect laryngoscopy. Some patients are difficult to examine by this means. Anatomical variations and/or a strong gagging reflex can make the procedure ineffective. Even when a topical anesthetic is used to deaden the gag, some patients, particularly children, are difficult to examine. Patience and an explanation of the fact that no pain is involved can be helpful. Figure 2–1 demonstrates indirect laryngoscopy.

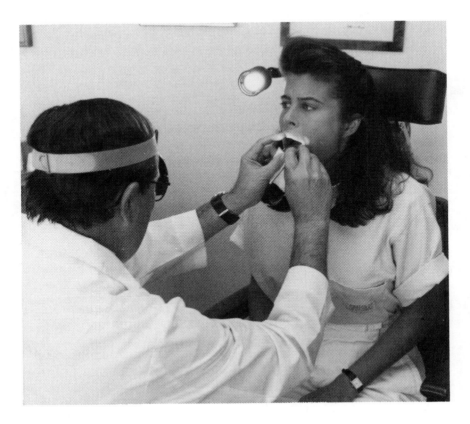

Figure 2–1 Indirect Laryngoscopy.

Endoscopy

The prefix *endo* refers to "within," so laryngeal endoscopy refers to any procedure that allows inspection within the confines of the larynx. Several variations of laryngeal endoscopy have been used in the history of laryngology.

Laryngoscopy. A number of instruments allow direct inspection within the larynx. With the patient asleep under general anesthesia, a metal tube can be placed into the throat to allow direct inspection of the larynx. Some are illuminated proximally and others distally, but the view is direct rather than from mirror reflection. These laryngoscopes had to be held in place by the examiner until, after some years, a suspension system was developed by Killian and perfected by Jako (Paparella & Shumrick, 1980) that allowed direct inspection and surgical access to the tissues of the larynx.

Microlaryngoscopic microscopes with binocular magnification now enable the surgeon to see fine changes in the status of laryngeal tissue.

Fiber Optic Endoscopy.   The development of fiber optics permits endoscopic examination through flexible tubing. Light travels along a bundle of hair-thin fibers from a cold light source, providing illumination at the end of the bundle. Another bundle of fibers carries the image being investigated back into a magnifying scope. Machida America, Inc., is one company that has developed flexible nasopharyngolaryngoscopes, models ENT-3L or ENT-4L, which allow direct inspection in close proximity of the nasal cavity, pharynx, or larynx, depending on how deeply into the body cavities the scope is inserted. A patient being examined with the flexible nasopharynlaryngoscope and an internal view of structures revealed are shown in Figures 2–2a and 2–2b, respectively.

Once the instrument is in place at the point of desired investigation, the examiner can manipulate the tip 100° in an upward or downward direction. This flexibility permits careful inspection of tissue at close proximity. The device is designed to be inserted into the nasal cavity, through the velopharyngeal port, into the pharynx, and finally into the laryngeal cavity. During the insertion process, inspection can take place along the entire route. Attachments are available for 35 mm single-lens reflex photography as well as videotape cameras.

Yanagisawa, Isaacson, Kmucha, and Hirokawa (1989) reported on the merits of various endoscopic techniques, including rigid and fiber optic methods. They strongly recommended video recording of the examination process, whichever method is used: "The addition of the video camera in nasopharyngeal observation greatly enhances the examiner's ability to assess structure, function, and disease by permitting review and comparison of images that once were preserved only in the examiner's memory" (pp. 17–18). Yanagisawa, Godley, and Muta (1987) provided information regarding the selection of the best video cameras for endoscopic documentation.

Fiber optic videolaryngoscopy is not without its pitfalls and limitations. Casper, Brewer, and Colton (1988) presented evidence of distortions in the video image and cautioned making judgments of anatomical or physiological integrity solely on the basis of fiber optic examination data. Shaw and Lancer (1987) provided a marvelous color atlas of upper respiratory tract structures in normal and pathological states, and the reader is encouraged to utilize this excellent reference.

Stroboscopy

The stroboscope permits an observer to view moving objects as though they are stationary or in slow motion. When a beam of light is focused on a moving

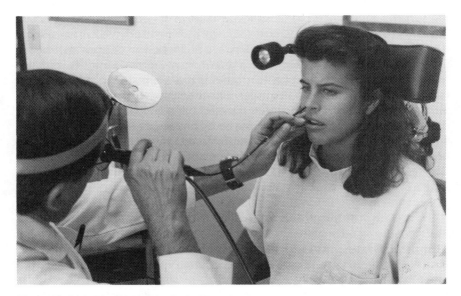

Figure 2–2(a) Flexible Fiber Optic Nasopharyngoscopy.

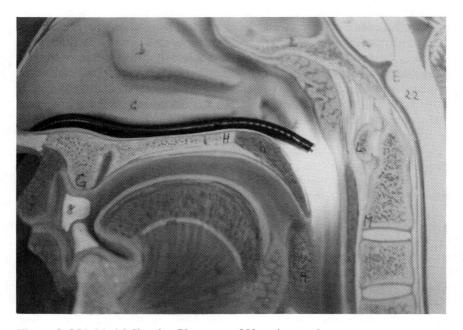

Figure 2–2(b) Model Showing Placement of Nasopharyngolaryngoscope.

object and interrupted in regular pulses, the observer views only the phase of movement exposed by the light. Movement patterns occurring between light pulses are not seen. People have seen the effect of stroboscopic light in discos as the beats of light illuminate the dancers' movements.

The vibrating vocal folds can be viewed in the same manner as each light pulse illuminates a point in the vibratory cycle. A microphone is placed on the client's neck to conduct laryngeal sound to a stroboscopic generator that filters and amplifies the sound and then determines the fundamental frequency (F_0) of the laryngeal sound. The fundamental frequency is transmitted from the generator via electronic pulses to a lamp that emits an intermittent beam of light at the identical frequency. This beam of light is introduced into the larynx via an endoscope or laryngeal mirror (indirect laryngoscopy) for examination. The endoscope can be attached to a video camera for videotape storage (videostroboscopy). The examiner controls a foot pedal that activates the system and permits alteration of the light beam frequency. If the light beam frequency is exactly the frequency of vocal fold vibration, the vocal folds will be seen at the same phase of vibration and will appear stationary. If the light beam is altered slightly out of frequency phase, then the vocal folds will appear as moving in slow motion. A loud speaker provides an audio model for the patient to match a specific frequency (pitch).

Stroboscopy (videostroboscopy) facilitates examination of the details of vocal fold movement that are not apparent under traditional indirect or direct laryngoscopy. It documents patterns of abnormal vibration and the sites of lesions. The assessment of the following vocal fold parameters has been discussed by Hirano, Feder, and Bless (1983):

- The nature of vocal fold edges during phonation

- Width of the open glottis and amplitude of vibration

- Fundamental frequency (F_0)

- Phases of vibration (opening, opened, closing, closed)

- Open quotient, speed quotient, speed index

- Regularity or periodicity of successive vibrations

- Symmetry of movement between the vocal folds

- Vibration of the mucosal tissue covering the vocal fold muscles

- Vibration patterns of the lower and upper lips of the vocal folds

- Extent of contact area between the vocal folds during closed phase

The use of the stroboscope and videostroboscopy of laryngeal structures is becoming standard practice in otolaryngology. Its value as a diagnostic tool is well documented in the literature. Sataloff et al. (1987) reported that in 161 of 515 cases examined by videostroboscopy, its use established or altered the diagnosis or management of the patients involved. Among the disorders diagnosed or altered were arytenoid dislocation (7 patients), hemorrhage (22), nerve paralysis (25), nodule (10), scar (33), and web (3). Numerous additional categories of diagnosis were presented. The videostroboscope has also been utilized by Izdebski, Ross, and Klein (1990) and McFarlane and Watterson (1990) to document laryngeal function in various forms of voice disorder.

Radiologic Examination

Several radiological techniques, traditional as well as advanced, are available for investigating the status of the vocal tract for voice production. These techniques range from standard lateral radiograms to advanced scanning forms.

Roentgenography. A standard means of photographing the body is by roentgen rays, more commonly called radiography or X-ray. Still or in-motion pictures can be taken. Motion picture radiography is called cineradiography when standard motion picture film is used or videoradiography when the image is stored on videotape. Fluoroscopy is a radiological technique that utilizes a fluoroscope in which the image is shown on a fluorescent screen covered with crystals of calcium tungstate. Videofluoroscopy is a common technique in radiologic motion study stored on videotape.

Angiography. Angiography is a radiological technique in which radiopaque contrast materials are injected into the blood vessels and exposed to X-rays, with the resultant image recorded on X-ray film. This technique permits inspection of the integrity and nature of the vascular system, including the head, neck, larynx, and vocal tract. Angiography, an invasive technique, is not without risk, so general anesthesia might be required, especially in the young or when pain is expected. Cerebral complications may result from clot or air embolization. Angiography is not a common technique in the study of the larynx.

Tomography. Tomography is a radiological technique in which a roentgenogram is taken of a layer of tissue at any given depth of the body. Frontal tomograms are used in laryngology to study the vibration patterns of the true and false vocal folds.

Computed Tomography (CT). Computed tomography, a specialized radiographic scanning technique, is based on the physical principle of the slight difference in radiation absorption coefficients in various normal and pathological soft tissues. These differences do not show up in standard radiography, appearing as only one shade of gray.

In CT scanning, the X-ray photons entering and exiting the patient are measured by crystal or gas detectors, and multiple density readings are taken as the X-ray source shifts and rotates around an axis. The computer then solves the equations of relative density detected as a result of the relative absorption factors of the various tissues. The results are displayed in two dimensions on a cathode ray tube (CRT) for direct interpretation or photographic recording.

CT scanning has been replacing angiography and pneumoencephalography as a diagnostic tool in looking for cerebral vascular disease and is a common process in producing images of the larynx (laryngograms).

Magnetic Resonance Imaging (MRI). The application of nuclear magnetic resonance physics to anatomical imaging has had a significant effect on medical practice. The designation nuclear magnetic resonance has been replaced by the less threatening designation of magnetic resonance imaging (MRI). Underlying this technology is the notion that various elements (including human tissues) contain randomly spinning protons which tend to align within a superimposed magnetic field. The process of magnetization enables tissue differences to be detected and utilized to generate maps (images) of those difference values in gray-scale-coded images. The images provide clear distinctions of various tissues along a gray-scale continuum.

MRI, which has been used to image laryngeal and surrounding structures, provides definite advantages over CT scanning techniques for diagnostic purposes. Hoover, Wortham, Lufkin, and Hanafee (1987) stated, "MR surpasses CT, especially in ability to differentiate subtle differences in soft tissue boundaries and tumor extension in the head and neck" (pp. 245–246). MRI techniques have also been used extensively in craniofacial management of patients who have, among other anomalies, orofacial clefting that affects the velopharyngeal and other speech-related structures. This procedure is commonly used with many patients seen at the Southwest Craniofacial Team, of which I am a member.

Xeroradiography. Another specialized technique is xeroradiography, which produces a laryngogram that shows striking enhancement of tissue edges. The xerolaryngogram is produced when transmitted X-rays from a conventional tube expose a cassette-enclosed positively charged aluminum plate photoconductor. In a dry printing process, a negatively charged toner powder is blown across the plate, producing a blue-white image. Dense tissue images such as bone are reflected as white, and less dense tissues such as cartilage and muscle as shades of blue. The edges of tissue demarcations of laryngeal cartilages can be particularly enhanced by this procedure.

Welch, Sergeant and MacCurtain (1989) reported the use of xeroradiography and other techniques in the study of male vocal registers of voice. This technology allowed the authors to determine patterns of vocal tract morphology that could not be determined by standard radiological techniques.

Ultrasound. Diagnostic ultrasound, which has been commonly used in obstetrics because it is safe and noninvasive, is now being utilized in laryngology, particularly in the evaluation of neck lesions. The technique is based on sound waves that are recorded as they are reflected (echoed) back from tissue surfaces in the body. High-frequency sound waves are used with frequencies between 2.5 and 10 million Hz. As sound waves pass through the skin and underlying tissue, different tissue densities produce varying impedance characteristics, causing them to be reflected, refracted, or transmitted. The sound transducer serves as both generator and receiver of returning echoes. The returning echoes are converted into electrical impulses (transduced) for display on an oscilloscopic screen.

Drug Treatment in Voice Disorder

Several pharmacotherapeutic treatments are used in the medical management of voice-disordered patients. These include antibiotic treatment of infections, symptomatic treatment of upper respiratory conditions in the form of antihistamines, anti-inflammatory and antiedematous treatment in the form of adrenocorticosteroids for tissue swelling, psychological or mood-modifying drugs, moisteners for dry mouth and throat and nasal crusting, and local anesthetics to eliminate gagging or nerve transmission.

It is beyond the scope of this book to cover the many drugs that are used by physicians in treating voice disorder. The speech–language pathologist will find that nearly every voice-disordered patient will require pharmaceutical treatment. I have consulted the *Physician's Desk Reference* (PDR; Barnhart, 1990) for most evaluations. The typical speech–language pathologist has insufficient background in biochemistry to understand the pharmacological effects of various medications and can get into trouble when attempting to explain such effects to a voice-disordered client. Although it is tempting to comment on the medications' effects on the voice, I feel that such comments should be left to the physician.

In taking a case history, it is appropriate to ask about the medications being taken. Most clients can provide a list, often with correct spellings. The speech–language pathologist should write down each medication in generic or trade form, and consult the PDR for further information about the drug. The PDR often mentions possible sequelae of a specific medication on the voice. In such instances, the referring physician should be asked to clarify the effect the medication might have on the voice.

Often, a speech–language pathologist working in a medical setting or directly with a physician will become, through experience, rather familiar with various medications in terms of usage, dosage, and voice sequelae. Until such experience is gained, it is best to recognize that some medications can affect the voice and to investigate each reported medication by looking in the PDR. Additional references that are available to help the speech–language pathologist in this process include books by Goudie and Emmett-Oglesby (1989), Haber (1987), and R. M. Miller and Groher (1990).

Martin (1988) wrote a fine tutorial on drugs and vocal function, which covers such topics as basic principles of drug action, biological variation, dose–response relationships, multiplicity of actions, placebo effects, and specific pharmacological medications as they relate to the voice. He discussed drugs that influence proprioception and hearing, drugs that stimulate or depress the central nervous system, anesthetics, drugs that influence airflow as in asthma, drugs that influence fluid content of the tissues of the vocal tract, drying agents, antihistamine effects, psychotropic medications, and various drugs that cause changes in the structure of the vocal folds. I highly recommend that the reader read and study this tutorial.

Surgery and the Voice Patient

Speech–language pathologists must be cognizant of surgical considerations in the treatment of voice-disordered patients, namely, the principles of anesthesia, laryngoscopic examination, biopsy, intubation (extubation), microsurgery, traditional "knife" surgery, and the newer techniques of laser surgery. Specific forms of surgery involved include Teflon laryngoplasty, Teflon pharyngoplasty, tumor or growth removal, and various techniques in cancer management. Only general surgical considerations are discussed here.

Phonosurgery

A growing and positive change in the attitude of many physicians who treat patients with voice disorder is to treat the voice as well as the larynx. When a physician examines a patient and discovers an abnormal change in the tissues of the larynx, particularly on the vocal folds, several treatment choices are available. One, of course, is to investigate surgically the nature of the tissue change in the form of biopsy. In some cases, this is an important course to take. From a voice disorder perspective, it is helpful when the physician realizes that surgery on the larynx is also surgery on the voice. Care must therefore be taken to determine whether the surgery needs to be done or whether a more conservative approach might be in order. Should surgery be necessary, it is helpful when the surgeon approaches the larynx from a concept of phonosurgery rather than laryngeal surgery.

Phonosurgery, as defined by von Leden, Abitbol, Bouchayer, Hirano, and Tucker (1989), is "surgery designed primarily for the improvement of

the voice . . . aesthetic surgery for the vocal system'' (p. 175). If this defini-
tion of surgery is accepted, such procedures as the surgical removal of vocal
nodules, of polyps and other tumors, and of Reinke's edema, whether done
by the knife or laser, would not be considered phonosurgery unless the surgeon
realizes that altering the vocal fold has the potential of altering the voice,
a concern that should be primary in the mind of the surgeon. Procedures that
fit directly into the concept of phonosurgery are those designed to position
the vocal folds into a better position for phonation; those designed to augment
the mass structure of the folds, such as Teflon injection; esophageal shunts;
or surgeries designed to change the position, length, or shape of the vocal
folds (von Leden et al., 1989).

Due to the growth in the concept of phonosurgery, a trend in laryngology
is to document the patient's voice prior to any surgery that has the potential
to alter the voice. This documentation could be done by a laryngologist or
by a speech–language pathologist who has the necessary equipment. This
documentation should include at least a high-quality audio recording of the
voice, and preferably an additional video recording of phonation. Additional
documentation is available using the equipment described in Chapter 3 (Berke
et al. 1989).

When a physician determines that laryngoscopic inspection with possible
biopsy is necessary, in most cases a general anesthetic is needed. The physician in charge of this process is the anesthesiologist, who produces the general
anesthetic effect by introducing into the patient one of several possible pharmacological agents.

Respiratory control is necessary and is accomplished by oral or nasal
intubation involving a plastic tube that is inserted through the nasal cavity
or oral cavity and into the larynx. A ballooning device on the tube allows
the anesthesiologist to inflate it to protect against aspiration during the surgery since the normal reflexive potential of the larynx is lost under anesthesia.
A respirator is attached to the intubation device, and respiration is thus
controlled.

Before the anesthesiologist intubates the patient, direct physical access
to the larynx is obtained by the insertion of a metal laryngoscope, such as
the Jako System. Close cooperation between the anesthesiologist and the surgeon is necessary since they often must share the same airway space at the
same time. With the patient anesthetized, laryngoscoped, and intubated, surgery
can begin. Throughout the surgical procedures, the anesthesiologist monitors
respiration, blood pressure, pulse, and degree of anesthetic effect; often an
electrocardiogram is used to check heart activity more carefully.

Visualization of the status of the larynx through the laryngoscope is aided
by the attachment of a binocular microscope. The surgeon can inspect the
tissue of the larynx and insert instruments through the laryngoscopic tube
for tissue manipulation and possible removal. These instruments have long
handles, such as the Jako forceps shown in Figure 2–3.

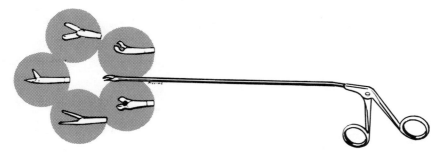

Figure 2–3 Jako Forceps for Microsurgery of the Larynx. Reprinted with permission from *Otolaryngology, Vol. 3: Head and Neck* (2nd ed., p. 47) by M. M. Paparella and D. A. Shumrick (eds.), 1980, Philadelphia: W. B. Saunders. Copyright 1980 by W. B. Saunders.

    Instruments that can be used, depending on the purpose of the surgery, include forceps, scalpels, probes, scissors, suction tip instruments, fiber optic probes for transillumination, needle holders for suturing, and special staining instruments. Each of these instruments is attached to a long handle so it can be introduced through the laryngoscope to reach the larynx. Long needle syringes are used for the injection of materials such as Teflon in the treatment of laryngeal paralysis (described in detail in Chapter 5). With these instruments, the surgeon can remove the tissue for biopsy that will be sent to the pathologist, who will determine its nature under microscopic analysis. If the purpose of the surgery is endolaryngeal removal of pathological tissue, rather than biopsy, this can be accomplished by using the same general surgical procedures.

Laser Microsurgery

Laser microsurgery is a relatively new technique involving the use of the carbon dioxide (CO_2) laser in the treatment of many laryngeal diseases. The CO_2 laser beam has a thermal effect that evaporates the water content and rapidly destroys soft tissue. The amount of destruction depends on the power setting of the beam and the duration of application.

    The CO_2 laser has advantages over traditional surgical techniques involving scissors and scalpels in that it produces minimal bleeding, with no visible postoperative edema or scarring. The CO_2 laser allows more critical demarcation of tissue since it is coupled to a surgical operating microscope. More information on the use of the CO_2 laser for the treatment of various lesions is provided in Chapter 4.

Other additional surgical techniques for voice disorders are described in chapters pertaining to specific disorders. Helpful references include Bailey and Biller (1985), Cody, Kern, and Pearson (1981), Myers and Suen (1989), and Tucker (1987).

Summary

This chapter focuses on presenting general descriptions of medical treatment for the voice-disordered patient. Few patients with voice disorders are not involved in significant medical treatment. The chapter covers the nature of medical specialties pertinent to voice, as well as general examination procedures available, including techniques of laryngoscopy, endoscopy, and radiological examination. General information regarding the importance of pharmaco-therapeutic treatment and general material on surgical techniques are also discussed.

3

Evaluation Procedures in Voice Management

A television commercial shows an automobile engine that from a distance looks normal in every respect. As the camera zooms in and the engine's individual parts become more clearly defined, the announcer describes the filth and contamination actually present in the carburetor as finally seen under the uncompromising scrutiny of the electron microscope.

Luckily, human characteristics are not submitted to the scrutiny of the electron microscope or everyone would be found "filthy and contaminated," ready for the proverbial junkyard. If vocal habits are scrutinized, one finds that many individuals have such pleasing voice characteristics that they attract attention and enhance a communication message. Others have such abnormal voices that listeners' attention is focused on the abnormalities at the expense of communication. Between these extremes lie the majority of persons whose characteristics fall on the various continua that comprise the normal voice.

The professional responsibility of physicians who treat voice-disordered patients and of speech–language pathologists is to identify and discriminate the voice characteristics that are sufficiently abnormal to require some form of treatment. This chapter is designed to help speech–language pathologists in this evaluation.

The voice evaluation process is made more difficult by the fact that some normal parameters cannot be determined easily or objectively (see Chapter 1).

Pitch, loudness, suprasegmentals such as inflection and stress, oral–nasal resonance balance, laryngeal valving functions of the glottal waveform, and general vocal tract resonance functions comprise some of the many parameters with which the speech–language pathologist must be concerned. Many of these factors can be identified and described objectively with the proper equipment; however, some aspects of vocal tract resonance and laryngeal tension are not so easily analyzed. Many times the voice modification decisions are based on perceptual judgments of well-trained speech–language pathologists. Therefore, the state of the art in voice therapy remains a combination of science and perceptual judgment.

The speech–language pathologist often becomes involved in the management of a voice-disordered patient by referral from a physician who has diagnosed the problem, done whatever was medically possible to alleviate abnormal symptoms or characteristics, and finally passed the client on for speech pathology services. In other cases, such as in schools, a child is screened out as having voice characteristics that appear abnormal, and a chain of events is begun to determine whether the disorder is significant enough to warrant management. In both types of cases, the speech–language pathologist must conduct a proper and thorough diagnosis or evaluation.

Medical Referral

One of the most troublesome concerns speech–language pathologists experience is knowing whether or when to refer for medical consultation when the voice case has not been evaluated and referred by a physician. This problem occurs often in schools. Many speech–language pathologists have been trained never to work with a voice case until there has been a medical examination of the larynx and the physician has referred the patient or student for voice therapy. In schools, this can become frustrating to the speech–language professional because medical referral requires parental support and usually a significant amount of money. A student may be identified as having a voice disorder and the referral process begun, only to be stopped by a parent who is unwilling to take the child to a physician; or the child may be referred to a physician, who reports "nothing wrong." Parents then ask, "Why the referral? Why the expense?"

Although there are no easy solutions to these problems, some recommendations are possible. Medical referral is an important part of voice management, and when deliberate and carefully thought-out processes are followed, significantly more referrals will be handled properly. However, this management of referrals requires hard work in developing professional relations with referral physicians.

Although some physicians are happy to work closely with speech–language pathologists; others may not be so cooperative. Thus, it is wise to seek doctors with cooperative attitudes or attempt to change the opinions of those with less cooperative attitudes. Moran and Pentz (1987) surveyed otolaryngolists in five geographical regions of the United States and found that most have a positive attitude about the role of voice therapy with their patients. Most are happy to work with a competent speech–language pathologist and will provide medical support for the voice therapy process.

A speech–language pathologist seeking good relationships should obtain an appointment with a physician (otolaryngologist) to whom referrals are likely. The speech–language pathologist should explain that, since referral is important in the management of voice clients, the purpose of the meeting is to determine or discuss how this can best occur. The following are typical questions that could be asked of the physician:

- How do you feel about referring all persistently hoarse children for a laryngoscopic examination?

- Who should not be referred?

- What happens when you examine a student who is persistently hoarse and your examination does not identify any vocal fold pathology?

- What do you say to the parents and child about the hoarseness? Does this disturb you?

- How do you feel that children with vocal nodules should be handled? With surgery? Vocal therapy? Both? In what order?

- What should I do with a child who has been screened as having a hoarse voice, but whom the parents will not take to a physician for examination because of expense? Are there clinics where these services can be obtained? Do you ever see patients and not charge them full fees?

The issues raised by the above questions are controversial, and both professions are somewhat divided over the answers. A focused position statement on the issue of voice therapy in the public schools was recently presented in *Language Speech & Hearing Services in Schools* (Kahane & Mayo, 1989; Sander, 1989). The speech–language pathologist should understand the polemics involved and form an opinion prior to meeting with the physician, but remain open to the physician's opinions. In any regard, this communication process between the two professionals will form the foundation of a good relationship and can help one decide which physicians are receptive to voice referrals. Open communication is essential for developing rapport, but is difficult over the phone; most physicians would be happy to meet the speech–language pathologist for lunch or dinner to discuss professional matters.

Parental support of the medical referral process is most important. Many problems must be overcome to gain that support and, once again, communication is essential. A note sent home usually produces success in only a few cases. A telephone call is much better. A personal appointment is best and is critical for referral follow-up. The speech–language pathologist should call the parents, set an appointment, and be prepared to convince them that their child has a voice disorder and that medical referral to establish etiology is necessary. It is hard to do this with words alone, and it is recommended that the speech–language pathologist use pictures, models, and tape recordings when possible. Some aids are commercially available.

F. B. Wilson and Rice (1977) have published a voice disorder kit that is excellent in helping to convince parents. The kit contains slides of normal and abnormal vocal folds plus taped samples of children and adults with various voice disorders. These items can be used to help explain in either a simple or a complex manner why there should be a medical referral. The student with the voice disorder also should be present during this explanation.

At the end of the presentation, the parents and involved student should understand what comprises a voice disorder, what its long-term and short-term consequences are, what the possible causes may be, why the medical referral is necessary to determine the specific reason, and whether medical treatment might be necessary before or during therapy. This communication process greatly increases the probability of a successful referral, particularly when good rapport has been established with the physician.

School or clinic policy often forbids referral to a specific physician. Instead, a list of all available doctors in the area who can provide the service is given to the parents or client, who then must make the decision as to whom the referral should be made. This makes little sense and can lead to disappointing results. It would be preferable to provide the names of several physicians who are likely to respond well and let the parents or client decide. In such cases, there is no bad choice. It also is wise to go through a family general physician when one is involved before referring directly to a specialist such as an otolaryngologist.

Screening and Identification

Students with voice disorders usually are identified in screening by a speech–language pathologist early in the school year or by teacher referral. To identify these students accurately, both the speech professional and the teacher must have a working knowledge of what normal voice is and is not. It is appropriate for the speech–language pathologist to hold a short workshop early in the school year to teach the faculty basic listening skills to help the identification process. Again, the Wilson and Rice (1977) kit is helpful in providing slides and taped examples of specific disorders.

Many teachers have little understanding of the voice and the bases of its disorders. A voice disorder workshop should be directed at general listening skills necessary to help identify the two most common areas of voice disorder found in schools: hoarseness and excessive nasality. Many other voice concerns could be taught, but it is wise to keep the instructional process simple and manageable.

The lecture should cover one disorder that causes hoarseness (e.g., vocal nodules) and one that produces excessive nasality (e.g., cleft palate). It is a good idea to show slides to illustrate the laryngeal and pharyngeal bases of these disorders, play taped samples of voice and speech characteristics, and provide practice in listening and judging recorded samples. The presentation should encourage considerable dialogue between the teaching staff and the speech–language pathologist and improve the process of teacher identification of students with voice disorder.

Problems in Voice Screening

When screening children in school, it is necessary to keep in mind that voice patterns and larynx conditions are highly changeable and capricious. Many severe voice disorders are a result of temporary conditions. A child may have a severe cold or allergic reaction that causes changes in the laryngeal structures that produce hoarseness. It is inappropriate to enroll such a child in voice therapy until more is known about the persistency and etiology of the vocal pattern. Since the same voice characteristics can be caused by temporary as well as by more persistent etiologies, it is necessary to follow up on screening to ensure that the child has a condition that requires remediation.

Questions should be asked of the child at the screening: "Does your voice always sound as it does today? Do you have a cold? How long has your voice sounded like this?"

The reliability of the answers may be questionable, but they can provide some insight as to whether the voice disorder is temporary or persistent. These same questions should be asked of the child's classroom teacher.

Regardless of the information thus gained, the speech–language pathologist should screen the child again 2 weeks later. Comparison of vocal patterns 2 weeks apart requires that at the initial screening a sample be taped of any child whose voice is abnormal. The student should state name, date, school, and count from 1 to 20. This is the only sample needed.

Whether to Refer to a Physician

When the persistency of voice disorder has been determined and the vocal pattern judged abnormal, the next question is whether medical referral is necessary. To be on the safe side, the speech–language pathologist could refer every child with any kind of voice disorder for medical clearance before initiating therapy; however, such a conservative approach is unnecessary. The primary concern is that a child might have a serious medical condition in the laryngeal structures requiring surgery or medicine rather than therapy. Such conditions do exist commonly and the concern is legitimate.

A question often asked is whether speech–language pathologists should be concerned about laryngeal cancer in children. The answer is simple: This condition is so rare in children that voice cases need not be referred just to be sure that the youngsters do not have cancer. However, other medical conditions that are not rare can be progressive and interfere with breathing, and the speech–language pathologist should be aware of these possibilities.

Juvenile papillomas (see Chapter 8) resemble wart-like growths in the larynx that can obstruct the airway. The vocal symptoms are not easily distinguished from those produced by a less threatening condition such as vocal nodules, but the treatment is radically different and entirely medical. Other conditions such as laryngeal web, polyps, laryngeal paralysis, and trauma all can produce similar voice symptoms. Medical examination of the larynx thus is necessary to determine the exact cause of the vocal symptoms.

Therefore, a safe but not necessarily conservative position on referral is that any child with a voice disorder stemming from abnormal functioning of the vocal folds that produces a difference in voice quality, or in any way makes breathing difficult, should be evaluated medically before management by a speech–language pathologist. Laryngeal symptoms of persistent breathiness, tension, hoarseness, diplophonia, strain, aphonia, stoppage of phonation in the middle of a word or phrase, or any combination of these factors requires medical attention before voice management when not associated with a cold or upper respiratory infection (discussed in detail in other sections).

Other characteristics such as high-pitched voice, slight nasality that probably is not associated with velopharyngeal insufficiency, a soft (insufficiently loud) voice, or an excessively loud voice not associated with other laryngeal symptomatology usually can be managed without medical referral as long as improvement occurs rather quickly. When progress is not rapid, the speech–language pathologist would do well to refer the patient to a physician so as to rule out organicity. Experience with persons having voice disorder can help shape the philosophy of each speech–language pathologist as to when medical referrals should be made. Before sufficient experience has been obtained, a speech–language pathologist should perhaps be more liberal in selecting those who need medical referral. It is better to err on the side of over-referral.

The Case History

The process of taking a case history in the evaluation of persons having voice disorder is very important. Information can be obtained that can help the speech–language pathologist determine factors related to organicity requiring medical attention or to stress or emotional maladjustment requiring psychological or psychiatric referral, as well as factors that provide prognostic value and insight about which therapeutic approach might be most successful. The taking of case histories requires excellence in interviewing so the client is made to feel comfortable in sharing information that might be considered private and rather intimate. Several excellent case history forms have been published (Boone & McFarlane, 1988; Colton & Casper, 1990; D. K. Wilson, 1987; F. B. Wilson & Rice, 1977). However, the proper form to guide the questioning is not sufficient for obtaining an excellent case history; much more is necessary.

Emerick and Hatten (1974) pointed out that the speech–language pathologist who has been trained to think objectively and scientifically often may find talking with a client or the parents of a child so difficult that case history forms replace personal interaction. They described a case history interview as "essentially a process, not an entity—a process of verbal and nonverbal intercourse between a trained professional worker and a client seeking . . . services" (p. 25). They discussed many of the mistakes commonly made by clinicians and offered constructive suggestions.

Hutchinson, Hanson, and Mecham (1979) suggested that a good interview should begin with open-ended, unambiguous, but not too specific questions. In a voice case history, such questions might include, "What is the problem you are having with your voice? Tell me how it developed."

The next important task for the speech–language pathologist is to listen to the information provided so that pertinent follow-up questions can be asked. One of the most common mistakes beginning speech–language students make in the case history process is to ask a general question listed on some form and not respond to the information provided, but merely proceed to the next listed question. Listening and responding by comment or further questioning demonstrate mature and well-developed skills in interviewing.

If the speech–language pathologist follows a form in taking a case history, it should be used toward the end of the interview as a safeguard to ensure that all specific questions have been asked. The interview should begin with general questions such as those suggested. The interview then can proceed with specific follow-up questions through the background of the disorder; onset and treatment history; related illnesses and medical aspects; day-to-day variability; social, vocational, and educational considerations; and finally the effect it is having on the client.

The speech–language pathologist then can go back over the case history form to ask specific questions that might have been overlooked. The form can be introduced by saying, "Let me go over this form to see if we have missed anything of importance. Let me see . . . Oh yes, what medications are you taking?"

The following specific areas should be investigated in any voice disorder case history:

- Nature of concern regarding the voice
- Date of onset of the disorder
- Known etiology
- Progression of the disorder since onset
- Treatment(s) sought
- Success of previous treatments
- Nature of general health and history of previous illnesses
- Association of onset with any physical ailments, emotional stress, or psychological disturbance
- Variation of vocal parameters throughout the day
- Voice fatigue factors
- Vocal habits during typical day
- Leisure time vocal habits
- Stability of vocational, social, and familial background
- Significant aspects of stress in vocational, social, familial, and marital life
- History of significant medicine usage, including current usage
- History of tobacco and alcohol consumption
- Litigation procedures pertaining to the disorder
- Pain associated with the voice disorder
- Voice disorder's effect on vocational, social, familial, and marital life
- Aspects of voice most distressing: pitch, loudness, quality, durability, stability
- Other considerations not specifically covered that the client feels might be important

These questions and areas of concern pertain to a general voice disorder case history. Obviously, many clients are referred for an evaluation because of a specific disorder, and much of this information would not be relevant. Examples include the person who is being seen shortly after a laryngectomy, or one referred because of vocal nodules, contact ulcers, or some other specific disorder. In such cases, only questions pertaining to that problem would be appropriate.

Some of the above topics of investigation in the case history are self-evident for inclusion; others may need clarification. One area of questioning is concerned with the history of tobacco and alcohol consumption. If alcohol consumption is merely social, there is little concern. The possibility exists, however, that excessive alcohol consumption can be related to concerns of alcoholism, general health, and behavioral control from a vocal abuse point of view. The relationship between smoking and laryngeal pathology is so clearly delineated that to ignore the evidence is foolish. I am so convinced of smoking's deleterious effect on voice that I would not enroll a client in voice therapy if smoking continues to be a problem. The specific evidence for such a position is provided in Chapter 4.

Another area of questioning is concerned with litigation matters. Laryngologists are facing an increase in medicolegal cases involving the voice. Von Leden (1988) reported that the most common areas of litigation involve aggressive surgery for vocal nodules, failure to diagnose a malignant tumor, injudicious injections of Teflon and other prosthetics, and iatrogenic injuries of the laryngeal nerves. He cautioned his otolaryngology colleagues to take elementary precautions, keep good records, obtain informed consent, be precise in surgery for benign lesions of the vocal cords, and make pre- and post-surgery audio recordings of patient voices. It is important that any speech–language pathologist working with patients involved in litigation recognize the importance of good record keeping practices and voice recording documentation.

Evaluation of Specific Voice Parameters

Following the case history interview, the speech–language pathologist must evaluate specific parameters of phonation to determine which, if any, are abnormal and contribute to the voice disorder. The evaluation process includes a description of instrumentation involved in objective measurement.

Pitch (Frequency)

The pitch of a human voice is a psychological or perceptual correlate of the physical dimension of frequency of vocal fold vibration. When exhaled air from the lungs reaches the closed vocal folds, pressure builds until it is sufficient to blow the vocal folds apart, setting them into vibration. The frequency of vibration establishes the perceived pitch. Stated more simply, a person's voice is high, low, average, appropriate, or inappropriate for a given age and sex depending on how many times per second the vocal folds vibrate when activated by exhaled air. There are complex anatomical, physiological, and acoustical bases for this process, as explained in Chapter 1 (see, e.g., A. E. Aronson, 1985; Bless & Abbs, 1983; Colton & Casper, 1990).

Frequency of vocal fold vibration is determined by the critical variables of (a) vocal fold length, (b) vocal fold mass, (c) vocal fold tension, (d) shape of the resonance system, and (e) airflow and subglottal air pressure factors. These variables interact in complex fashion to determine voice pitch. Age and sex differences are apparent and are reflected in pitch.

The speech–language pathologist is not capable of determining the status of the vocal folds with regard to length, mass, and tension except by analyzing the pitch of the voice; only subjective judgments about the actual size characteristics of the vocal folds can be made. Therefore, the client's pitch is critical to evaluate. Key questions to ask include: Is the pitch appropriate for the age and sex of the person? Is it too low? Too high? Monopitched? Is there sex confusion when others hear the voice without seeing the speaker? Is the pitch a factor of vocal abuse/misuse?

Essentials of Pitch Evaluation. To be comfortable with pitch evaluation, the speech–language pathologist should be generally knowledgeable about the pitch spectrum of the human voice and how it relates to the musical scale. The following are some basic concepts relating these two areas:

- The range of tones produced by the human voice can be compared with the musical tones (notes) on a piano, pitch pipe, or any musical instrument.

- Piano notes, for example, range from 27 Hz (lowest note) to 4186 Hz (highest note).

- All the notes (tones) between these frequency values on the piano can be divided into octaves.

- An octave represents a doubling of the frequency of vibration, so a tone of 100 Hz doubled to 200 Hz would constitute an increase of one octave.

- Each octave is divided into eight whole tones, with each tone represented by a letter of the alphabet: CDEFGABC. Each C begins a new octave.

- From C to D is one whole tone step. C sharp (C$\sharp$) represents a halftone step up. That same C$\sharp$ can be represented as a halftone step down from D, in which case it would be designated as D flat (D$\flat$).

- The octave in the middle of the piano scale contains the commonly known note of middle C, which corresponds to a frequency of 262 Hz. (The term middle C derives from the fact that it is the note that divides the treble and bass clefs and is common to both clefs.) Any C note in an octave below middle C is designated as C_1, C_2, C_3, depending on the octave below middle C in which it is found. C_1 is stated as C one octave below middle C, D_2 as two Ds below middle C.

- A note falling above the octave in which middle C is found carries the designator above the letter, such as C^2, F^3 or A^1. These examples are stated as C two octaves above middle C, F three above the F in the middle C octave, and A one above the A in the middle C octave.

- Some references show a different octave designating system in which the lowest octave is the first (1), the next octave up the scale is second (2), third (3), fourth (4), fifth (5), and so on. In that system, middle C is in the fourth (4) octave and the middle C note would be designated as C_4. That system is not used here.

- Each note or tone in the musical scale can be indicated by its alphabetical note (CDEFGABC) in the octave it represents, such as A_2 or B^2, or by its actual numerical frequency, such as 110 Hz or 1975 Hz, respectively.

Table 3–1 compares tones with the frequency and musical scale values in the human voice range.

In the evaluation, the speech–language pathologist's task is to determine the client's habitual pitch level and how it relates to the pitch that would be optimal. The habitual pitch is the modal or average level heard in a continuing sample of speech, the level around which normal pitch inflections occur, the one heard most commonly as a person talks—the central tendency of pitch. The optimal pitch is the one best suited for the length, mass, and tension factors in the client's larynx and is the level at which the larynx functions most efficiently.

TABLE 3–1
Frequency and Musical Scale Values

Note	Frequency (Hz)[a]	Note	Frequency (Hz)	Note	Frequency (Hz)
A_3	55	A_1	220	A^1	880
B_3	62	B_1	245	B^1	988
C_2	65	C	262	C^2	1046
D_2	73	D	294	D^2	1175
E_2	82	E	330	E^2	1318
F_2	87	F	349	F^2	1397
G_2	98	G	392	G^2	1568
A_2	110	A	440	A^2	1760
B_2	123	B	494	B^2	1975
C_1	131	C^1	523	C^3	2093
D_1	147	D^1	587	D^3	2349
E_1	164	E^1	659	E^3	2637
F_1	175	F^1	698	F^3	2794
G_1	196	G^1	784	G^3	3136

[a]All decimal points are rounded.

Under the best of conditions, the habitual pitch level used (the most common) should be the same as the optimal (the best suited), but this often is not the case. The speech–language pathologist thus must evaluate both the habitual and optimal levels to determine whether they are the same or different and, if different, whether the variance is clinically significant.

Pitch can be evaluated with complex and elaborate equipment or with a sample pitch pipe that can be purchased for a few dollars at any music store. One instrument is the Visi-Pitch 6087 DS (Figure 3–1) produced by Kay Elemetrics Corporation. The instrument provides a digital readout of the fundamental frequency of vocal fold vibration (F_0), as well as an oscilloscopic rendering of phonation. When the client speaks into a microphone attached to the Visi-Pitch, the F_0 of the voice is extracted; up to 8 sec of voice can be stored on the oscilloscope. A cursor then can identify the specific F_0 for any point along the 8 sec. The device has a split screen for stored comparisons. These measurements also can be obtained from a quality tape recording. The instrument provides analyses of relative intensity (loudness) changes in the voice, voice onset time (VOT), quality variations, glottal attack patterns, intonation, timing and stress functions, and vibrato. (Many of these functions are described later.)

A pitch pipe (Figure 3–2) is a miniature harmonica-type instrument that produces any of 13 specific tones in an octave when blown upon by a person. The tones include sharps and flats, which are the halftone steps mentioned

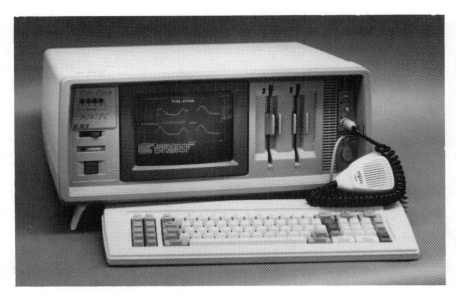

Figure 3–1 Visi-Pitch Voice Analyzer.

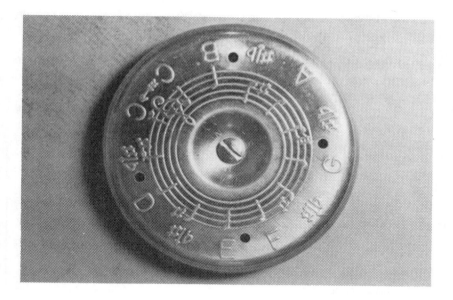

Figure 3–2 A Pitch Pipe.

earlier. Since a pitch pipe is restricted to the notes or tones in a specific octave, the user must be prepared to make octave adjustments when using it. The pitch pipe is seldom used in speech–language pathologist's evaluations since instrumentation for such evaluations is so readily available; however, in school systems and less well-equipped facilities, a pitch pipe or piano may be the only means available for pitch evaluations.

Habitual and Optimal Pitch Levels

The human voice is capable of producing tones which can be closely matched to notes or tones on the musical scale using a pitch pipe or piano, or which can provide a digital frequency F_0 display when the appropriate instrument is used. The following are verbal instructions a speech–language pathologist can use in eliciting a client's habitual pitch levels.

Habitual Pitch. After the speech–language pathologist has listened long enough in conversation to recognize the client's habitual pitch level, the next task is merely to isolate the habitual (modal) pitch so it can be measured. An instrument such as the Visi-Pitch is used to isolate the pitch of the voice. The cursor can be used to produce a ''goodness of fit'' that should isolate the habitual pitch rather closely. The speech–language pathologist must merely determine that the isolated sample on the oscilloscope or the CRT is representative of the client's typical speaking voice. If so, the digital readout or the average on the computer readout (computed statistics) is the habitual pitch.

Basal pitch.   To determine the basal pitch, have the client start at the determined habitual pitch and hum down the scale until a tone is produced that is low but does not involve glottal fry. This likely represents the basal pitch. Measure this pitch with the instrumentation.

Ceiling pitch.   To determine the ceiling or highest pitch possible, have the client hum up the musical scale until the highest note emerges that does not sound strained. With instrumentation, it is easy to have a client produce a glissando or sliding pitch. This can be modeled by the speech–language pathologist. Merely measure the highest point in the pitch to obtain the ceiling.

Range.   Subtract the ceiling frequency from the basal frequency to determine the vocal range in frequency. Normal values for a healthy larynx would be in the order of two to three octaves. Remember, an octave is a doubling of the frequency. If a female client had a basal frequency of 150 Hz and a ceiling of 600 Hz, she would have a two-octave range of pitch: $150 \times 2 = 300$ Hz (1st octave) $\times 2 = 600$ Hz (2nd octave). Thus, her pitch range could be expressed in actual hertz ($600 - 150 = 450$ Hz), or in octaves (two octaves), which would be a better expression of her vocal range. It is easier to compare pitch range in octaves than actual frequency since two persons, one male and the other female, might have the same frequency range in hertz and reflect very different laryngeal conditions. In the example above, our female client had a range of 450 Hz, representing a two-octave range. A male with a range of 450 Hz with a basal frequency of 80 Hz would have closer to 2½ octaves of range: $80 \times 2 = 160$ Hz (1st octave) $\times 2 = 320$ Hz (2nd octave) $+ 130$ Hz left over into the third octave.

Optimal Pitch.   Finding the habitual, basal, and ceiling pitches is only the first step in determining the appropriateness of the client's pitch. The speech–language pathologist then must determine the optimal pitch, the one best suited for the client's voice structure. The optimal pitch should not be interpreted as a single level, but rather as a range below which the client should seldom speak except on downward pitch inflections at the end of a phrase or sentence. Therefore, when optimal pitch level is discussed here, it is with this range concept in mind, and the optimal pitch should be considered as the lowest pitch in that range.

The optimal pitch usually is about three or four whole tones from the bottom of the range. The following are steps the speech–language pathologist should follow in locating this pitch:

- Have the client hum the tone that was established as the habitual pitch level, for example, A#$_1$ (230 Hz).

- Have the client start at this habitual pitch and hum down the scale in whole tones until the lowest tone possible has been produced that does not involve glottal fry. This is the basal tone.

- Have the client hum up the musical scale in whole tones until a tone about four tones above the basal has been reached. This should be close to the optimal tone if not exactly it.

- Determine when the optimal pitch has been reached by noting that the client's voice suddenly becomes a little louder without increased vocal effort. The client should report that this tone is easier to produce than those below it.

- Decide that the optimal tone or pitch has been found when the client's repeated attempts to produce a tone in whole steps from the lowest one up four notes produces the same tone that increases suddenly in loudness and is easier to produce. This tone then can be measured on an instrument such as the Visi-Pitch.

The speech-language pathologist must keep in mind that the optimal pitch level is a subjective level at which voice production seems easiest and most efficient for the client. It usually is found about four tones above the basal. This is not to say that it is the only optimal pitch, but merely that it is the lowest tone that should be used habitually as the optimal pitch, with normal pitch inflections up and down from it. The client should be able to speak comfortably in a narrow range of pitches beginning not much lower than the determined optimal pitch. Habitual use of the optimal pitch level takes much less effort to produce the normal pitch inflections and loudness changes necessary to provide dynamic characteristics of voice.

The concept of optimal pitch is controversial in that attempts to experimentally establish its validity and reliability have been somewhat unsuccessful, particularly when optimal pitch is associated with the ability to increase significantly the intensity of the voice (Colton & Casper, 1990; Stone, 1983). I agree, however, with Perkins (1983) that it is clinically appropriate to determine whether a voice client is using a pitch level that is devoid of constriction. Such a pitch requires a high or vertical pitch focus. When this is achieved, vocal abuse associated with pitch is eliminated. Therefore, comparing a client's habitual pitch with some construct of what might be optimal makes clinical sense.

As indicated previously, the human voice frequency range is approximately three octaves. An octave contains 8 whole notes or tones, so most adults have a speaking range of about 24 tones. Since the optimal pitch usually is about 4 tones above the basal of that 24-tone range, this means that a person typically has much more potential for pitch inflection upward than downward when speaking at the optimal pitch. If the habitual pitch level is too low compared with what would be optimal, there is increased risk that the person will be speaking very near the basal pitch, which is hard on the larynx. (This is discussed in detail in Chapter 4 in the section on vocal abuse/misuse.) This potential for vocal abuse and misuse makes it important to determine the habitual and optimal pitch levels in clients with voice disorder.

Additional Methods of Finding Optimal Pitch

Several other methods of finding the optimal pitch level have been reported in the literature. Fairbanks (1960) described a method in which the client is asked to phonate the entire vocal range, including a falsetto. The total range of all musical notes is counted. For adult males, the optimal pitch level would be found one-fourth of the range from the bottom.

Several less objective methods of finding the optimal pitch include having the patient sigh loudly or say "uh-huh" in a spontaneous manner or grunt in a natural manner. It is likely that these methods produce a tone close to the optimal level.

It should be pointed out, however, that many persons when sighing, saying "uh-huh," and grunting will do so with considerable pitch inflection. Depending on the extent of a sigh, or perhaps how relaxed a person is when producing it, the sigh may involve a frequency range of nearly one octave from beginning to end. In such a case, which note of the sigh constitutes the optimal pitch? It is generally accepted that the highest note produced is closest to the target optimal pitch.

Pitch Range

Fundamental frequency range has been used extensively as an index of vocal health. The F_0 difference between the lowest tone produced and the highest tone constitutes the range, which can be expressed in absolute frequencies, tones or semitones, or octaves. Several authors have presented data on vocal range (Baken, 1987; Boone & McFarlane, 1988; Cotton & Casper, 1990; D. K. Wilson, 1987) and found the typical range of children and adults to be between two and three octaves. My clinical experience indicates that a typical range is usually closer to two octaves than three. The range is determined by the lowest and highest frequencies chosen for comparison, and these frequencies are affected by several variables, including time of day, whether the voice has been used and properly prepared for testing, and the method of eliciting the high and low frequencies. Reich, Mason, Frederickson, and Schlauch (1989) tested 40 normal children under five conditions of eliciting maximal and minimal F_0 and found significant differences under each condition among the same children. The condition that elicited the widest range was the fast glissando method.

Vocal Quality

Chapter 1 describes the parameters of normal voice quality, including characteristics of the glottal waveform and resonance contributions. This section deals with voice quality in the clinical sense. It demonstrates how the speech–language pathologist can evaluate a person's voice quality with instruments, as well as by listening skill and perceptual judgment.

Voice quality can be a confusing dimension for many speech–language pathologists since the descriptive terms often used have little scientific basis or semantic uniformity. Such abstract terms as mellow, rich, harsh, raspy, piercing, twangy, throaty, hoarse, and spastic are difficult to measure or describe. Nevertheless, the speech–language pathologist must be prepared to evaluate specific voice characteristics that determine the overall quality so as to identify parameters that require modification.

Voice quality is determined either at the vibrating vocal fold level or by the shaping and resonating of sound produced by the vocal folds in the chambers of the pharyngeal, oral, and nasal cavities. When quality is affected negatively at the vocal fold level, it is because the folds are not vibrating properly as a result of some organic or functional condition in the larynx. Resonance processes cannot mask the negative effect produced by the vocal folds when they are vibrating abnormally.

Hypofunctional and Hyperfunctional Voice

For normal voice quality to occur, the vocal folds must be able to meet at laryngeal midline to approximate along their entire length with just enough medial compression to impede the exhaled airstream, causing them to vibrate. There is a delicate balance between this approximation and resistance to airflow and the subglottal air pressure necessary to produce voice vibrations.

Several conditions in the larynx might affect the balance negatively. The vocal folds might vibrate with too little approximation, allowing excessive air to escape through the glottis, in which case the voice will sound excessively breathy, meaning there is excessive airflow through the glottis during phonation. On the other hand, too much approximation can result in a voice marked by excessive tension. These conditions, respectively, cause voice quality to be hypofunctional (too little approximation) or hyperfunctional (too much approximation).

Hypofunctional and hyperfunctional extremes occur often. An extreme of hypofunctional approximation is no voice at all, a condition called aphonia. An extreme of hyperfunctional approximation produces a voice quality so tense that airflow from the lungs cannot overcome the resistance of the taut vocal folds, producing a quality that sounds spastic.

Between these extremes is a continuum of the gradients of laryngeal vibration. The voice qualities reflected in this continuum are described next in sufficient detail to allow the speech–language pathologist to be comfortable with each one. Exhibit 3–1 illustrates this continuum of vibration function at the vocal fold level.

Aphonia

The hypofunctional condition of aphonia results from some forms of psychogenic voice (nonorganic) disorder in which nothing is structurally wrong with the vocal folds, but the client produces no voice or sound at all. It also is found in recently laryngectomized persons. Other than laryngectomees, aphonic individuals are those who for psychological reasons make no attempt to produce voice or are so weak from illness or neurological disease that voice production is not possible.

Whisper

Whisper, which is on the hypofunctional end of the continuum, is easy to understand and identify because everyone has had an occasion to use it deliberately in such instances as in the library, in church, or behind someone's back. However, the person who at all times can only whisper has a serious voice disorder. It could be caused by organic disease or psychological maladjustment.

The quality described as whisper voice is produced by vocal folds that are so far apart during speaking attempts that only articulated airstream is heard. This articulation of sounds without voice support is the distinguishing characteristic between the whisper quality and aphonia. In other words, the consonant sounds articulated by the tongue, teeth, or lips are heard in the whisper quality, but no voice supports them.

My opinion is that whisper quality usually is a psychogenic (nonorganic) voice disorder, since an organic condition seldom produces true whisper other than in cases of severe and advanced neuromuscular disease. In most instances, whisper represents a functional turnoff of phonation.

The glottal and supraglottal configurations supporting whispering have been generally described for clinical purposes (A. E. Aronson, 1985; Boone

Exhibit 3–1 Continuum of Vocal Fold Approximation

Hypofunction	*Normal Function*	*Hyperfunction*
Aphonia . . . Whisper . . . Breathiness . . . Normal Tension . . . Excessive Tension . . . Spasticity		

Note. Reprinted with permission from *Clinical Management of Speech Disorders* (p. 114) by D. E. Mowrer and J. L. Case, 1982, Austin, TX: PRO-ED. Copyright 1982 by PRO-ED.

& McFarlane, 1988), but only recently objectively delineated. Solomon, McCall, Trosset, and Gray (1989) used fiber optic endoscopy on 10 normal subjects under various conditions of whispered speech. They described vocal fold configuration, glottal size, and airway constriction of supraglottal structures and found significant differences between low-effort and high-effort whispering. Individual subject differences, however, tended to be considerably larger than any systematic patterns of whisper type. One significant finding pertains to the recommendation of whisper to accomplish vocal rest: The authors generally found vocal fold approximation during running speech whispering, which would be counterproductive to the recommendation of whispering as a form of vocal rest.

Breathiness

Breathiness is a mixture of voice with an excessive escape of air during speaking attempts. On the low end of the continuum, it is almost like a whisper except that slightly more voice is heard. Breathiness ranges from the near whisper to nearly normal voice. The significance of these subtle degrees of breathiness and an understanding of their causes are important factors in the clinical management of many voice disorders.

Excessive Tension

On the hyperfunctional side of the normal vibration pattern (described in Chapter 1) is phonation, which includes excessive overaddduction or medial compression of the vocal folds. This quality is heard perceptually as excessive tension. Like breathiness, tension exists on a continuum from slight (beyond normal approximation) to a degree that essentially stops the passive vibration of the vocal folds.

Tension is a common factor in many organic and nonorganic voice disorders, and the subtle variations often heard from client to client are important in distinguishing various voice disorders. Tension is a factor of excessive glottal resistance to airflow and subglottal pressure and often is described as a factor of overpressure. The greater the tension or overpressure factor, the greater the factors of airflow and subglottal pressure needed to cause vibration.

The above categories of vocal fold approximation from hypofunctional to hyperfunctional aspects have been described perceptually. Hillman, Holmberg, Perkell, Walsh, and Vaughan (1989) are among many who have attempted to quantify vocal characteristics. Using noninvasive aerodynamic and acoustic recordings, measures of transglottal pressure, average glottal airflow, glottal resistance, vocal efficiency, vocal intensity, and fundamental frequency were obtained on 15 voice patients with nodules, polyps, contact ulcers, and nonorganic dysphonia. The results from these voice patients were compared with normative data on 45 subjects from an earlier study by these same authors. Although the authors reported their findings to be preliminary, they were able to discriminate objectively various conditions of hyperfunctional voice and correlate them to specific disorder conditions. Organic manifestations of vocal hyperfunction from nodules and so on were accompanied by abnormally high values for the glottal waveform parameters of airflow, which reflected high vocal fold closure velocities and collision forces which produce vocal trauma. The opposite flow and acoustic parameters were found among the nonorganic voices, resulting in increased unmodulated airflow, forces less likely to cause vocal trauma. Other researchers have obtained surface electromyographic signals in an attempt to quantify the vocally hyperfunctional patient (Redenbaugh & Reich, 1989).

Spasticity

When vocal tension from too much approximation of the vocal folds or overpressure is so great that even increased effort is not sufficient to overcome the resistance, voice is stopped and vocal spasticity occurs. In most cases, vocal spasticity is an intermittent phenomenon during voice production, rather than a complete stoppage at all times. Typically, the person with a spastic voice quality manifests periods of excessive tension with periodic episodes of spasticity.

Combination of Factors in Dysphonia

In addition to the voice quality parameters just described, which represent variances along the phonation continuum from hypofunction to hyperfunction, several characteristics involve combinations of factors. These include hoarseness, breathiness, tension, and diplophonia.

Hoarseness

Many different organic conditions affecting the vocal folds can produce the perceptual quality described as hoarseness (Boone & McFarlane, 1988). Hoarseness is a voice quality characterized by a rasping, grating, sometimes husky sound, frequently accompanied by voice breaks and/or diplophonia (double pitch). This description is typical of the perceptual usage of this term.

However, Yanagihara (1967) attempted to describe the components of hoarseness more objectively by ranking perceptual judgment samples of hoarseness as to slight, moderate, or severe degrees. Sonograms (spectrograms) were used to identify the acoustic parameters that distinguished the severity ratings. The acoustic properties of hoarseness were determined mainly by the interactions of three factors:

1. Noise components in the main formant of each vowel sampled

2. High-frequency noise components above 3000 Hz

3. Loss of high-frequency harmonic components

The greater the severity of hoarseness, the more prominent and exaggerated these factors become. On the basis of these findings, Yanagihara advocated a classification of four types of hoarseness using sonogram tracings:

Type I: The regular harmonic components in the sonogram are mixed with the noise component, chiefly in the formant region of the vowels.

Type II: The noise components in the second formants of /ɛ/ and /i/ predominate over the harmonic components, and slight additional noise components appear in the high-frequency region above 3000 Hz in the vowels /ɛ/ and /i/.

Type III: The second formants of /ɛ/ and /i/ are totally replaced by noise components, and the additional noise components above 3000 Hz further intensify their energy and expand their range.

Type IV: The second formants of /ɑ/, /ɛ/, and /i/ are replaced by noise components, and even the first formants of all vowels often lose their periodic components, which are supplemented by noise components. In addition, more intensified high-frequency noise components are seen.

V. I. Wolfe and Steinfatt (1987) utilized, among other measures, Yanagihara's (1967) sonogram tracing types to discriminate objectively normal from abnormal phonation among 51 patients with diverse laryngeal pathologies and found spectrographic noise to be the best single predictor of abnormality.

In addition to the objective classification of hoarseness advocated by Yanagihara (1967), several authors have described acoustic characteristics involved in hoarseness, including vowel roughness (Emanuel & Whitehead, 1979), quasi-periodicity or aperiodicity of vocal fold vibratory pattern (Lieberman, 1963), and abnormal frequency perturbation (jitter) patterns (Murry & Doherty, 1980).

It seems clear from the descriptions of hoarseness that many different characteristics are involved that have been described perceptually and acoustically. Many different organic conditions affecting the vocal folds can produce that quality.

When a person has a cold and accompanying laryngitis, the voice becomes hoarse. Hoarseness also is caused by upper respiratory infections; allergies in the larynx; growths on the vocal folds, including cancer; vocal abuse/misuse; and numerous other conditions (described later). Because the etiologies of hoarseness are so varied, the patterns of voice quality described as hoarseness similarly are varied.

Breathiness

Most varieties of hoarseness result when some condition of the vocal folds prevents normal approximation and symmetrical vibration. For example, folds swollen from an infection usually are not affected uniformly. The mass characteristics of each fold therefore are different. In addition, the vibrating edge of each fold may be rough and uneven, resulting in incomplete approximation while speaking. This results in increased unobstructed airflow through the glottis during phonation, and breathiness is the perceptual characteristic heard.

Tension

Tension is often heard perceptually in hoarseness. Tension is introduced when the person attempts to overcome breathiness. These factors of breathiness and tension, coupled with vocal folds that vibrate aperiodically because of mass differences, form the bases of hoarseness. Some types of hoarseness involve a wet quality when excessive mucous secretions are present on the tissue of the folds. Other forms sound excessively dry when there is insufficient lubrication of those tissues. Hoarseness in its many forms can range from slight to severe.

Diplophonia

Another characteristic commonly heard in dysphonia is double pitch, called diplophonia in the literature (A. E. Aronson, 1985; Boone & McFarlane, 1988; Colton & Casper, 1990). Reasons for diplophonia include the following:

- One vocal fold's having different mass characteristics from the other vocal fold and therefore vibrating at a fundamental frequency that is sufficiently different to produce the perception of two pitches

- The action of the ventricular folds in vibrating simultaneously with the true vocal folds, producing two pitches

Diplophonia often is heard in cases of unilateral vocal fold paralysis in which the nerve supply to one vocal fold is disrupted for some reason. Without innervation, the approximation potential of the paralyzed fold is disrupted, which after a considerable period of time will cause tissue atrophy. The lessened mass of the paralyzed vocal fold will cause it to vibrate faster when it is in a position to be influenced by exhaled air. The faster rate of vibration will be perceived as a higher pitch being produced by the paralyzed vocal fold than by the normal one.

Instrumentation in Voice Quality Evaluation

Some instruments available for the speech–language pathologist in evaluating voice parameters that determine quality include the spectrograph, the electroglottograph, aeromechanical (flow and pressure) instrumentation, and a good audio recorder. The clinical voice laboratory is becoming an expected facility in training programs in speech–language pathology as well as in the clinical offices of otolaryngologists. An excellent description of the basic instrumentation needed for such a laboratory is found in Gould (1988).

Spectrograph

The sound or speech spectrograph has been described by Lieberman (1977) as probably the single most useful device for the quantitative analysis of speech. It was developed at Bell Telephone Laboratories in connection with work on analysis–synthesis speech transmission systems.

Common instruments are the Kay Electronic Company Digital Sona-Graph 7800, which is a DC-16k Hz Spectrum Analyzer, which produces spectrographic, fast Fourier transform, waveform, amplitude, and other analysis displays in real time. The DSP Sona-Graph's memory stores 2 MB of sampled data, which translates to about 50 sec of speech sampled at 20k Hz. An example of a digital sonagraph is shown in Figure 3–3.

Electroglottograph

One of the most precise instruments available for glottal waveform analysis is the electroglottograph, also called the laryngograph. An example of such an instrument is the Kay Elemetrics Laryngograph. The laryngograph

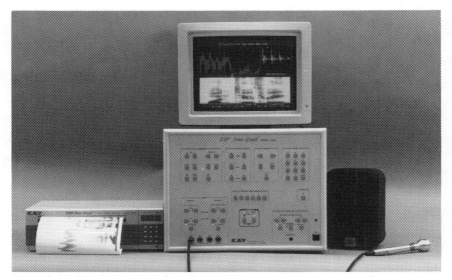

Figure 3–3 Digital Sound Spectrograph.

transducers, positioned on the surface of the user's neck, detect changes in voltage across the vocal folds during the vibratory cycle. The duration, velocity, and degree of closure of the vocal folds are visually represented. These results are displayed on a monitor, oscilloscope, or graphic printout. The laryngograph system works with VisiPitch, IBM PC, or Sona-Graph. The waveform data can be compared with acoustic and airflow data for further quantification of vocal parameters (Baer, Titze, & Yoshioka, 1983; Karnell, 1989; Scherer, Gould, Titze, Meyers, & Sataloff, 1988; Titze, Baer, Cooper, & Scherer, 1983).

Aeromechanical Instrumentation

Basic to understanding phonation under normal and abnormal conditions is the concept of how airflow and air pressure relate to vocal fold vibration. Several attempts have been made to measure the efficiency of the vocal folds in opposing the flow of air through them to cause vibration, a process called laryngeal airway resistance.

Smitheran and Hixon (1981) described a method of calculating laryngeal airway resistance from the ratio of translaryngeal pressure to translaryngeal airflow. The aeromechanical instrumentation necessary to measure these factors included an air pressure transducer coupled to an amplifier, a filter and storage oscilloscope system for pressure measurements, and a pneumotachometer coupled to a second but matched differential air pressure transducer, amplifier, and storage oscilloscope system for the measurement of airflow. From measurements obtained through these channels directed through a mask, the ratio representing laryngeal airflow resistance was calculated. Data on 15 normal subjects were provided with a mean laryngeal airflow resistance of 35.7 cm H_2O/LPS (liters per second).

Smitheran and Hixon's data compared favorably with earlier studies of laryngeal airway resistance that involved puncturing of the trachea with a hypodermic needle to measure tracheal pressure. The present method is non-invasive and therefore superior.

Woo, Colton, and Shangold (1987) utilized phonatory airflow with 150 patients having various laryngeal diseases and compared them with 60 persons having normal voices. They were able to discriminate categories of dysphonia etiology (paralysis, polyp, cancer, vocal nodules, etc.) on the basis of mean flow (unphonated) compared with alternating flow (modulated by vocal folds in phonation), as well as other frequency spectra data.

Normal values of laryngeal airflow are between 100 and 150 cc/sec (or ml/sec). Laryngeal pathology significantly alters normal values. For example, a patient with laryngeal paralysis manifests poor laryngeal valving, and excessive air escapes during phonation, producing airflow values from 300 to 400 cc/sec. The perceptual correlate of excessive airflow is increased breathiness in the voice.

When a pneumotachometer is not available, an estimate of laryngeal airflow can be obtained using a measure called phonation quotient, which correlates quite well with actual measurements of flow. The phonation quotient is calculated by dividing the vital capacity by the maximum phonation duration. Normative data on this procedure would suggest a phonation quotient of around 145 ml/sec for males and 137 ml/sec for females (Prator & Swift, 1984). Hirano (1981) reported extensive data on phonation quotient values for various ages, but the data compare favorably to Prator and Swift's values.

Instrumentation for Loudness Measurement

With many disorders of phonation, it is necessary to quantify the loudness potential of the voice. The Kay Visi-Pitch (see also Chapter 1) has a loudness (intensity) function as well as pitch analysis function and can measure the two simultaneously. In the intensity-only mode, the Visi-Pitch displays voice intensity variations on the oscilloscope. The oscilloscope screen is subdivided into four grids for each of the lower and upper sections of the screen. Each vertical division represents a 10 dB increase in intensity within the intensity mode. This measurement is of relative intensity, since it provides no absolute value of sound pressure. Absolute intensity can be measured with a sound level meter.

Instrumentation for Resonance Evaluation

Many voice disorders involve functional or organic dysfunction of the velopharyngeal mechanisms, resulting in abnormal vocal tract resonance. When velopharyngeal dysfunction occurs in speech, the vocal quality usually involves excessive nasal resonance, called hypernasality. Devices and instruments have been developed to detect and measure the airflow and air pressure bases to this abnormal resonance.

One instrument designed to measure the velum's effectiveness to effect an air seal between the oral and nasal cavities is the PERCI-IIC (Palatal Efficiency Rating Computed Instantaneously) produced by MicroTronics Corporation (P.O. Box 339, Carrboro, NC 27510). PERCI-IIC measures the air pressure differential between the oral and nasal cavities and nasal airflow during the production of speech sounds, words, and phrases. These measurements are then utilized to electronically calculate the orifice area and airway conductance. With appropriate pressure and airflow transducers, PERCI-IIC provides a selectable digital readout of peak differential pressure, airflow, orifice area, and airway conductance for evaluation or therapeutic feedback purposes.

The technique is noninvasive and can be used successfully with patients as young as 3 years of age. Since PERCI-IIC measurements are made during speech, the assessment problems of nonspeech functions such as blowing or sucking need not be considered.

The aeromechanical instrumentation described earlier also is valuable in the evaluation of oral–nasal coupling when separate pressure transducers measure oral and nasal sound pressure and flow (Baken, 1987; Dickson, Barron, & McGlone, 1978; Hixon, Bless, & Netsell, 1976). Additional methods of detecting nasalization include the use of accelerometers (Lippman, 1981) and nasal manometers (Hess, 1976).

Instrumentation for Respiration Measurement

The speech–language pathologist must be prepared to evaluate the respiratory system as part of a voice evaluation. In most cases, the dysphonic client has more than sufficient respiratory support for phonation and any abnormality in respiration involves coordination of effort rather than sufficiency. Respiration is considered so important to speech and singing that nearly an entire edition of the *Journal of Voice* (Sataloff, 1988) was devoted to this topic.

Sufficiency of Respiration

Under normal conditions, the human respiratory system provides more than sufficient air for normal phonation. The vital capacity of a person's lungs is measured by the amount of air that can be exhaled after as deep an inhalation as possible. The displaced air in such an effort ranges from 4.6 liters in young males to 3.1 liters in young females. The vital capacity is used as an index of lung capacity, although rarely does a person use the entire vital capacity in functional respiration.

Tidal volume is the amount of air inhaled and exhaled during any single respiration cycle. Zemlin (1988) stated that 750 cc is a typical mean tidal volume value for young adult males with a 95% range from 675 to 896 cc. For adult females, the range is from 285 to 393 cc, with a mean value of 339 cc.

Two additional respiration values beyond vital capacity and tidal volume are important in the phonation evaluation process. Inspiratory reserve volume is the amount of air that can be inhaled after a tidal volume inhalation; expiratory reserve volume is how much can be exhaled after a tidal exhalation. The inspiratory and expiratory reserve volume values are large in healthy adults, ranging from 1,500 to 2,500 cc and from 1,500 to 2,000 cc, respectively. All of these respiration values exceed the minimal requirements for normal phonation.

In phonation, these volume respiration values must be translated into pressure and flow values to be meaningful. In other words, the respiration system must be able to generate sufficient pressure and flow to drive the vocal folds in vibration. During conversational speech, the level of this pressure typically ranges between 5 and 10 cm H_2O.

Airflow through the glottis during phonation is around 100 cc/sec; the exact value depends on the magnitude of subglottal pressure and the opposition that the larynx provides to the flow (Baken, 1987; Hirano, 1981; Netsell & Hixon, 1978).

How can the speech–language pathologist measure these values in the voice evaluation? If only a simple screening procedure is needed to ensure that a client has minimal respiration support for phonation, and elaborate instrumentation is not available, Hixon, Hawley, and Wilson (1982) have provided a simple method. It requires a tall (12 cm or more) transparent drinking glass nearly filled with tap water, a regular drinking straw held to the inside of the glass by a large paper clip, and a strip of common surgical adhesive tape with centimeter markings on it about as long as the glass is tall. The straw is submerged 10 cm into the glass. The subject blows into the straw. If bubbles are produced and if they can be sustained for 5 sec, the minimum of 10 cm H_2O pressure over time has been obtained and the client passes the screening test.

Wet Spirometer (Respirometer)

Figure 3–4 shows a wet spirometer, an instrument commonly used for measuring lung capacities. Essentially, a wet spirometer consists of a gas chamber floating in a tank of water. When the subject blows air into the gas chamber, it rises. Its ascent is dependent upon the quantity of air exhaled. A recording

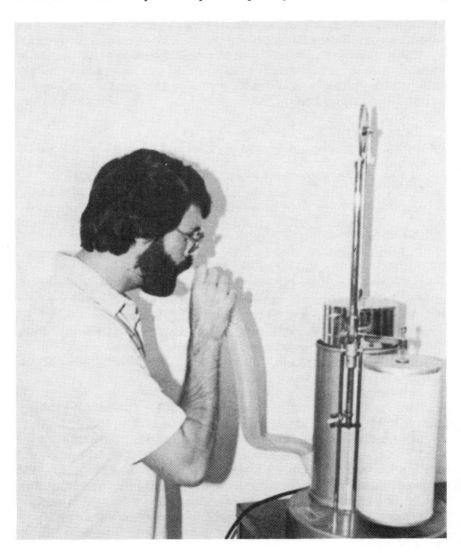

Figure 3–4 A Wet Spirometer in Use.

pen marks the extent of the chamber's movement on a kymograph recording drum that rotates to mark breathing changes over time.

Chest and Diaphragm Movement

Several researchers have studied respiration volumes by measuring changes in chest wall, rib cage, abdomen, and lung dimensions during breathing. Hixon, Goldman, and Mead (1973) used electromagnetic transducers (magnetometers) placed on the body so one sensing coil could sense the strength of a magnetic field generated by a coil mate. Two generator-sensor pairs were used, one pair to sense rib cage diameter changes, the other for abdominal diameter changes. Measurements were obtained on normal subjects in upright and supine body positions. The authors concluded the following:

1. Expiratory effort in the upright body position during conversational speech involves both the rib cage and abdominal regions, and in the supine position only the diaphragm region.
2. The abdomen occupies an especially important role during running conversation by supporting and increasing the diaphragm's inspiratory efficiency so that interruptions for inspiration during speech are minimal.

A system that utilizes diameter changes in the rib cage and abdominal regions to quantify respiratory volumes is provided by Respitrace. This is a plethysmographic (size measurement) system consisting of two coils of wire (called respibands) that encircle the rib cage and abdominal compartments. The expansion and contraction of these coils during breathing cause changes in the oscillating frequency of the circuits within the Respitrace electronic system. After the signals are calibrated for volume, recording values will be equivalent to air volumes inhaled and exhaled.

More information is provided in Chapter 4 regarding the training of improved respiration for speech. Excellent general references for understanding respiration patterns in women and men, respectively, are by Hodge and Rochet (1989) and Hixon, Watson, Harris, and Pearl (1988).

Maximum Phonation Duration

The ability to sustain phonation to a maximum duration is clinically relevant information as part of a voice disorder evaluation (Boone & McFarlane, 1988). Ptacek and Sander (1963), investigating a statement by Fairbanks (1960) that adults should be able to phonate from 20 to 25 sec, reported that they found females generally unable to reach that level and that both males and females experienced differences in maximum phonation duration, depending on pitch and loudness factors.

Tait, Michel, and Carpenter (1980) accepted the 20 to 25 sec duration for adults and provided data on children 5, 7, and 9 years of age using /s/ and /z/ prolongation as the database. They found no distinct pattern of maximum phonation duration differences between males and females in 5- and 7-year-olds. However, males consistently produced longer maximum phonation durations than females in the 9-year-old group. Unlike sex, age appeared to have an influence, increasing with years. In addition to maximum phonation duration values, s/z ratios were figured and reported in mean and median form. Table 3–2 provides mean values for maximum phonation duration on /s/, /z/, and s/z ratios for 5-, 7-, and 9-year-old children.

Eckel and Boone (1981) provided data on s/z ratios of dysphonic patients with laryngeal pathology, dysphonics without laryngeal pathology, and normals covering a wide age range and including both sexes. Although they reported no statistical difference among the three groups in ability to sustain /s/, those with pathology had lower duration times for /z/ than subjects in the two other groups. The computed s/z ratios also were significantly higher for the dysphonic subjects with laryngeal pathology (ratios of 1.40 obtained 95% of the time compared with approximate ratios of 1.0 for the nonpathology and normal groups). Eckel and Boone concluded that the s/z ratio has clinical relevance in determining laryngeal efficiency.

The reliability of the s/z ratio was tested by Fendler and Shearer (1988), who tested 78 normal children on occasions separated by 1 week. Two clinicians each tested one-half of the children the first week, and the opposite children 1 week later. Test–retest statistics indicated no significant differences between the testers and subject performance. In other words, children who tended to have either longer or shorter s/z durations did not vary in the retest condition. Test–retest reliability of the s/z ratio was found to be consistent between tests and clinicians doing the testing.

TABLE 3–2
Maximum Phonation Durations for Children 5, 7, and 9 Years of Age

Age	Sex	N	Mean /s/	Mean /z/	s/z Ratios
5	M	6	7.9	8.6	0.92
5	F	9	8.3	10.0	0.83
7	M	6	9.3	13.2	0.70
7	F	8	10.2	13.1	0.78
9	M	15	16.7	18.1	0.92
9	F	9	14.4	15.8	0.91

An additional caution should be expressed about the usage of the s/z ratio and maximum phonation durations. Hufnagle and Hufnagle (1988) reported data on 123 dysphonic children, 69 with vocal nodules and 54 with no obvious vocal fold pathology, but with vocal dysphonia. No significant difference was found between the ratios of children with nodules and those with no obvious pathology, and the ratios tended to be similar to values expected in normals (range: .84 to 1.03). However, the durations of /s/ and /z/ were shorter than expected for normals (range for /s/, 4.69 to 5.74 sec; for /z/, 5.94 to 6.53 sec). The authors cited respiratory support as a significant factor in their findings, but concluded that the s/z ratio does not discriminate the presence of mass lesions in dysphonic children.

The maximum phonation duration data and s/z ratios reported in the above studies on children and adults seem to support the notion that considerable information can be gained about a client's laryngeal efficiency from these simple tests. However, the speech–language pathologist must keep in mind the data of Stone (1983) indicating that maximum phonation durations, which he called maximum phonation times, are highly variable under conditions of pitch level, presence of performance feedback, and number of trials. In fact, Stone's subjects continued to increase maximum phonation times up to 15 trials. Stone's data should at least caution the speech–language pathologist to limit the significance of maximum phonation durations and s/z ratios when viewed as isolated measures.

Schmidt, Klingholz, and Martin (1988) also reported similar variability of maximum phonation durations among singers as a function of pitch, sound pressures, and vowels utilized.

Perceptual Rating Scales

Perceptual ratings of normal and abnormal voices have received considerable attention in the literature on voice disorder. Perceptual judgment of voice is a controversial method. Some authorities find perceptual judgment so invalid and unreliable as to be meaningless, and believe that only objective and instrumentally based measurements should be used to discriminate voices. At the opposite extreme of that position is the voice clinician who relies only on perceptual judgment of voice without objective assessment. However, in the many voice evaluations that occur daily in clinics, hospitals, private practices, and school systems, it is likely that a combination of perceptual judgment and objective assessment is the standard. I think that highly experienced judges are rather good at discriminating parameters of voice with validity and reliability, characteristics that can be taught (see Bassich & Ludlow, 1986), but objective assessment provides highly valuable support for those judgments.

Despite the addition of new instruments to the voice laboratory at Arizona State University, I continue to use my ears in the evaluation process.

Valuable information can be obtained from critical listening and perceptual ratings of various parameters of voice as part of the overall evaluation process. Two commonly used perceptual rating scales are the Voice Profile (F. B. Wilson & Rice, 1977) and the Gelfer Rating Scale (Gelfer, 1988).

The Wilson and Rice Voice Profile

In the Wilson and Rice scales, voice patterns are profiled according to three major parameters (pitch, laryngeal opening, and resonance) and two minor parameters (intensity and vocal range) (see Exhibit 3-2). Factors identified as being abnormal are rated on a voice severity rating scale from 1 (*barely perceptible*) to 7 (*significantly interferes with communication*).

Ratings on pitch are based on perceptual rather than measured judgments regarding the appropriateness of the client's pitch in relation to sex and age. If the client's pitch seems appropriate in this respect, it is judged as 1; if it seems high for age and sex, it is judged as +2 or +3, depending on severity. A +3 pitch judgment indicates that the pitch is socially demeaning and, in the case of a male, could cause sex confusion when heard over the phone. If the client's pitch seems inappropriately low for sex and age, it is judged as −2 or −3, depending on severity. A −3 indicates that the pitch is socially demeaning and, in the case of a female, also might cause sex confusion over the phone. A −3 pitch judgment also indicates that the client's pitch, regardless of age and sex, is sufficiently low to constitute a factor of vocal abuse.

The other laryngeal cavity rating parameter in the Voice Profile is related to vibration patterns of the vocal folds, the actual glottal tone. It is based on the notion that vibration patterns can deviate from normal in the direction of hypofunction (undervalving) or hyperfunction (overvalving). Perceptually, the range of judgment is from an "open" position of phonation to a "closed" position.

If a client's voice indicates that the vocal folds are meeting at midline with normal medial compression, the judgment is 1. A −2 judgment indicates that there is too little medial compression; the perceptual correlate is breathiness. If there is so little medial compression that no phonation occurs and the speech is supported only by whisper, the judgment is −3. A −4 indicates that no sound is heard, such as immediately after laryngectomy or with complete aphonia. In the hyperfunction direction, a +2 indicates overadduction of the vocal folds during phonation; the perceptual correlate is excessive tension. A +3 judgment indicates that the tension is sufficient to stop phonation, such as in a spastic dysphonic voice.

Some organic voice disorders present perceptual combinations of these features. For example, vocal nodules may prevent complete glottal closure,

Exhibit 3–2 Form Used for Voice Profile

VOICE PROFILE

NAME: _____ AGE: _____ SEX: _____

(circle one)

VOICE RATING: 1 2 3 4 5 6 7

LARYNGEAL CAVITY
PITCH

RESONATING CAVITY
NASALITY

INTENSITY
  −2   1   +2
soft   loud

high
+3
+2
open −4 −3 −2 1 +2 +3 closed
−2
−3
low

hypernasal
+4
+3
+2
throaty −2 −1 +2 frontal
−2
hyponasal

VOCAL RANGE
  −2   1   +2
monotone   variable
pitch

		YES	NO
INTERMITTENT DIPLOPHONIA		_____	_____
DIPLOPHONIA		_____	_____
AUDIBLE INHALATION	*Indicate presence or absence of acoustic feature by (✓)*	_____	_____
PITCH BREAKS		_____	_____
ERRATIC PHRASING		_____	_____
IMMATURE RESONANCE		_____	_____

MARKING SYSTEM

Primary Feature X   Secondary Feature / e.g. +2

Intermittent Feature *(int)*   Noted Feature / e.g. +2 /

Note. Reprinted with permission from *Voice Disorders: A Programmed Approach to Voice Therapy* by F. B. Wilson and M. Rice, 1977, Hingham, MA: Teaching Resources Corp. Copyright 1977 by F. B. Wilson.

producing a -2 (breathy) feature in combination with an effort to compensate for the breathy feature with excessive tension, a $+2$. This -2 and $+2$ combination is a common perceptual profile in voice disorders with varied etiology.

The main resonance parameter in the Voice Profile involves perceptual judgment in relation to a balance between oral and nasal resonance. Under normal conditions of velopharyngeal closure, complete separation of the oral and nasal cavities occurs during speech except in the production of the nasal consonants /m/, /n/, and /ŋ/. When a client's voice indicates this normal balance of velopharyngeal functioning, a 1 judgment of resonance is given, meaning the velopharyngeal port is closed except during the production of these nasal consonants.

Individuals often display resonance characteristics in which the presence of nasal consonants causes an assimilation of nasality to surrounding consonants and vowels, in which case a $+2$ (assimilation nasality) is given. This is a relatively insignificant deviation from normal. When nasality is heard in all vowel sounds, the rating is a $+3$, indicating significant velopharyngeal dysfunction. A more severe indication of velopharyngeal dysfunction causes nasality on all vowel sounds and nasal air emission on pressure consonants, such as /s/, /z/, and /t/. This combination of nasality on the vowels and nasal air emission on the pressure consonants is rated as a $+4$ (hypernasal).

Several organic conditions in the nasal cavity can affect normal functioning in resonation in the direction of hyponasality, a condition in which there is too little participation of the nasal cavity in resonance. For example, if a client has a severe cold or nasal allergy, during the production of the nasal consonants, the velopharyngeal port opens normally but nasal resonation is restricted because of congestion in the cavity. This dampening of nasal resonance is rated as -2 (hyponasal). The main effect of such a resonance change is that the nasal consonant /m/ sounds more like /b/, the /n/ like a /d/, and the /ŋ/ like a /g/.

In addition to the hypernasal–hyponasal resonance features, abnormal resonance focus in the throat (-2) or in the front of the oral cavity $(+2)$ can be rated. These features are more difficult to evaluate because perceptual features of frontal and throaty resonance are less identifiable.

Use of the Wilson and Rice Voice Profile also requires judgment on a parameter of intensity, with -2 for a voice that is too soft, 1 normal, and $+2$ too loud for communication circumstances. Pitch variability also is rated on the vocal range parameter, with -2 indicating deficient pitch variation (monotone), 1 normal variability, and $+2$ extreme and unusual variation.

Primary features in a client's voice profile are marked, as Exhibit 3–2 shows, with an x, secondary features with a / mark through the feature, and, if a feature is intermittent, the abbreviation (int) is used. When a feature is noted but is not significant enough to be considered as a primary or secondary factor, it is identified with half a slash mark. After the four parameters of voice are rated, the speech–language pathologist indicates on the form the presence or absence of diplophonia, audible inhalation, pitch breaks, erratic phrasing, and immature resonance. The severity of primary features is indicated by rating them on a 1 to 7 scale (7 being *most severe*).

The Wilson and Rice system can be learned through a training package available through Teaching Resources Corporation. The package includes audio recordings to illustrate the ratings system, as well as forms and slides of various laryngeal pathologies that correspond to audio descriptions of each pathology shown. When the perceptual ratings of this Voice Profile or any similar system are coupled with objective information from instrumental measurement of voice parameters, a thorough evaluation of a client's voice can be accomplished.

Gelfer Rating Scale

A more recently developed rating scale which shows promise utilizes a set of bipolar perceptual rating scales that can be used to relate listener perceptions to physiological and acoustic measures. Using measures of confidence, several parameters of voice were eliminated until the following aspects remained, which could be evaluated by speech–language pathologists:

High Pitch	__1__2__3__4__5__6__7__8__9__	Low Pitch
Loud	__1__2__3__4__5__6__7__8__9__	Soft
Strong	__1__2__3__4__5__6__7__8__9__	Weak
Smooth	__1__2__3__4__5__6__7__8__9__	Rough
Pleasant	__1__2__3__4__5__6__7__8__9__	Unpleasant
Resonant	__1__2__3__4__5__6__7__8__9__	Shrill
Clear	__1__2__3__4__5__6__7__8__9__	Hoarse
Unforced	__1__2__3__4__5__6__7__8__9__	Strained
Soothing	__1__2__3__4__5__6__7__8__9__	Harsh
Melodious	__1__2__3__4__5__6__7__8__9__	Raspy
Breathy Voice	__1__2__3__4__5__6__7__8__9__	Full Voice
Excessive Nasal	__1__2__3__4__5__6__7__8__9__	Insuff. Nasal
Animated	__1__2__3__4__5__6__7__8__9__	Monotonous
Steady	__1__2__3__4__5__6__7__8__9__	Shaky
Young	__1__2__3__4__5__6__7__8__9__	Old
Slow Rate	__1__2__3__4__5__6__7__8__9__	Rapid Rate
I Like/Voice	__1__2__3__4__5__6__7__8__9__	Don't Like/Voice

This scale has many parameters to judge. Some appear redundant, and one point of confusion is apparent. Most of the parameters judged are arranged so that low-number judgments (i.e., 1 to 3) indicate normalcy of voice and high-number judgments (i.e., 7 to 9) indicate abnormalcy. However, this is not always the case. Low-number judgments on the parameters of "high pitch," "breathy voice," "excessively nasal," and "slow rate" would not indicate normal aspects of voice. Thus, each parameter would require individual analysis rather than relying on an overall profile to discriminate normal from abnormal characteristics of voice. Gelfer (1988) provides extensive information regarding the development and testing of this scale.

It is important that the speech–language pathologist who utilizes perceptual rating scales recognize the inherent weaknesses of perception and the need for extensive experience in voice judgment (Bassich & Ludlow, 1986). I also hope speech–language pathologists move more toward objective assessment to complement and enhance the validity of perceptual voice judgments.

Case Example of Voice Evaluation

The following evaluation was conducted at the Arizona State University Speech and Hearing Clinic. It is presented here in abstracted form.

Background and Case History

Tom J., who is 12 years old, was referred by an otolaryngologist. The physician's statement indicated that Tom had vocal nodules bilaterally, as well as generalized edema of the vocal folds. The otolaryngologist also was concerned about the possibility of a personality factor behind the vocal abuse since Tom had displayed instances of "aggression." The boy was referred for a complete evaluation of vocal habits and possible therapy to eliminate any traits that had caused the voice disorder.

Tom was accompanied to the evaluation by his mother, who provided information on his background. She said that Tom, as the youngest of three boys, constantly seemed to come out on the losing end of family arguments. Mrs. J. conceded that the whole family had a tendency to be aggressive and competitive in daily interactions and that Tom constantly had to yell and speak intensely just to compete with his dominating brothers. Most arguments occurred with the brother just older than Tom.

Athletics played an important part in Tom's life. He was large for his age and well coordinated, making him a natural leader in team sports. Because of this leadership, Tom was constantly yelling instructions at other boys on his team. The vocal abuse/misuse that was centered on his family interactions and sports activities constituted important factors in the pathogenesis of his vocal nodules.

As a result of the information obtained in the case history, the following specific items of vocal abuse/misuse were identified:

- Intense verbal interaction with family members, especially his brother

- Intense verbal arguments with his friend, Jerry

- Intense yelling and screaming on the playground and as an athletic team leader

- Constant clearing of his throat in an abusive manner

- Hard or abrupt onset of voicing, especially when yelling or screaming

- A tendency to call people to him from a distance rather than make an effort to get closer to those being sought

- Miscellaneous instances of vocal abuse when playing army, motorcycle sounds when riding his bicycle, and in general outdoor playing activities

Tom's voice was evaluated perceptually on the Voice Profile with the following ratings:

- Pitch: +2 (too high)

- Laryngeal Opening: +2 (tense) and −2 (breathy); Severity: 4 (1–7 scale)

- Resonance: 1 (normal)

- Intensity: +2 (too loud)

- Vocal Range: −2 (restricted pitch variability . . . monotone)

A formal evaluation of Tom's pitch revealed the following values (all measurements done with Visi-Pitch):

- Habitual Pitch: $F_0 = 349$ Hz (F above middle C on musical scale)

- Optimal Pitch: Could not be estimated because of excessive hoarseness

- Pitch Range: 314 Hz to 420 Hz (D# to G# in middle C octave); highly restricted pitch range

- Vocal Efficiency: Prolongation of /a/: 6 sec (2 trials); prolongation of /s/: 11 sec; /z/: 7 sec; s/z ratio: 1.57 (abnormal)

- Spectrographic Recordings: Sonograms reveal Yanagihara Type IV (second formants are replaced by noise components; first formant not periodic and supplemented by noise component)

- Respiration: Not formally evaluated but subjectively felt to be normal

- Baseline Audio Recording: A baseline sample of Tom's voice was taken as he stated his name, the date, the time, counted from 1 to 20, and read a paragraph

Clinical Impression

Tom represents a classic case of vocal abuse/misuse, resulting in bilateral vocal nodules and laryngeal edema. Several instances of continuing vocal abuse were identified and listed (as above). His vocal quality, as judged perceptually and documented spectrographically and on audio recording, is consistent with the diagnosis of vocal nodules. His pitch is high and probably reflects extreme laryngeal tension. Vocal efficiency measurements of /a/ prolongation and an s/z ratio of 1.57 indicate significant laryngeal dysfunction and inefficiency. His restricted pitch variability is compatible with his diagnosed condition.

The treatment procedures for Tom involve the systematic elimination of the identified forms of vocal abuse. No attention should be given to lowering his pitch since his high pitch seems to be a function of the tension in his voice. Audio recordings should be taken during each therapy session and analyzed for evidence of improvement. (More specific recommendations on similar cases are presented in Chapter 4.)

Summary

Several evaluation procedures have been described, including voice screening; medical referral; case history taking; and vocal parameter evaluation of pitch, loudness, quality, resonance, and vocal efficiency using perceptual scales and instrumental devices. Not all of these processes and procedures must be followed in the evaluation of every voice-disordered client. However, the speech–language pathologist should be familiar with each procedure so as to be able to select the proper ones for each case.

4

Voice Disorder from Vocal Abuse

One of the most dramatic examples of how the delicate tissues of the larynx can be abused was captured on film by Moore and von Leden (1958). During one segment, a person's cough was filmed in high-speed cinematography (5,000 frames per second) but projected at the normal rate of 16 frames per second. The ultraslow motion shows what happens to the vocal folds and surrounding laryngeal tissues during this brief cough.

For what seems like several minutes, the tissues of the larynx are tossed about as though caught in a hurricane. The arytenoid cartilages are in chaotic and frenzied motion, matched by the turbulent actions of the vocal folds. The entire larynx is adversely affected by this aerodynamic turmoil. It is impossible to watch this coughing episode without realizing how vulnerable laryngeal tissues are to this and other forms of abuse.

Considering that during normal phonation, the vocal folds are vibrating from one to several hundred times each second (depending on the pitch of the voice), it is surprising that tissue trauma from all this action does not occur more commonly. Furthermore, considering the great numbers of fans heard screaming at sporting events, it is even more surprising that thousands of people have not damaged their vocal folds by abnormal vocal behavior.

Although the total is not great, a number of individuals have developed voice disorder from vocal abuse. Vocal abuse is found at all ages and in most segments of society. Children yell and scream on the playground, and adults yell and scream at sporting events. Children enjoy making strange and loud toy and animal noises during play, and adults enjoy singing in styles and environments that foster vocal abuse. Loud and aggressive children verbally intimidate and bully other children, and these same verbal characteristics can be found in many adults.

When children grow into adulthood, many enter professions with highly demanding verbal requirements: teaching, law, professional singing and acting, auctioneering, sales, and the ministry. Many of the verbal activities in these professions are incompatible with good vocal hygiene and can damage the delicate tissues of the larynx, producing a voice disorder caused by vocal abuse or vocal misuse. This chapter provides speech–language pathologists with information for evaluating and remediating voice disorder cases resulting from various types of vocal abuse.

The two most common and significant voice disorders that result directly from vocal abuse/misuse are vocal nodules and contact ulcers.

Vocal Nodules

The most common voice disorder resulting from vocal abuse or misuse, and the most common cause of hoarseness in children, is a condition of vocal nodules or vocal nodes (Benjamin & Croxson, 1987). Vocal nodules are also called "singer's nodules," "screamer's nodules," "cheerleader's nodules," "parson's nodules," and "teacher's nodules" (Lancer, Syder, Jones, & LeBoutillier, 1988), markers which indentify the etiology of this voice disorder.

Nodules are benign (nonmalignant) growths of extra tissue that develop at the margin or junction of the anterior and middle thirds of the glottal length, including intermembranous and intercartilaginous portions (Figure 4–1; compare with normal vocal folds in Figure 1–9). Nodules are typically found bilaterally, but a few cases of unilateral nodules have been reported (Lancer et al., 1988; McFarlane & Watterson, 1990). Because vocal abuse is the primary etiology of vocal nodule pathogenesis, it is difficult to explain how vocal abuse can cause only one vocal fold to develop a nodule and the other fold remain uninvolved, but this appears to be the case in instances of unilateral vocal nodules. One must be careful, however, not to incorrectly identify a cyst or some other type of growth as a vocal nodule.

Nodules have been compared with corns or calluses on toes and hands that develop from excessive rubbing and physical abuse. Vocal nodules develop in children as well as adults, and a sex ratio of 2:1 to 3:1 (male to female) has been reported (Kay, 1982). McFarlane and Watterson (1990) reported significant variation in the size and location of vocal nodules in both children and adults, including an instance of quadruple vocal nodules (two nodules

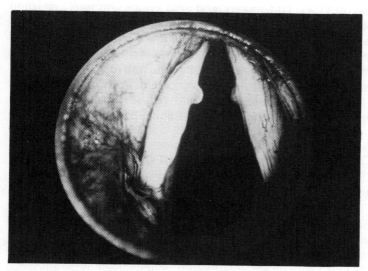

Figure 4–1 Vocal Folds with Nodules. Reproduced with permission from *Voice Disorders: A Programmed Approach to Voice Therapy* by F. B. Wilson and M. Rice, 1977, Hingham, MA: Teaching Resources Corp. Copyright 1977 by F. B. Wilson.

on each fold) in a 38-year-old female. The majority of their adult cases were female, both singers and nonsingers.

The reason vocal nodules develop at this location rather than elsewhere on the folds can be understood by reviewing the nature of vocal fold vibration. The anterior two-thirds of the glottal opening is composed of muscular tissue that vibrates during phonation. The posterior third is composed of cartilaginous tissues (arytenoids) that do not vibrate during phonation. Therefore, the junction of the anterior and middle thirds, where nodules develop, represents the midpoint of vocal fold vibration. During the vibratory cycle, it is at this junction the excursion from midline is widest and the vocal folds contact with greatest energy during normal or abnormal phonation. It is logical and consistent with known principles of voice science that vocal nodules should develop at this location when phonation is abusive.

The pathogenesis of vocal nodules occurs in two stages, acute and chronic. The acute nodules are soft, reddish, vascular, and edematous, and they resemble laryngeal hematomas. They often are surrounded by generalized edema of the entire vocal fold tissues, and the entire glottis appears erythemic (reddish). The surrounding edema and erythema usually appear only in the acute stage of development. In the chronic stage, the nodules are hard, white, thickened, and fibrosed, but contain little edema in the nodule or in the surrounding tissue (Cotton & Casper, 1990).

Kleinsasser (1986) reported that microlaryngoscopy reveals vocal nodules to be hyperplastic, acanthotic (thickened), squamous epithelial growths with markedly thickened basal membrane. The submucosal connective tissue of Reinke's space does not show any fibers connecting or fixing the epithelium to the vocalis muscle. Hirano and Kurita (1986) found that vocal nodules are always located in the superficial layer of the lamina propria and do not invade the muscular tissue. They cautioned that any surgical attempt to remove them should be strictly limited to this layer.

Arnold (1980) reported that in chronic vocal nodules, the thickened epithelium becomes altered by acanthosis (hypertrophy), keratosis (horny growth or calluses), pachydermia (abnormal thickening), and metaplasia (change in the type of cell), and advanced lesions may show precancerous changes, including leukoplakia (white patches). Case (1981) reported one instance in which biopsied tissue diagnosed to be benign vocal nodules was found later to contain malignant cells requiring a laryngectomy.

Voice Characteristics with Nodules

The voice is affected in several ways when nodules occur. Its quality is altered dramatically. The most common complaint is that the voice is raspy, hoarse, and breathy. Speech–language pathologists use these same terms to describe the voice characteristics, although these are perceptual judgments that often lack objective criteria.

The Voice Profile (F. B. Wilson & Rice, 1977) for the person with vocal nodules typically is +2 (tension), −2 (breathy), and intermittent −3 (whisper) on the laryngeal opening parameter. The severity of this +2/−2 judgment can range from 1 to 7. Aperiodicity and diplophonia can result from the mass differences in the two vocal folds.

The main factors involved in producing these perceptible characteristics are breathiness, overpressure (medical compression) of the vocal folds perceived as voice tension, and asymmetrical vocal fold vibration. Two reasons can account for the breathiness:

1. The nodular mass on the vibrating edge of each vocal fold prevents complete approximation from occurring. This allows excessive air to escape during phonation through the glottal chinks anterior and posterior to the contact between the nodules.

2. Constant abuse of the voice structures produces irritation in the tissue, particularly in the posterior area around the arytenoid cartilages. This irritation can add a slight pain factor in phonation, causing the client to avoid hard approximation of the arytenoid cartilages at the onset of and during phonation, which also allows excessive air to escape and further causes the voice to be breathy.

The excessive overpressure (tension) factor usually is caused by the client's attempt to exert increased effort to overcome the incomplete approximation of the vocal folds. This increased effort is the basis of the tension. Because a nodule on one fold rarely matches the mass size of the nodule on the opposite fold, each vocal fold vibrates in a slightly different phase, resulting in aperiodicity. All of these factors contribute to the voice quality heard in clients with vocal nodules.

More objective voice measurements of dysphonia can be derived from spectrographic analysis. M. Cooper (1974), who analyzed 155 patients undergoing voice rehabilitation for various dysphonias, including vocal nodules, reported that spectrograms discriminate the dysphonias (hoarseness) from the improved voice qualities following treatment. He used the spectrographic classification system developed by Isshiki, Yanagihara, and Morimoto (1966). Cooper recommended that the spectrograph be used as standard documentation of voice acoustics in the clinical management of voice-disordered patients.

Further voice characteristics of clients with vocal nodules include reduced maximum phonation durations and abnormal s/z ratios (Eckel & Boone, 1981; Rastatter & Hyman, 1982; Tait, Michel, & Carpenter, 1980). Although the results of these studies reveal some inconsistencies, Rastatter and Hyman are less enthusiastic about the s/z ratio as an indicator of vocal nodules and other laryngeal pathology than are Eckel and Boone, the maximum phonation durations for /z/ typically are shorter than for /s/, and the ratios of persons with nodules is greater than 1.40. The speech–language pathologist should at least consider short maximum phonation durations and s/z ratios over 1.40 as an indication of laryngeal inefficiency, without having to make a diagnosis of vocal nodules.

Pitch Factors

The pitch of individuals with vocal nodules usually is too low, considering the age and sex involved. Early literature in speech and language pathology suggested lowering the habitual pitch level clinically, since one factor of causation was a high pitch (Van Riper & Irwin, 1958; West, Kennedy, & Carr, 1947). However, it now is rather universally recognized that vocal nodules lower the voice because of extra mass of the folds, which reduces the fundamental frequency vibration, and further reduction is likely to contribute to the abuse.

Some persons may attempt to compensate for the vocal nodules by increasing the tension in the folds, thus causing an increase in the pitch, but the typical pattern usually is found to be too low. This low-pitched characteristic should be considered as both an etiological and a by-product factor. The person with nodules may not be attempting consciously to lower the pitch, so it probably is occurring because of the mass factor, but this must be determined clinically. Clinically raising the pitch should be done only when an etiological factor is involved (discussed in the next section).

Pitch control and stability also are problems for persons with vocal nodules. Upward or downward pitch breaks can occur at the onset of phonation on a regular basis. They reflect a highly unstable laryngeal mechanism. Mattson (1980), in a report on the pitch changes over 10 months of a single subject (a cheerleader) with vocal nodules, found significant fluctuation of habitual pitch. These changes occurred between morning and night voice, before and after cheerleading, and particularly the day following extensive cheerleading. On one occasion, this subject's pitch changed from an habitual level of A_1 (220 Hz) to F_1 (174 Hz) overnight as a result of cheerleading the previous night. Many similar pitch fluctuations were revealed during the 10-month span. This same subject experienced significantly reduced vocal durability from morning to night, another common characteristic of many persons with vocal nodules.

Etiology of Vocal Nodules

Although there are some exceptions (Kay, 1982), the etiology of vocal nodules is thought to be vocal abuse or misuse (A. E. Aronson, 1985; Boone & McFarlane, 1988). Several specific forms of vocal abuse and associated causal factors must be considered, including the following:

- Yelling and screaming

- Voicing with a hard glottal attack

- Singing in an abusive manner (as a professional or an amateur)

- Speaking in a noisy environment

- Coughing and excessive throat clearing

- Grunting as in exercising and lifting

- Calling others, such as friends, children, or pets, from a distance

- Using inappropriate pitch levels in speaking or singing

- Speaking in an abusive or excessive manner during allergy or upper respiratory infection episodes

- Vocalizing under conditions of muscular tension

- Smoking excessively (including marijuana) or speaking in a smoky environment

- Speaking excessively or abusively during menstrual periods
- Vocalizing excessively
- Speaking with inadequate breath support
- Laughing hard and abusively
- Vocalizing excessively while taking aspirin, which can increase the potential of hemorrhage of vocal fold blood vessels
- Cheerleading and pep club activities
- Vocalizing toy and animal noises
- Engaging in athletic activity involving yelling, such as in coaching or serving as a football quarterback
- Possessing an aggressive personality
- Arguing with peers, siblings, and others
- Reversing phonation
- Talking in night clubs
- Talking in arcades

This compendium seems comprehensive, yet the speech–language pathologist will find unique and individual forms of vocal abuse that do not appear on any traditional list. (Most of the listed types are discussed below.)

Yelling and Screaming

Yelling and screaming are so common that they appear normal in many circumstances. Children of all ages seem to yell and scream constantly in both organized playground activities, such as sporting events (Little League baseball, football), or in unorganized play in the backyard or street. During school recess, as most teachers can attest, children seem to release their contained emotions and energy through their voices as much as by running and jumping. Some children are more vocal than others and become the "generals" of the playground, constantly yelling instructions to others in an attempt to establish and maintain a leadership role. Verbal arguments develop over trivial matters and end in yelling matches that involve no verbal logic, only loudness of voice. One wonders why nearly all such children do not hurt their voices and develop vocal nodules.

Adults also yell and scream. Both males and females, for example, can become emotionally involved in sporting events and cheer and boo with gusto. Parents of children in organized games scream at kids on the field, umpires, referees, coaches of opposing teams, and anyone else considered a threat to victory. Many adults who become coaches of youth teams find themselves yelling constantly at the players. This is particularly noticeable in youth football, in which the players' ears are partially covered by helmets, making it even more difficult for coaches to communicate without yelling. Again, one wonders why every coach of a youth team does not have vocal nodules—especially coaches of losing teams.

When a child or adult has been referred or screened out for voice therapy because of vocal nodules, speech–language pathologists must take care to explore all possibilities of yelling and screaming as causal factors.

Hard Glottal Attack

Even though vocal nodules develop at the junction of the anterior and middle thirds of the glottis, swelling and inflammation in the posterior region around the arytenoid cartilages are not uncommon. One factor that could explain this is the tendency for some clients to begin phonation abruptly, a process called the hard glottal attack or *coup de glotte* (attack of the glottis).

In hard glottal attack, phonation is begun with a forceful closure of the arytenoid cartilages. Such slamming together does not cause vocal nodules, but can account for generalized swelling in the entire glottal region. Clients should be made aware of this tendency and should be helped to modify such behavior.

Singing in an Abusive Manner

One of the most vocally demanding professions is that of a professional singer. Regardless of the style of music—the classical music of the opera, in which the performer is well trained in vocal usage, or the more popular style involving the big-time business of recording and touring or the small-time nightclub circuit, in which performers may have little or no vocal training—the demands for vocal effort are great. A growing body of literature addresses the issue of singing and laryngeal concerns (McFarlane & Watterson, 1990). Much of the literature on professional voice concerns comes from The Voice Foundation and its official journal, the *Journal of Voice*. Several articles from this journal are invaluable to speech–language pathologists working with singers (e.g., Hixon, Watson, Harris, & Pearl, 1988; Leanderson & Sundberg, 1988; Sataloff, 1988). Some of the more general vocal concerns of the professional singer are reviewed by Teter (1977):

1. Singing excessively high or low in pitch

2. Singing excessively loudly

3. Using an exaggerated glottal stroke (hard glottal attack)

4. Attempting to sing during respiratory infections

5. Using laryngeal irritants such as tobacco, alcohol, and other drugs

6. Singing without adequate voice training or warmup before performance

Even singers who are well trained in musical pedagogy can develop laryngeal tissue changes as a result of their singing. Singers of the great arias and choral selections face the most challenging of musical scores. Not only are the high and low tones often near the upper or lower limits of a singer's range, but the notes must be hit precisely. For example, in Mozart's aria "Arie der Koigin der Nacht" (Queen of the Night), the soprano must rapidly change the pitch of her voice in 8th and 16th notes, jumping vocally in the following note sequence: D, C, D, E, F, F, C, G, G, G, C, A, F, A, C, F, C, D, B^b, C, F, C, F, A, C, F, C, D, B^b, C. Anyone familiar with this musical transition of vocal pitch marvels that Mozart could write it and that even well-trained singers can sing it. To accomplish this vocal task, however, the singer must have precise and rapid control over laryngeal adjustments. It is obvious when the singer is off by just a few hertz in this precise and demanding sequence. The singer must be well trained, and her larynx must be in superlative shape. Any swelling or abnormal change in her vocal fold tissues would make such singing essentially impossible.

Vocal productions that are near to or that exceed the vocal capabilities of a performer can be presumed to be deleterious to the performer's laryngeal tissues. Coleman (1987) provided a method that a singer can use to determine whether a given musical score falls within his or her performance limits. This phonetogram method can help a performer avoid those scores with damage potential.

When working with a singer who has vocal nodules, the speech–language pathologist's analysis must involve viewing the performer in action both on and off stage. Modification or elimination of behaviors that are not related directly to the performance can make a difference in the singer's durability. Abuses that are not part of the act are the only ones over which the singer has much control without taking away the means of employment. It is highly unlikely that the typical nightclub performer will have the talent or means to become a trained singer and advance to a better performance situation. By observing the singer in the actual work setting, the speech–language pathologist can discover abuses that can be modified rather easily, but can make a significant difference in vocal durability.

The speech–language pathologist is more likely to work with a nontrained singer who has developed vocal nodules than with a classically trained one. The less-trained singer will often choose music that challenges the vocal range and potential of his or her voice, and all of the concerns of the well-trained singer apply. When an untrained singer is successful and popular, even with a singing style and vocal quality that are unacceptable to the well-trained singer, the speech–language pathologist will have little success if an attempt is made to change the style and vocal quality that foster such success. Rather, the speech–language pathologist must be prepared to help the nontrained successful singer modify those aspects of vocal behavior that can be modified without sacrificing the successful singing style.

Several other factors must be considered when working with professional singers, particularly those on the nightclub circuit. Duration of vocal performance is a major factor in the development of nodules. In the typical nightclub gig, the singer must perform up to four sets of 40 to 50 min each, typically starting at 9 P.M. and ending at 1 A.M. During the breaks between sets, management often encourages the performer to mingle with the audience. The mingling is wonderful for socialization and public relations for management, but deleterious to already traumatized vocal folds.

The typical nightclub crowd is noisy, with constant chatter, laughter, clinking glasses, and jukebox music during breaks. Singers must compete with this noise as they mingle and are forced to almost yell simply to communicate when what they need most is vocal rest. The larynx is not given time to recuperate before another intense musical set begins. These between-set conversations can be more abusive to the voice than the actual singing since amplifiers can reduce vocal strain during singing.

Even the child or adult who enjoys amateur singing must be evaluated to determine whether this is a contributing factor to the development of nodules. People often sing with the radio, while doing housework or other activities around the home, and while in the shower. These all bring joy to the heart but trauma to the vocal folds when done in an abusive manner. Many people are members of church, youth, or community choirs, and those activities can contribute to vocal abuse.

In my experience, amateur singing seldom constitutes a significant factor in the pathogenesis of vocal nodules; however, when a person has developed nodules from other causes, amateur singing can constitute a sufficient abuse factor to maintain the nodules. Therefore, speech–language pathologists should recommend that most amateur singing be halted temporarily during the weeks of therapy.

Professional, well-trained singers such as those in the opera are less likely to experience vocal abuse. Such singers learn to use the vocal mechanisms well and avoid techniques and conditions that may be harmful. Hirano (1980) and Large (1980) provided excellent discussions on the topic of voice research in singing. Excellent studies on the voice care of the professional singer were written by Sataloff (1981, 1983, in press). Feder (1983) wrote of a specific anatomical abnormality of the vascular tissue in the larynx that can vocally handicap the professional singer or actor.

One rather important laryngeal concern for all singers, regardless of extent of training or singing style, is the general position in the neck of the larynx during singing. Shipp (1987) provided extensive information showing that singers with classical vocal training maintain a vertical laryngeal position at or below the resting level of the larynx, whereas untrained singers typically position their larynges higher, well above the resting position, particularly as vocal pitch is raised. Shipp reported that maintaining a low position during singing results in (a) facilitating a vocal fold vibratory pattern that produces substantial energy in the higher portion of the resonance spectrum, (b) a greater opening of the vocal tract enhancing vocal resonation, (c) a greater easing of transitions of voice from one vocal register to another, and (d) a reduction of vocal fold contact or closure forces that might be considered a vocal abuse factor.

Speaking in a Noisy Environment

When a person is forced to speak in a noisy environment, several things happen to the larynx and speech system. First, a high ambient noise level makes it difficult to monitor how loud the conversation is, so the individual is unlikely to eliminate the excessive vocal effort. Second, to be heard above the noise, the person generates greater lung airflow, to which the vocal folds respond with greater resistance that is equivalent to what is perceived as laryngeal tension. Although the resistance is quantifiable and measurable, the instrumentation necessary to do so does not work well in a noisy environment such as a nightclub or a factory.

An easy way to demonstrate the effect of a high ambient noise level on conversation involves making a tape recording of the noise in a nightclub (the quality of the recording is not important). The speech–language pathologist then plays the recording at a noise level typical of a nightclub, and engages the client in conversation. The widely known Lombard effect will cause the client's voice to become more intense (loud), usually in direct proportion to the loudness level of the tape. The speech–language pathologist can demonstrate what is happening to the client's voice by suddenly turning off the tape recorder in the middle of the person's speech. The client usually will notice that the voice has been nearly shouting and generating considerable tension to compete with the noise. The impact of this demonstration can be helpful in convincing a client with vocal nodules how important it is not to compete with a noisy environment.

Coughing and Throat Clearing

The speech–language pathologist can use the example of the cough photographed and shown in ultraslow motion discussed earlier to communicate the deleterious effect of coughing and throat clearing on the larynx. Coughing, of course, occurs when the protective valving mechanisms of the larynx are stimulated by a foreign irritation. It is a reflex act and hard to control or eliminate when caused by an upper respiratory infection or allergy.

Antihistamine–decongestant medicines are helpful in reducing this reflex act, and clients with vocal nodules should be encouraged to solicit the help of a physician when an upper respiratory infection or allergy is present. As in the case of the hard glottal attack, coughing and excessive throat clearing are unlikely to cause vocal nodules, but can act as generalized irritants to the larynx and can add a vulnerability factor to other forms of vocal abuse. Therefore, it is important that the speech–language pathologist discuss the effect of coughing and excessive throat clearing and provide modification support. This can include physician referral as well as instruction on cough and throat-clearing modification.

The manner of coughing and throat clearing can be modified when a person is taught to do them with less intensity and glottal explosion. Zwitman and Calcaterra (1973) discussed the "silent cough" method of eliminating the abusive aspects by teaching the client to push air from the lungs in blasts, being careful not to produce sound whenever the urge to cough or clear the throat occurs. Even reflex coughing during upper respiratory infection can be modified in this manner. Most throat clearing is not reflexive, and behavior modification can be helpful in eliminating it. The speech–language pathologist should point out that most clearing of the throat is unproductive in terms of actually removing the stimulating mucus from the glottis and that swallowing quickly after a small air blast is more likely to clear the area of the mucus than is a loud, phonated grunt.

Grunting as in Exercising and Lifting

Grunting is a significant form of vocal abuse and often is overlooked. Anyone who has been on the sidelines of a football game can attest to the grunting that goes on during blocking and tackling. Fortunately, those engaged in this strenuous vocal activity usually are large and strong and their larynges are frequently strong enough to resist the abuse involved.

However, many of the general public's activities involve the same kind of laryngeal trauma. Daily exercise and lifting involve glottal closure under pressure in order to contain air in the lungs to stabilize the chest cavity so skeletal muscles can function efficiently. Push-ups, pull-ups, lifting of weights, hard tennis serves or volleys, heavy lifting, and jumping usually involve hard closure of the glottis. Clients should be informed of this potential form of vocal abuse so they can analyze their behavior with regard to it.

Calling Others from a Distance

Men, women, and children who develop vocal nodules often are surprised to discover how often they yell from room to room or yard to yard to communicate with other people or pets. It seems to be easier to yell than to walk closer for communication. However, walking—a simple activity—can help both the cardiovascular system and the vocal folds and can eliminate significant abuse to laryngeal tissues. The speech–language pathologist should encourage clients to make the extra effort to decrease distance before communicating verbally, especially when there is noise in the environment, such as in a house with the radio or television playing.

Using Inappropriate Pitch Levels

Pitch characteristics of vocal abuse clients merit considerable attention. The speech–language pathologist must evaluate the basal, habitual, and optimal pitch levels in such individuals, and modify any significant disparity found between habitual and optimal levels. One of the most common forms of vocal abuse in clients with vocal nodules or contact ulcers (discussed later) is speaking at a habitual pitch level that is too low.

Since the average optimal pitch level is about four whole notes from the basal level, any tendency for a person to speak at a pitch level lower than optimal will place the habitual pitch very close to the basal level. At or near the basal level, the larynx does not function efficiently in phonation, so considerable tension and effort must be expended to initiate voice. For a high pitch to be abusive, it would have to approach the upper limits of the vocal range, a level rarely approached by most people. However, a high-pitched and tense voice is also considered abusive.

In singing, it is common for untrained but professional vocalists to attempt to use tones at the extreme limits of their range, either too high or too low. Falsetto singing does not need to be abusive, but in pop music, where it is common, it often is. Falsetto singing that is abusive is more often falsetto screaming and has affected many professional singers adversely.

One of the first signs that a singer's larynx has been damaged by vocal abuse is loss of control on high tones, including falsetto. However, singers usually do not try to transpose the pitch or range requirements of certain songs to fit their voice range, but rather work harder to achieve the target pitch as written. In the long run, this is counterproductive to good vocal performance and is abusive to the laryngeal tissues.

Abusive Speaking During Allergy or Upper Respiratory Infection

When the delicate tissues of the larynx are inflamed by allergy or upper respiratory infection, they are more vulnerable to vocal abuse. Even normal communication during these episodes can harm the tissues, but when verbal use is intense, prolonged, at inappropriate pitch levels, or in any other way abusive, the negative effect is compounded. Therefore, it is important to determine whether such inflammations exist when the individual is evaluated.

A medical examination is required to distinguish between inflamed tissues resulting from allergies or upper respiratory infections, but the adult client's own impression as to whether either is present can be helpful. In any case, medical attention is necessary, and the client should be encouraged to seek such service. Rubin (1988) provided extensive information regarding the effects on the voice of allergy, diet, chemical reactions, stress, and hormonal influences such as premenstrual syndrome, supporting the notion of medical intervention in such cases.

Vocalizing Under Muscular Tension

The speech–language pathologist must give considerable attention to the evaluation of excessive muscular tension in the laryngeal area during phonation as a vocal abuse factor. Biofeedback through electromyography (EMG) can be used to monitor objectively the involvement of both intrinsic and extrinsic laryngeal muscles during phonation; this also provides excellent behavior modification feedback when excessive tension is detected. Prosek, Montgomery, Walden, and Schwartz (1978), reporting on the use of EMG biofeedback in the treatment of hyperfunctional speakers, showed success in the elimination of tension in 3 of 6 speakers.

Subjectively, the speech–language pathologist generally can determine whether excessive tension is present by palpating the extrinsic laryngeal muscles (sternocleidomastoid, mylohyoid, sternohyoid, masseter, etc.). If tension is found in the extrinsic muscles during phonation, it also is likely to be present in a hyperfunctional manner in the intrinsic musculature. Such tension contributes to the overall pattern of vocal abuse.

Smoking or Speaking in a Smoky Environment

Several authors have reported on the abusive effects of smoking on the larynx (Colton & Casper, 1990; Kirchner, 1986; Myers & Suen, 1989). Tobacco smoke is sometimes an allergen, but it is always an irritant to respiratory tract tissue. Nicotine constricts the peripheral blood vessels, reducing blood flow. The usual effect of excessive smoking is a lowering of the fundamental frequency of the voice. This is particularly noticeable in women (Gilbert & Weismer, 1974).

The irritating effects of smoking on the vocal folds are so substantial that it is not unreasonable for the speech–language pathologist to expect the client with vocal nodules or other abuse conditions to significantly cut down or eliminate smoking to establish a good prognosis for therapy. As with many factors, smoking—even excessively—does not cause vocal nodules, but does add a significant vulnerability factor.

Marijuana smoking also is a significant factor in many cases. Although marijuana (canabis) is an ancient drug, its use as a significant part of our society has occurred only since the early 1960s. Many marijuana smokers report dry mouth and throat, raspiness in the voice, and difficulty with pitch change (Gilman, Goodman, & Gilman, 1980).

In my experience with professional singers, particularly those who tour extensively and sing traditional rock and roll, marijuana is commonly used and has a deleterious effect on singing control, particularly in reaching high notes at low intensities. The singer who has vocal nodules will experience an even more significant effect from tobacco and marijuana smoke. Therefore, marijuana use should be discouraged in clients with vocal nodules.

Speaking Abusively in Menstrual Periods

The effect of menstrual cycles on vocal changes in some women is clear. Although these changes may be subtle and not experienced by all women, the speech–language pathologist should alert female clients to be cautious about excessive vocalization during premenstrual and menstrual periods. It may be necessary to document in a specific client whether voice quality and pitch seem to change just before menstruation. If so, it would indicate that tissue edema is sufficient to establish a vulnerability factor on the effects of abuse on the vocal folds.

Abitbol et al. (1989) studied 38 women during the ovulation and premenstrual phases of two monthly cycles. They found that estrogen–progesterone level alterations associated with these cycles caused laryngeal water retention, edema of the interstitial tissue, and venous dilatation causing vocal hoarseness and vocal fatigue in 22 of the 38 women. All of these women were vocal performers (classical, jazz, vocal teachers, and actors). Only 5 of the women smoked cigarettes. These women were studied with synchronized acoustic, visual (videostroboscopy), and glottographic instrumentation. This study, along with others (Higgins & Saxman, 1989; W. Rubin, 1987), provides significant documentation that hormonal changes in women can affect the larynx and the voice, particularly in women who perform vocally.

Excessive Vocalizing

It is not necessarily the amount of vocalization that becomes abusive, but the nature of it. When a person has vocal nodules, however, it can be helpful to suggest the elimination of nonessential communication during the early weeks of therapy. Certainly, the speech–language pathologist must judge whether such a suggestion would add such stress to the client as to be counterproductive, but the elimination of superfluous talking should at least be considered. Ohlsson, Brink, and Lofqvist (1989) provided a means of objective assessment of phonation time by means of a "voice accumulator." This is high technology at work to document that some people talk more excessively than others.

Inadequate Breath Support

The volumes of respiration necessary for phonation support were discussed in Chapter 3, along with a description of instrumentation needed for objective evaluation of the human respiration system. At this point, I provide a more clinical description of the breath support necessary for the phonation and articulation processes of speech. Boone (1988) provided practical steps for improving breath support for speech by explaining to the client that inspiratory–expiratory respiration is a continuous ongoing movement and by suggesting drills to maximize those processes in speech and singing. He emphasized speaking in simple terms (bigger, smaller, expiratory control, renewed breath, etc.), rather than in the complex terms of respiratory measurement (vital capacity, inspiratory capacity, expiratory reserve volume, etc.). His four-step approach provides a practical solution to many respiratory problems encountered in voice therapy, and the reader is encouraged to investigate this reference.

One benefit of formal singing or acting training is the realization of how important breath support is for proper laryngeal function, including specific instructions for proper breathing. When the larynx is supported well by proper breathing, it is as though vibration is occurring with little effort. Without such support, the larynx must be tense and must work hard to produce the vibration.

It is important for the speech–language pathologist to evaluate clients with vocal nodules to determine whether breath support is adequate. This is not a major etiological consideration in vocal nodules therapy as it is with some neurologically based speech disorders, but the speech–language pathologist should be prepared to evaluate a person who may be utilizing the respiration system poorly in phonation and speech. The following describes normal breath support for phonation and how to evaluate respiration beyond the instrumental processes discussed in Chapter 3.

Good breath support for phonation requires a sufficient inhalation of air but rarely requires a maximum effort such as in measuring vital capacity. A deep inhalation beyond tidal inhalation is all that is required. This occurs with the abdominal muscles essentially relaxed to facilitate the contraction of the diaphragm. The diaphragm is a dome-shaped muscle surrounding a central tendon that separates the abdominal cavity, which contains the stomach, intestines, and visceral organs, from the thoracic cavity, which contains the lungs, heart, and mediastinum. When the diaphragm contracts, by virtue of its shape and skeletal attachments, it pulls itself downward and forward, expanding the vertical dimensions of the thoracic or pulmonary cavities and therefore enlarging the lungs in that direction. This expansion draws air into the lungs and inhalation (inspiration) occurs.

For inhalation sufficient to support running phonation and speech adequately, the diaphragm must be able to contract without excessive resistance. Resistance is less when the abdominal muscles have decreased tonicity. As the diaphragm contracts, its movements displace the visceral organs in a forward and lateral direction, distending the abdominal wall.

The functions of the diaphragm during inhalation are complemented by musculature that lifts the rib cage to produce lung expansion in an anterior direction. In other words, deep inhalation requires that the stomach and visceral organs be displaced in a forward direction at the same time as the chest wall is expanding. If the client puts a hand on the stomach during proper inhalation, the inspiration should push the hand forward slightly. The deeper the inhalation, the farther the hand should move forward.

Following the inhalation cycle, the air is exhaled by essentially a reversal of the inhalation process. The diaphragm relaxes and pulls itself back to its precontraction position and the muscles that lifted the rib cage relax, allowing the rib cage to be lowered. These relaxation processes have the effect of decreasing the dimensions of the lungs, squeezing out their air through the open glottis. If phonation is to occur during this exhalation cycle, the glottis is closed and the exhaled air vibrates the vocal folds.

The early stage of exhalation is essentially passive, with tissues (diaphragm and rib cage) merely returning to their precontracted state. Air inhaled into the inspiratory reserve volume and tidal air are exhaled by this passive process. Beyond tidal exhalation, the process of exhalation becomes active, involving the contraction of the abdominal muscles to compress the abdominal cavity by displacing the visceral organs up against the diaphragm, which in turn compresses the lungs to force exhalation.

This compression is aided by the compression of the rib cage by muscles antagonistic to rib elevation (intercostals, transversus thoraces, serratus posterior inferior, and abdominal muscles). These compression forces have the effect of decreasing the vertical and anterior dimensions of the chest wall cavity to complete the exhalation involved in the expiratory reserve volume. The abdominal muscles also facilitate rapid and efficient contractions of the diaphragm for quick inhalation without significant interruptions in speech flow during running conversation.

The following are indicators that the client with vocal nodules has inadequate breath support for phonation:

- Phonation is attempted before adequate inhalation.

- Phonation is started after considerable exhalation has occurred, forcing voice and speech with little respiratory reserve.

- Poor reciprocity is exhibited between the muscles of inhalation (inspiration) and exhalation (expiration).

This information on breathing for speech is important in treating the typical client with vocal nodules or similar vocal abuse disorder such as contact ulcers. It is based on the assumption that breathing is essentially normal and devoid of pathology and merely needs to be maximized to support better the phonation and articulation processes of speech. The references on respiration mentioned in Chapter 3 must be considered in viewing this general information about breathing.

Laughing Hard and Abusively

The speech–language pathologist never wants to be accused of suggesting that a client eliminate the joy of a good laugh, but laughing is an altered form of phonation and some of its forms can involve considerable abusive stroking of the glottis. This concern for laughing patterns usually is not very significant in the treatment of vocal abuse, but some attention may need to be directed at modifying abusive laughter during the early weeks of therapy or following surgical removal of vocal nodules.

Cheerleading and Pep Club

Perhaps the classic example of vocal abuse in school-age children is organized cheerleading and pep club activities. In most junior and senior high schools, students are encouraged to abuse their vocal folds physically to improve school spirit and support the team. It is almost as though the chosen cheerleaders have been elected to sacrifice their voices on the altar of team victory. Organized cheerleading also is found in Little League baseball and Pop Warner football programs.

For several years, several graduate students in speech–language pathology and I studied the effects of cheerleading on the voice and vocal folds. Several high school and university cheerleaders were investigated longitudinally through basketball and football seasons.

The first study involved 10 varsity basketball cheerleaders at Arizona State University. Before the beginning of the 1977 basketball season, 8 female and 2 male cheerleaders were examined medically by an otolaryngologist and found to have normal larynges. Baseline voice recordings were obtained on each. Before and after home basketball games during the season, voice recordings were made of each subject.

At the end of the season, each person was medically evaluated by the same otolaryngologist. Both male cheerleaders had developed vocal nodules. One significant finding was that the voice recordings that were judged by three independent experts and also were used to obtain spectrographic measurements were not specific in identifying the presence of the vocal nodules; only the medical inspection identified them. This study was significant in that subjects with identified normal larynges were involved in a vocally abusive activity that resulted in a 20% incidence of developed vocal nodules. Observation of the cheering styles of the 2 males revealed an abusive pattern that was significantly different from that of the 8 females who did not develop vocal nodules (Case, Beaver, & Nenaber, 1978).

A further study involved voice and laryngeal characteristics of high school cheerleaders and an additional group of those at the university. These groups were followed longitudinally through a football season. Each cheerleader was evaluated by an otolaryngologist at the beginning and the end of the 1978 football season, as well as periodically throughout the season. Each subject's voice was recorded at the time of each medical examination. The voice recordings also were used for listener judgments and spectrographic analyses.

In the high school group, initial medical examinations revealed that none of the 9 subjects (all female) had laryngeal pathology. After this initial examination, the 9 participated in a week-long cheer camp, then were examined medically again. Four of the 9 subjects had laryngeal pathology (i.e., early vocal nodules and laryngeal edema) that the otolaryngologist attributed directly to vocal abuse. The cheerleaders reported that the cheer camp was an intense and vocally abusive experience that involved constant yelling in both formal and informal cheering sessions.

The listener judgments and spectrographic analyses were in agreement with the medically diagnosed status of the subjects' larynges—100% when no pathology was present and from 68 to 79% when pathology was present. These findings indicating the presence of pathology among many of the subjects made it more difficult to obtain agreement. Both false positives and false negatives were obtained; that is, medical inspection revealed pathology when listener judgment or spectrographic analysis indicated a normal larynx, or vice versa. By the end of the football season, even with some counseling from the authors of the study, 2 of the subjects continued to have vocal nodules, as confirmed by medical inspection.

The 12 football cheerleaders studied at Arizona State University presented a different pattern. They were evaluated medically the day before the first football game. An otolaryngologist examined each cheerleader's larynx and took a medical case history. Voice recordings for listener judgments and spectrographic analyses also were obtained.

Surprisingly, 9 (5 males, 4 females) of the 12 were found to have laryngeal pathology related to vocal abuse—a 75% prevalence. It had been hoped that in examining the cheerleaders prior to the first game, the larynges would be normal. However, the captain of the squad indicated that for several weeks the members of the squad had been practicing their yells intensely, and it was obvious that this was responsible for the high prevalence of laryngeal pathology.

The research team felt an obligation to inform the team members of the condition of their larynges and the probable causes of the pathology. This was done with slides and discussion about the development of vocal nodules. By the end of the football season, only 7 (4 males, 3 females) of the 12 cheerleaders continued to have laryngeal pathology from vocal abuse (58%).

In this study, probably because of the high prevalence of preexisting laryngeal pathology, agreement between spectrographic analyses and medical inspections and between listener judgment of voice quality and medical inspections was lower than in the previous studies (56 and 64%, respectively) (Case, Thome, & Kohler, 1979).

Since many of the cheerleaders in these studies developed pathology but others did not, it was important that the distinguishing causal factors be determined. By observation and subjective judgment, the following behavior seemed to be excessive in the cheerleaders who developed the nodules and other laryngeal pathologies:

- Cheering without good abdominal breath support

- Cheering with an energy focus in the larynx

- Cheering with excessive tension in the neck and larynx

- Using hard and abrupt onset of voice (hard glottal attack)

- Cheering during colds, infections, or severe allergy attacks

- Cheering at an inappropriate pitch level (too high or too low)

- Excessive individual cheering in addition to the group yells

In addition to the above factors, researchers have identified factors that must be considered when working with cheerleaders to prevent vocal difficulty. Perhaps one of the most important factors is to screen out those cheerleading applicants who predictably will have vocal difficulty. Campbell, Reich, Klockars, and McHenry (1988) have developed a screening protocol that could easily be incorporated into the selection process. Many factors were found to be important considerations, even when not statistically significant:

- Frequency of day's end sore throats and tired voices

- Severity of progressive aphonia and dysphonia on noncheering days (e.g., history of vocal difficulty even when not cheerleading, presence of excessive muscular tension in speech mechanisms, inadequate breath support)

- Severity of acute vocal problems at cheerleading camp

- Frequency of coughing and throat clearing

- Amount of loud talking when not cheerleading

- A-scale personality factors, such as aggressive personality

Based on this list and other additional factors that would be obvious to one who understands the vocal demands of cheerleading, improved selection of cheerleaders could reduce the prevalence of laryngeal and vocal difficulties experienced by this high-risk group. (For additional information on cheerleading and voice, see Reich & McHenry, 1987; Reich, McHenry, & Keaton, 1986.)

Considering the high prevalence of laryngeal pathology in cheerleaders, it seems important that the school speech–language pathologist evaluate cheerleaders to determine whether vocal abuse is affecting their voice quality and laryngeal structures. It also is suggested that the cheerleaders and pep squads be advised before practices on cheering techniques that are less abusive, in accordance with the principles outlined.

Vocalizing Toy and Animal Noises

Verbal dramatics often are important parts of children's play. Bears growl, lions roar, monsters make weird noises, airplanes scream as they dive in combat, machine guns and rifles make sharp bangs, and bicycles become motorcycles—all in the children's voices. Numerous play activities seem to require children to mimic sounds, thus abusing the larynx.

The speech–language pathologist, when working with a child with vocal nodules, should explore these verbal activities thoroughly. Some children engage in many such activities, others in only one or two but often and routinely. For example, the child who makes only motorcycle sounds when riding a bicycle, but does so often, can abuse the larynx sufficiently to produce nodules even when good vocal hygiene is practiced in all other circumstances (Johnson, 1976).

Athletic Activity Involving Yelling

The high school athletic coach, particularly in football, basketball, and wrestling, is in a high-risk profession for vocal abuse and the development of vocal nodules. The wrestling coach, for example, constantly yells instructions during a match in an atmosphere of extreme noise and emotional tension. A typical wrestling match involves three rounds of 2 min each, and it is not unusual for the coach to be yelling throughout each round, telling the wrestler to execute one move or another to gain points or avoid being pinned. Hand signals or gestures will not work since the wrestler's eyes usually are buried in his opponent's armpit. Only the voice can be used to communicate. This occurs match after match until often, by the end of the meet, the coach is voiceless, and the next morning it is worse.

It is a great challenge for the speech–language pathologist to help the athletic coach solve the dilemma of vocal abuse while still functioning effectively as a coach. To accomplish this, the pathologist must carefully consider with the client ways of modifying the communication process to eliminate as much of the abuse as possible.

Aggressive Personality Factor

Aronson (1985) classified vocal nodules as a psychogenic voice disorder because abuse or misuse most often is not the primary etiology. Rather, abuse is an intermediate link in the chain of causes that begins with an emotionally determined tendency to vocalize in an aggressive manner. This attitude is shared by Toohill (1975), who reported that 62 of 77 children with vocal nodules were described by their parents as screamers, incessant talkers, or loud talkers who were aggressive, hyperactive, nervous, tense, frustrated, or emotionally disturbed. Throughout the literature, children with vocal nodules have been described as having these personality characteristics, as well as greater feelings of inadequacy, poorer relationships with parents and siblings, and greater difficulty controlling themselves in verbal relationships.

Some of these factors have been verified in my clinical experience, but not to the degree reported by Aronson and Toohill. The possibility that a client with vocal nodules has a significant personality disturbance as a contributing factor in the etiology of the disorder certainly must be considered; in such cases, referral to a psychologist or psychiatrist is in order as an adjunct to vocal abuse therapy.

Arguments with Peers, Siblings, and Others

The aggressive personality factor often manifests itself in constant arguments with other people, peers, and siblings. To a certain degree, this is a normal part of social and family life unless it occurs in the extreme. The client with vocal nodules (or, if a child, family members) must be interviewed about the prevalence of such behavior.

In children, this often is such a meaningful factor in voice abuse that it is wise to include peers and significant others in the early therapy sessions to enlist their help in avoiding such confrontations. If a sibling or significant peer is not willing to cooperate in avoiding verbal arguments, it is hard to convince the client to become verbally passive when conflict arises.

Reverse Phonation

Phonation in inhalation produces a sound that many youngsters call donkey voice. The abusive nature of this form of phonation seems likely, but has not been verified by research. Luckily, it does not occur often in the verbal repertoire of most children. However, if a client uses such a style in verbal games or play activity, it should be eliminated since it probably is not a healthy form of phonation, even in play.

Nightclub Social Talking

Many of the factors related to nightclub social talking have been discussed already: talking in a noisy and smoky environment, loud and abusive laughter, and talking to people from a distance. One additional factor in the behavior of persons who frequent nightclubs for socialization is the consumption of alcohol.

Alcohol, as a depressant of the central nervous system, also acts to inhibit restraint. The client with vocal nodules who engages in nightclub social behavior and consumes alcohol increases the probability of vocal abuse or misuse without being able to monitor competently the amount of verbalization (vocalization), its loudness, the pitch used, the degree of laryngeal tension involved, the abruptness of phonation onset, the breath support involved, and most of the other significant factors involved in good vocal hygiene.

An additional concern is that alcohol has an irritant effect on the mucous membranes of the body (including the larynx) that may produce considerable inflammation of body tissues (Gilman et al., 1980), adding a vulnerability factor of no small significance. Young adult clients with vocal nodules must be advised against nightclub behavior during the treatment period and must reduce it significantly as a permanent change in life-style.

Arcade Talking

The game arcade is the nightclub of the teenager, except for the absence of alcohol. Although some young people become so involved in game playing that they do not talk, others use the arcade for socialized activities, particularly when they are in a group. The loud ambient noise level and general excitement of the arcade constitutes a dangerous place for the young person with vocal nodules who is trying to eliminate vocal abuse and misuse.

Evaluation and Therapy Procedures in Vocal Nodules

Persons with vocal nodules receive the services of speech–language pathologists either by screening or teacher referral in school, or by physician referrals in clinics, centers, and private practice. When a student is screened or referred by a teacher, the speech–language pathologist first must determine the nature of the problem and the possible causes and effects. The only information available initially is that the student has a hoarse or raspy voice. The etiology of the vocal systems is not known until a medical inspection is conducted. That process should begin as soon as it has been established that persistent voice disorder exists.

Once the medical confirmation of vocal nodules is obtained, the formal evaluation of the student can proceed. There is no clear distinction between evaluation and therapy processes in cases of vocal nodules. However, the management protocol in Exhibit 4–1 should help the speech–language pathologist working with cases of vocal nodules.

Session 1

The first order of business is to obtain a case history. Exhibit 4–2 is a case history form that can be used in the evaluation of children with vocal abuse, and Exhibit 4–3 is a similar form for adults. As indicated on both forms, information beyond the case history is required as part of the evaluation process. Most of the information needed is self-explanatory once the material in this chapter and in Chapter 3 is understood.

In the evaluation of persons with vocal nodules, the most significant process is to identify each form of vocal abuse so that each can be systematically eliminated. Exhibit 4–4 (Vocal Abuse Checklist) can be helpful in this process. Separate lists for adult and child are not provided, so the items must be considered selectively. By direct questioning and clinical observation, the speech–language pathologist should be able to determine which of the factors listed require clinical attention. The speech–language pathologist also should ask the client to describe a typical day from morning to night in sufficient detail to help identify any peculiar abuse forms not listed.

After all abuse forms have been identified, the speech–language pathologist can rate the client's voice perceptually, using some system such as the

Exhibit 4–1 Vocal Abuse Protocol

Evaluation and Session 1

Case history (form provided [Exhibits 4–2 and 4–3]): Obtain medical clearance
Identify all abuses (form provided [Exhibits 4–2 and 4–3])
Evaluate vocal parameters (Wilson's Voice Profile)
Evaluate pitch:
- Habitual
- Basal
- Ceiling
- Optimal

Obtain s/z ratio and other measures of vocal efficiency such as /a/ prolongation, initiation of voicing.
  Record on tape.
Obtain spectrographic baseline and audio recording ("My Grandfather") for serial documentation
Establish hierarchy of vocal abuses
Determine nature of reinforcement
Teach hypofunctional form of phonation and assign its use for 3 to 4 days
Provide counting mechanism for datakeeping of all departures from hypofunctional voice
Make next appointment

Session 2

Check data card on departures from hypofunctional voice
Provide reinforcement if appropriate
Make serial recording and compare. Discuss aspects of improvement by noting pitch change (usually
  higher) and vocal efficiency
Modify hypofunctional voice to be a more normal form of phonation with less laryngeal tone focus
Target vocal abuses to be eliminated
Determine whether time (all abuses eliminated during) or specific abuses are to receive attention
Determine time for phone contact
Formalize datakeeping process for abuse targets (form provided)
Make new appointment

Session 3

Continue same procedures as in Session 2
Give client opportunity to discuss difficulties
Choose new abuse forms or time periods until such expansion eliminates all abuse
Continue serial recordings and comparisons
With Children: Engage in real-life opportunity to see how child behaves vocally
Consider benefits of group therapy

Wilson and Rice Voice Profile. The significant parameters from that profile can be marked on the case history form.

Following the perceptual rating, the speech–language pathologist should evaluate the client's pitch objectively by determining the habitual, basal, ceiling (optional), and optimal levels. This can be done with an instrument such as the Visi-Pitch or a pitch pipe, as outlined in Chapter 3. This process can help

Exhibit 4–2 Vocal Abuse Case History (Child)

Name: _____ Birth Date: _____ Age: ___ Sex: ___ Date: _____
Address: _____ City: _____ State: _____
School: _____ Home Phone: _____ Parents: _____
Medical Examination Information: _____

Date of medical evaluation: _____ Done by: _____
Date of current evaluation: _____ Done by: _____
Information provided by parent: ___ child: ___ teacher: ___ other: _____

Background Information:
Onset of voice disorder: _____

How has voice disorder changed since its onset: _____

Briefly describe any treatment received: _____

When is voice best: _____
When is voice worst: _____
How easily does voice tire: _____
Briefly describe child's general health status: _____

Previous serious illnesses: _____

Medications being taken now: _____

Prevalence of allergies: _____
Previous surgeries: _____
Fine motor coordination (describe): _____

Tonsillectomy: _____ If yes, when: _____
Adenoidectomy: _____ If yes, when: _____
History of hearing loss: _____
History of significant upper respiratory infections: _____

Has anyone noticed or commented on negative aspects of your voice: _____ If yes,
describe:_____

What aspects of your voice disorder concern you the most:
Pitch: None _____ Slightly _____ Moderately _____ Significantly _____
Loudness: None _____ Slightly _____ Moderately _____ Significantly _____
Quality: None _____ Slightly _____ Moderately _____ Significantly _____
Durability: None _____ Slightly _____ Moderately _____ Significantly _____
Consistency: None _____ Slightly _____ Moderately _____ Significantly _____

Exhibit 4–2 continued

Do you have trouble being heard: _____ If yes, describe circumstances: _____

Are you ever mistaken on the phone as being the opposite sex: _____

Rate the following on a scale from (1) insignificant factor to (7) significant factor:

Circle Answer

Easily upset	1	2	3	4	5	6	7
Prone to anger	1	2	3	4	5	6	7
Yells when angry	1	2	3	4	5	6	7
Talks constantly	1	2	3	4	5	6	7
Argues constantly	1	2	3	4	5	6	7

Fill out Vocal Abuse Checklist [Exhibit 4-4] Done: _____
How well do you understand what the larynx (voice box) is and how it produces sound: Very well: ___ Sort of: ___ Not at all: ___
Other significant factors not covered: _____

Current Evaluation:

Voice Profile (Wilson): Circle Number

Laryngeal Cavity Opening:	Open -4 -3 -2 1 $+2$ $+3$ Closed
Pitch Rating:	Low -3 -2 1 $+2$ $+3$ High
Resonating Cavity Rating:	Hyponasal -2 1 $+2$ $+3$ $+4$ Hypernasal
Intensity Rating:	Soft -2 1 $+2$ Loud
Vocal Range Rating:	Monotone -2 1 $+2$ Variable Pitch
Overall Severity Rating:	Mild 1 2 3 4 5 6 7 Severe

Habitual pitch: _____ Basal pitch: _____ Ceiling pitch: _____
Optimal pitch: _____ Diplophonia: _____ Vocal Fry: _____
MPD (Maximum Phonation Duration): /a/ ____ Trial 1 ____ Trial 2 ____ Trial 3 ____
s/z Ratio: /s/ ___ ___ ___ ; /z/ ___ ___ ___ ; Ratio: _____
Vocal tremor: _____ Thyroid cartilage movement: _____
Extrinsic laryngeal tension: _____ Audible inhalation: _____
Pain associated with phonation: _____ Where: _____
Evidence of dysarthria (describe): _____

Coup de glotte: _____ Pitch breaks: _____
Evidence of glandular dysfunction (describe): _____

Breath support for phonation (describe): _____
Spirometer readings: Wet/dry: _____
Aeromechanical (describe processes and findings): _____

Spectrographic analysis done: _____ Describe: _____

Exhibit 4–2 continued

Laryngoscopic information:	Indirect: _____	Direct: _____	Fiber optic: _____

Describe: _____

Hypofunctional voice taught: Yes: ___ No: ___

Assigned to use how long: _____

Baseline audio recording for serial comparison obtained:

Yes: ___ No: ___ Summary of evaluation: _____

_____

_____

_____

Reports to be sent to: _____

_____

Referral to (when appropriate): _____

_____

for: _____

Therapy recommended: No: ___ Yes: ___ When to begin: _____

the speech–language pathologist determine whether the client's pitch needs to be modified in some way as part of abuse elimination.

When the pitch has been evaluated, the speech–language pathologist can proceed to obtain maximum phonation durations for /s/, /z/, and /a/, and to calculate an s/z ratio.

Documentation of the client's voice profile with spectrography, electroglottography, aeromechanical measurement, videostroboscopy, or some similar process, can be done next. It also is very important to obtain a quality audio recording of the client reading a passage such as "Arthur, The Young Rat" or the "Rainbow Passage," which are commonly used by speech–language pathologists in such recordings. This recording will constitute a baseline of the client's voice at the time of evaluation and will be used for serial comparison throughout the therapy process.

At the completion of the objective measurement of the voice, the process becomes therapeutic. It is important that the client have a clear concept of the nature of vocal nodules, how they develop, and how they are treated. Therefore, the speech–language pathologist must explain their pathogenesis, using slides and models as illustrations. Few of my clients with vocal nodules have understood specifically what the larynx is, what vocal folds are, how phonation occurs, and, perhaps more importantly, how vocal nodules appear and affect the voice.

The Wilson and Rice (1977) kit provides excellent slides and audio recordings for this. Excellent color photos of vocal nodules and other laryngeal pathologies are also found in the books by A. E. Aronson (1985) and Colton and Casper (1990). Pictures of normal vocal folds compared with ones damaged

Exhibit 4–3 Vocal Abuse Case History (Adult)

Name: _____ Birth Date: _____ Age: ___ Sex: ___
Address: _____
City: _____ State: _____ Zip: _____ Phone: _____
Referred by: _____ Diagnosis: _____
Information provided by client: _____ Parent(s): _____ Other: _____
Evaluated by: _____ Supervisor: _____

Background Information:
Reason for this evaluation: _____
_____
_____

When did you first experience voice disorder: _____
_____

How has it progressed since onset: _____
Explain treatment received to date: _____
_____

How does voice change from morning to night: _____
_____

Do you experience vocal fatigue: _____
_____

General health history: _____
_____

Medications being taken now: _____
_____

Smoking history: _____
Alcoholic consumption history: _____
Prevalence of allergies: _____
   Treatment: _____
   Medications: _____
Vocation: _____
   Nature of work: _____
   Noise level at work: _____
Educational background: _____
Hobbies and leisure activities: _____
_____

Sporting activities: _____

How has voice disorder affected your life:
Socially: None _____ Slightly _____ Moderately _____ Significantly _____
Work: None _____ Slightly _____ Moderately _____ Significantly _____
School: None _____ Slightly _____ Moderately _____ Significantly _____
Explain: _____
_____

What aspects of your voice disorder do you find most distressing:
Pitch: None _____ Slightly _____ Moderately _____ Significantly _____
Loudness: None _____ Slightly _____ Moderately _____ Significantly _____
Quality: None _____ Slightly _____ Moderately _____ Significantly _____

Exhibit 4–3 continued

Durability: None ————— Slightly ——— Moderately ——— Significantly ———
Consistency: None ————— Slightly ——— Moderately ——— Significantly ———

How much do you understand what the vocal folds are, how they work to produce voice, and how your voice disorder has developed:
Not at all: ——————— Slightly: ——————— Moderately: ———————

Rate the following factors on a scale from (1) insignificant to (7) significant:

		Circle Answer				
Stress on the job	1	2	3	4	5	6	7
Stress at home	1	2	3	4	5	6	7
Prone to anger	1	2	3	4	5	6	7
Express anger vocally	1	2	3	4	5	6	7
Ease when speaking	1	2	3	4	5	6	7
Ease socially	1	2	3	4	5	6	7
Talkative nature	1	2	3	4	5	6	7

Fill out Vocal Abuse Checklist [Exhibit 4–4] Done: ————
Other factors not covered: ——————————————————————
——
——

Current Evaluation:

Voice Profile (Wilson): Circle Number

Laryngeal Cavity Opening: Open   −4   −3   −2   1   +2   +3   Closed
Pitch Rating: Low   −3   −2   1   +2   +3   High
Resonating Cavity Rating: Hyponasal   −2   1   +2   +3   +4   Hypernasal
Intensity Rating: Soft   −2   1   +2   Loud
Vocal Range Rating: Monotone   −2   1   +2   Variable Pitch
Overall Severity Rating: Mild   1   2   3   4   5   6   7   Severe

——

Habitual pitch: ———— Basal pitch: ———— Ceiling pitch: ——————
Optimal pitch, if determined: ———— Diplophonia: ——————————
Vocal fry: ———— Pitch breaks noted: ——————————————————
s/z Ratio /s/: ——— seconds; /z/: ——— seconds; Ratio: ——————————
(Normal: 1.00; Dys: 1.50±)
Prolongation of /a/: Time: ——— seconds; Vocal onset efficient: ——————
Vocal tremor: ——————— Thyroid cartilage movement: ——————————
Extrinsic laryngeal tension: ————————————————————————
Audible inhalation: ——————————————————————————————
Pain associated with voice: ——————————————————————————
Describe tone focus: ————————————————————————————
Describe breath support for phonation: ——————————————————————

——

Aeromechanical information: ————————————————————————
——
——

Exhibit 4–3 continued

Spectrographic information: _____

Indirect laryngoscopy information: _____

Stimulability (hypofunctional voice): _____

_____

Summary of evaluation: _____

_____

_____

Vocal abuses targeted for immediate elimination: _____

_____

_____

Baseline audio recording (serial) obtained: Yes: _____ No: _____

Reports to be sent to: _____

Referral to: _____

Therapy recommended: No: _____ Yes: _____ To begin: _____

by vocal abuse can be most dramatic and provide a great source of motivation to the client. This is an important aspect of the management process.

Hierarchy of Abuses. The next step in the evaluation–therapeutic process involves ranking the abuses identified as significant in a manageable hierarchy, ranging from those the client feels are the easiest to modify to those that are most difficult. It is important that the ranking be based on the client's opinion, not the speech–language pathologist's. Exhibit 4–5 shows a hierarchy of a hypothetical client (a university professor) with vocal nodules.

Each of the abuses in the hierarchy must be eliminated if the body is to heal itself of the vocal nodules. Some of the abuses may be so difficult for the individual to modify that a separate hierarchy may need to be established. For example, changing his habitual pitch level to C_1 may be a great challenge to the hypothetical professor who has heard himself speak at a different pitch for many years. Exhibit 4–6 represents a hierarchy for changing pitch in the example of the hypothetical professor.

Reinforcement. The use of reinforcement in modifying behaviors generally, and speech in particular, has been well documented in the literature (Mowrer, 1982). Mowrer described principles of reinforcement in detail to help the speech–language pathologist use them in programming the therapeutic pro-

Exhibit 4–4 Vocal Abuse/Misuse Checklist

Name _____

___ Playground yelling	Explain _____
___ Toy and animal noises	Explain _____
___ Cheerleading	Explain _____
___ Cheer or pep club	Explain _____
___ Inappropriately low pitch	Explain _____
___ Inappropriately high pitch	Explain _____
___ Aggressive personality	Explain _____
___ Hard glottal attack	Explain _____
___ Abusive professional singing	Explain _____
___ Amateur singing	Explain _____
___ Coughing	Explain _____
___ Clearing throat	Explain _____
___ Speaking in noisy places	Explain _____
___ Grunting (exercise, etc.)	Explain _____
___ Calling pets, distance	Explain _____
___ Calling family members/friends	Explain _____
___ Persistent upper respiratory infection	Explain _____
___ Allergy	Explain _____
___ Prolonged talking	Explain _____
___ Laryngeal tension	Explain _____
___ Smoking	Explain _____
___ Marijuana	Explain _____
___ Alcohol	Explain _____
___ Speaking in smoky places	Explain _____
___ Vocally demanding job	Explain _____
___ Excessive speaking during menstruation	Explain _____
___ Breath support	Explain _____
___ Abusive laughter	Explain _____
___ Yelling at sporting events	Explain _____
___ Coaching	Explain _____
___ Athletic participant	Explain _____
___ Talking when using lawn mower or other noisy equipment	Explain _____
___ Motorcycle noise on bike	Explain _____
___ Nightclub social talking	Explain _____
___ Calling from room to room	Explain _____
___ Talking at arcade, etc.	Explain _____
___ Reverse phonation (donkey)	Explain _____
___ Verbal arguments with friends or peers	Explain _____
___ Aerobic instructor	Explain _____
___ Other factors	Explain _____
___ Performance	Explain _____

Exhibit 4–5 Hierarchy of Abuses in Vocal Nodule Cases

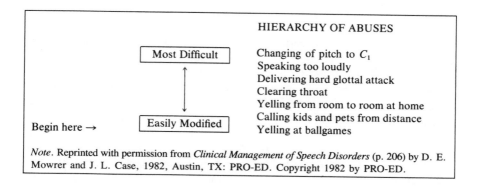

HIERARCHY OF ABUSES

Most Difficult

Begin here → Easily Modified

Changing of pitch to C_1
Speaking too loudly
Delivering hard glottal attack
Clearing throat
Yelling from room to room at home
Calling kids and pets from distance
Yelling at ballgames

Note. Reprinted with permission from *Clinical Management of Speech Disorders* (p. 206) by D. E. Mowrer and J. L. Case, 1982, Austin, TX: PRO-ED. Copyright 1982 by PRO-ED.

Exhibit 4–6 Pitch Change Hierarchy in Vocal Nodule Cases

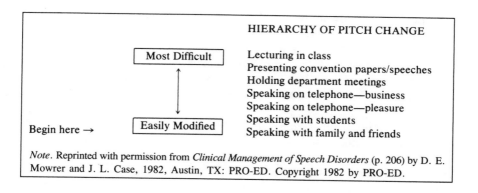

HIERARCHY OF PITCH CHANGE

Most Difficult

Begin here → Easily Modified

Lecturing in class
Presenting convention papers/speeches
Holding department meetings
Speaking on telephone—business
Speaking on telephone—pleasure
Speaking with students
Speaking with family and friends

Note. Reprinted with permission from *Clinical Management of Speech Disorders* (p. 206) by D. E. Mowrer and J. L. Case, 1982, Austin, TX: PRO-ED. Copyright 1982 by PRO-ED.

cess. Case (1982a) explained how these principles can be part of the therapy process in a vocal nodules case. Toward the end of the evaluation–therapeutic process with a child, the speech–language pathologist should discuss with the parents the concept of reinforcement and determine what type should be used. This might involve short-term reinforcement, as well as more significant reinforcement after a medical examination has confirmed that the vocal nodules are gone.

Principles of behavioral modification using techniques of operant conditioning are utilized in the treatment of vocal nodules by a number of authorities, including Drudge and Philips (1976), Johnson (1976, 1983), and F. B. Wilson and Rice (1977). An additional therapy program designed for public schools that utilized datakeeping without clear indication of reinforcement was described by Deal, McClain, and Sudderth (1976).

These various programs include procedures for identifying and reducing abuses, with tight reinforcement schedules either for eliminating the abuse or counting the target behaviors accurately. By choosing the proper reinforcement—whether it is money, a token economy, verbal praise, the opportunity to carry out activities the client enjoys, or whatever—the individual is motivated to count and eliminate abusive verbal behaviors. The precision with which behaviors are counted, charted, and reinforced distinguishes programs that are based on truly operant conditioning from those that merely involve reward or reinforcement.

In either case, it is a good idea to include the concept of reinforcement for following therapy suggestions, however precisely this is done. Before the end of the first therapy session, the speech–language pathologist should determine the role of reinforcements, select specific ones toward which the student will work, and establish criteria for attaining them.

Temporary Hypofunctional Phonation. Toward the end of the first evaluation–therapy session, the client should be taught to produce voice in a nonabusive, hypofunctional manner. This is neither whisper voice nor vocal rest, but a breathy and soft voice typical of how one person might talk to another during a movie, in a library, or in a quiet conversation that no one else is to hear. This voice pattern must be demonstrated by the speech–language pathologist.

Neither significant vocal rest nor whisper is recommended. Although whispering is unlikely to harm the vocal folds because of the lack of vocal fold contact during this activity, it is often accompanied by excessive effort that causes tension in the laryngeal system. Colton and Casper (1990) reviewed some interesting literature regarding various configurations of whispering and indicated that speech–language pathologists have been too concerned about having clients avoid whispering. I generally agree, but often clients have extensive laryngeal tension as part of phonation, and any speech behavior that encourages rather than discourages such excessive effort should be avoided.

The speech–language pathologist should explain that this soft hypofunctional voice is temporary but should be used exclusively of any other type for the next few days. There are two primary reasons for this recommendation:

1. It puts the brakes on normal speaking patterns in a dramatic way.

2. It offers the vocal folds a significant rest from constant vocal abuse and maximizes the probability that in a few days a serial audio recording will

demonstrate that voice improvement is occurring when compared with the baseline.

Datakeeping. An important component of vocal nodule therapy is the counting and elimination of vocal abuse forms. Figure 4–2 shows a datakeeping card that can be given to a client to tabulate vocal abuse forms. For example, this card could be presented at the conclusion of the first session with instructions for the client to tabulate all departures from the hypofunctional voice. Later, the card can be used to count other abuse forms as the speech–language pathologist moves up the hierarchy of established abuses. Figure 4–3 shows two cards on a client who counted two forms of vocal abuse, throat clearing and yells in the dorm.

Once the client is assigned the datakeeping card to tabulate all departures from the hypofunctional voice, the first session is over, and an appointment is made for another session in 3 or 4 days.

Session 2

The format for the second session is essentially the same as the therapy part of the first meeting. The client is asked about the previous few days in which hypofunctional voice was to be used exclusively:

• How easy was that to accomplish?

• What does the datakeeping card show in terms of numbers of departures?

• What problems were encountered?

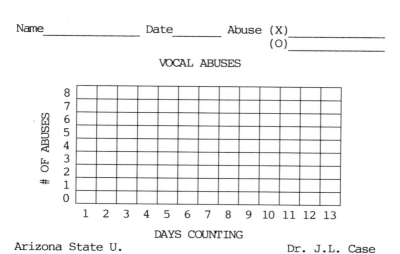

Figure 4–2 Vocal Abuse Blank Data Card.

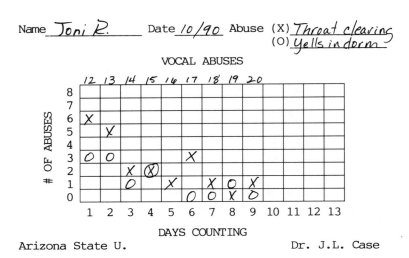

Name _Joni R._ Date _10/90_ Abuse (X) _Throat clearing_
                                    (O) _Yells in dorm_

Figure 4–3 Completed Vocal Abuse Form.

The answers to these questions will help the speech–language pathologist determine how well things are going generally. A new voice recording is made to compare with the baseline. If the hypofunctional voice has been used for most communication and there has been a general reduction in vocal abuse, a positive change is often evident. This improvement might be heard in more efficient onset of voicing or a slight natural rise in pitch. These are two of the voice improvement aspects most generally noted during the early days of therapy.

In this session, the speech–language pathologist must decide whether to continue having the client use the hypofunctional voice or begin "normal" phonation. Should the decision be made to move toward normal phonation, the client should be taught to produce voice with good breath support, reduced laryngeal effort, and resonance focus in the mask of the face. This technique of voice production is explained in Chapter 5. In addition to teaching a new form of phonation, the speech–language pathologist should add the goal of eliminating the next abuse(s) on the hierarchy. The decisions should be based on how well the client is doing. A specific program of abuse elimination is not recommended; instead, clinical judgment should form the basis for such decisions. By the end of the second session, however, the following should have been accomplished:

• Client report on progress obtained by discussion and checking data

• Voice recording made and compared

- Hygienic voice production taught
- Reinforcement provided when appropriate
- Aspects of difficulty discussed
- New abuse forms chosen for elimination
- New data cards provided for counting
- Encouragement provided for future effort

When these factors have been accomplished, an appointment is made for the next therapy session.

Additional Sessions

Additional sessions follow the same format as Session 2. In each, a recording is made of the client's voice and compared with baseline and previous recordings. Each session should reveal improvement in voice quality and efficiency, that is, efficient onset without pitch breaks, improved s/z ratios, longer maximum phonation durations, and so forth. If breathiness was present in the baseline recording, a reduction should be noted with each session. When little or no improvement is noted, there usually is an identifiable reason such as overlooking or not controlling some significant abuse.

Considerable time should be spent in therapy sessions discussing the significance of vocal nodules as deterrents to good voice quality, efficiency, and duration. The speech–language pathologist also should help the client identify factors in everyday living that make it difficult to control vocal abuses— sibling contentions, forgetfulness under social pressure, peer influences, job pressures, and so on. Some of these factors might be easy to correct once support is given, whereas other factors may not be.

The speech–language pathologist must take time to listen and understand how difficult it is for a client to change deeply rooted behaviors. If siblings or peers are factors, the client should invite them to therapy sessions so the process can be explained to them. Often a sibling or peer who does not have a voice disorder can be extremely helpful in the therapy process by serving as a gentle reminder to the client about good vocal hygiene.

When vocal nodules are large enough to affect voice in any significant way, it usually takes about 3 months of careful control to allow the body to heal itself and the nodules to disappear. After 3 months, the client should return to the otolaryngologist or other physician to determine the status of the larynx.

It should not be a surprise to find significant improvement in the physical status of the vocal folds even when there is a residual dysphonic voice quality. Several times I have sent clients back to the referring physician for visual inspection of the vocal folds and received reports that the nodules were gone even when slight dysphonia remained.

Group Therapy

A small number of clients with vocal nodules can constitute a homogeneous population for group therapy. Even though each individual might have different vocal abuses, the general cause is the same. Clients can spend time discussing difficulties in eliminating the abuses and strategies for dealing with them, encouraging each other when voice improvement is heard, and generally helping each other realize that none of them is a unique individual simply because of vocal nodules. The speech–language pathologist must ensure that age is considered in the grouping so that children and adults are not together. A school grouping can be effective in managing several students, particularly after the first few sessions of individual therapy.

Telephone Therapy

The speech–language pathologist can provide support between therapy sessions either by telephoning the client to discuss progress or by having the client call in at regular intervals. These calls can occur before, during, or after a period of particular difficulty for the client. A call reminding the individual to be aware of certain difficulties can be most supportive.

Calls to parents or others important to the client also can provide client support, as well as feedback to the speech–language pathologist. The call need not be long; merely an effort to touch base to offer support is adequate. This is particularly helpful during the first few days of therapy when the client is attempting to break long-term abusive vocal habits.

Teacher Participation in Therapy

When a client with nodules is being seen by a speech–language pathologist in school, it is important to remember that classroom teachers can function well as therapy associates. Teachers are in verbal interaction with the students much of the time. When provided with information about vocal abuse and general principles of therapy, teachers (with student approval) can report to the speech–language pathologist about a pupil's vocal behavior, and watch for vocal abuse in the classroom, on the playground, during lunchtime, and immediately after school. These teachers are overloaded with work and must not be expected to be responsible in any primary way for monitoring the child, but they can act as support persons.

The speech–language pathologist also should alert the classroom teacher as to activities from which the student with vocal nodules should be excused during the therapy—participation in plays, singing, and recitations that might be vocally abusive. Peer teasing can become a problem, and a cooperative teacher can thwart such tactics quickly.

In coping with the oral or verbal communication that is such an important part of daily classroom activities, an understanding teacher can help a student with vocal nodules control target behaviors. It is the responsibility of the speech–language pathologist to solicit such support and to demonstrate appreciation when it occurs since it is not the teacher's duty to provide this extra service.

Psychogenic Aspects of Vocal Abuse

A. E. Aronson (1985) advised that children and adults who develop vocal nodules or contact ulcers often have significant emotional disequilibrium in their lives which contribute to their voice disorders. In the case of children, the speech–language pathologist must spend time exploring this possibility with the patient and his or her parents and other family members. The child must be provided an opportunity to vent frustrations and emotional concerns. This can be done in individual therapy or in group dialogue. Time must be provided for the child to express feelings of anger, fear, anxiety, interpersonal and familial frustrations, and any other feelings that are of psychosocial concern. Parents can also be provided opportunity to receive counseling regarding their roles in these matters.

In adults, these psychogenic aspects of vocal abuse often are as critical as the abuse forms themselves. In some cases, the psychogenic basis for vocally abusive behavior may overwhelm an attempt to eliminate the abuses. Counseling must be provided by the speech–language pathologist who feels comfortable with such matters and processes, or a professional referral should be made. Referral can be concomitant with or preceding vocal abuse reduction.

Phonosurgery for Vocal Nodules

Surgery for vocal nodule removal remains controversial as a treatment mode. Recent research has demonstrated that surgery for nodule removal must be confined to the cover of the vocal fold, including the epithelial layer and the superficial layer of the lamina propria (Hirano & Kurita, 1986). The concept of phonosurgery is a marked departure from traditional laryngeal surgery for vocal nodules. The surgeon who approaches the task as representing surgery on the voice (phonosurgery) rather than surgery on the larynx will more likely approach the procedure with an attitude of conservative surgery and phonatory documentation and care. I think that much surgery has been done on the larynx and voice with little presurgical documentation of the voice in the form of audio and video recordings or acoustic baseline measurements. This is particularly true of vocal nodule surgery. Hirano (personal communication) stated that a surgeon would seldom approach the ear of a patient without careful presurgical audiometric baseline measurement for postsurgical comparison; however, the larynx and the voice have not received the same documentary attention. Hopefully, this is changing in the field of otolaryngology as a result of the work of the Voice Foundation and its symposia, Care of the Professional Voice (Cornut & Bouchayer, 1989; Sataloff, in press).

An excellent example of a phonosurgical approach to the management of voice disorder is described by Cornut and Bouchayer (1989) and Hirano (1990). Hirano documented the phonosurgery for 101 adult singers of various singing styles and training levels. Videostroboscopic and audio recording baseline measurements were done before and after surgery. Following the surgery, patients underwent 7 days of vocal rest until the postoperative checkup. Several months of voice therapy were then provided, after which the patients were able to resume singing exercises under the direction of a personal teacher. This all followed a decision regarding surgery which took into account several factors, including whether the lesion could be reversed without surgery. Hirano used forceps rather than a laser and described a careful technique directed toward preservation of the voice while surgically managing the case.

Adults often develop vocal nodules that become so large and fibroid that the physician decides to remove them surgically. However, it must be kept in mind that surgery removes not a disease but merely a symptom, since vocal nodules constitute an organic change (symptom) in the larynx developing from vocal abuse/misuse (cause). Nothing inherent in the best of endolaryngeal surgery can in any way eliminate the cause or stop the development or recurrence of the disorder. Therefore, without careful postsurgical management, the disorder will likely redevelop and nodules will reappear unless the cause is eliminated.

During the last decade, laser surgery has permitted endolaryngeal operations on various diseases, including vocal nodules. Without attention to the causal factors of vocal abuse/misuse, however, the nodules will reappear despite the most precise of surgical techniques. With elimination of causative factors, surgical results can be dramatic; without it, the postsurgical voice is not different from the presurgical voice after a few weeks, and often is worse. The following case, perhaps atypical, represents this concern.

Case Example of Poor Surgical Management

R.R., a female professional singer, was referred by a laryngologist who reported postsurgical return of vocal nodules. R.R. traveled with her husband, performing in lounges and private parties across the nation. During one extended tour through Florida, R.R. developed a prolonged hoarseness that interfered with her singing. A laryngologist diagnosed her as having singer's nodes (vocal nodules) and recommended surgical removal. Inasmuch as she had a 1-week hiatus between jobs, the surgery was scheduled.

R.R. reported that she checked into the hospital, underwent tests, had the surgery, and checked out the next day without speaking in any detail with the surgeon who performed the operation. "He gave me no recommendations and I assumed the problem had been taken care of and that I could resume my singing . . . I started the tour again and soon my hoarseness returned, only worse. I haven't been able to sing since," she said (clinic record).

When R.R. arrived in Arizona, she contacted another laryngologist who referred her to me. He reported that R.R. had large bilateral vocal nodules and generalized swelling of her entire vocal folds. Since she still was traveling, it was suggested that she obtain voice therapy to eliminate her vocal abuse as soon as she could be available for several weeks. She said that would be impossible in the foreseeable future. She left the clinic, disappointed that there was no easy solution to her problem.

Hopefully, this example is not representative of surgery for vocal nodules, but, without careful postsurgical management, the results R.R. experienced are not unexpected. Under any circumstances, surgery must be followed by as much postoperative control over patient behavior as possible. The surgeon can be aided significantly by a speech–language pathologist who understands the recovery process and who can help the client avoid abusing delicate tissue during the healing process. This provides the best opportunity for positive results from the surgery but requires the closest of relationships between physician and speech–language pathologist.

After surgery, the physician must inspect the healing at intervals and inform the speech–language pathologist when progress is sufficient to allow therapy for voice restoration. The pathologist then can begin to introduce phonation gently in the recovery process. The start should involve a highly breathy and easily produced vocal effort, similar to soft sighs—mostly breathy with a little voice. This should be done only a few times, followed by a break. If possible, the vocal folds should be inspected medically after this first attempt to determine whether there were any negative results (i.e., edema, erythema, etc.). If not, after a short rest, the same procedure can be repeated and somewhat expanded with a number of phonation efforts, but without increasing the intensity of voicing. The voice should remain breathy and gentle as in a sigh. This procedure should continue, with gradual increases in the number of phonation attempts, always followed by rest periods.

Periodic medical inspection is an important part of this early therapy. With such medical support, the speech–language pathologist can judge how quickly to move the client toward normal phonation. Once the laryngeal tissue can withstand normal and nonabusive phonation, the therapy process should continue by systematic identification and elimination of all vocal bad habits if that has not been accomplished already.

This procedure is tedious and circumstances might make it difficult to accomplish, particularly the medical inspections, but, without this postsurgical care, there is a great probability that the client soon will suffer a relapse and nodules will develop again on the vocal folds. It is not enough for a surgeon to place a patient on a few days of vocal rest after surgery and expect that the nodules will not return. Vocal habits must change.

Sorensen (1982) discussed the application of laser surgery in the therapy of benign laryngeal disease, including polyps, cysts, granulomas, hemangiomatosis, papillomatosis, and Reinke edema. Sorensen offered several advantages over traditional surgical techniques, as well as a description of potential hazards from using lasers in microlaryngoscopy:

Advantages

- Excellent precision is obtained by vaporizing tissue under continuous observation of the effect.

- The visual field is not impeded by the instruments, and the effect occurs exactly at the point of the aiming beam.

- The lesions usually are blood free since the laser coagulates blood vessels well.

- Postoperative reaction to surgery is nearly nonexistent. Patients are free from pain and edemas do not occur.

- The minimal tissue reaction produces rapid epithelialization of the wound surface and scar contractures are minimized.

Hazards

- There is an increased risk of fire and tracheal burns.

- Accidental burns can occur outside the laryngoscope because of reflections from the scope or instrument. Reflection burns can be minimized by using unpolished instruments.

- The target tissue must be kept within the direct light of the laser beam when the pedal switch is activated. If the patient moves, the size of the spot changes, control of the vaporized area is diminished, and accidental burns can occur.

- Large quantities of smoke and vapor arise and must be removed by continuous suction in order to maintain the visual field.

- Too deep a burning in the arytenoid region can produce perichondritis (inflammation of the tissue that covers the surface of the cartilage) or tissue necrosis (breakdown), so caution is imperative.

Hirano (1990) recommended that surgery for vocal nodules be done with forceps and only in extreme cases since most cases can be resolved by therapy. Kay (1982) indicated that surgical removal of nodules and voice therapy were not effective as a management procedure in 42 cases of vocal nodules. However, details regarding the nature of the surgery and therapy procedures were not well defined, so interpretation is difficult.

Other Approaches to Therapy

Methods of management of children and adults with vocal nodules are described by Andrews (1986); A. E. Aronson (1985); Boone (1980, 1982); Boone and McFarlane (1988); Greene (1980); Holbrook, Rolnick, and Bailey (1974); Johnson (1983); D. K. Wilson (1979); and Wilson and Rice (1977).

One of the best-organized programs is Johnson's (1976, 1983) Vocal Abuse Reduction Program (VARP). The VARP is designed to identify and systematically eliminate vocal abuses as they occur in specific high-risk situations, and applies to children as well as adults. It can be applied to the elimination of nodules, polyps, contact ulcers, and acute edema. High-risk times for children include morning and afternoon school recesses, trips home from school, lunch periods, bike riding, and the time immediately after school. The VARP is based heavily on data (counting and charting of abuses), and reinforcement is contingency managed by the speech–language pathologist. The most significant reinforcement is provided when laryngeal inspection by the referring physician reveals that the vocal nodules or other pathology involved have been eliminated.

Case Example of Vocal Nodules Management

Susan A., 22 years old, was referred by an otolaryngologist who reported bilateral vocal nodules and generalized edematous vocal folds. A case history interview revealed that Susan had started working recently as an aerobic dance instructor at a health spa. She also was training to become a cosmetologist. Both of these activities involved extensive voice usage.

The speech–language pathologist observed her aerobics class and noticed that for 45 min she was constantly yelling instructions to her class members over loud rock music. Often she was doing exercises that involved glottal closure (sit-ups, leg lifts, etc.), emitting a loud yell with each exercise. For example, she would yell, "Sit-ups, let's go—one, two, three, four . . . Come on, work! . . . seven, eight . . ." Each yell involved a hard glottal attack and, because of the physical strain, considerable laryngeal tension.

She reported that she often led two classes each work night. During the day, Susan spent several hours in a large cosmetology class, working on hair styles of women and men, surrounded by other students, all of them talking loudly with their customers. At the request of the speech–language pathologist, she provided a tape recording of the class, which revealed that the large room lacked acoustical treatment so, with some 50 persons all talking at the same time, the ambient noise level was extremely high. Susan spent about 5 hours daily in this noisy environment.

In her leisure time, Susan often went to a nightclub with her boyfriend. She was a one-pack-a-day smoker and a light beer drinker. Additional abuse forms involved an allergy factor that caused her constantly to clear her throat and cough, living in a house with three other women who all yelled from room to room to communicate with each other, constant singing with her radio in the car and at home, and hard and prolonged laughter. She was always on the go, and it seemed to the speech–language pathologist that for Susan it was always "vocal time."

Susan's abuses were ranked in the following hierarchy:

1. Aerobics instruction (most difficult to change)

2. Cosmetology communication

3. Smoking

4. Singing with radio

5. Yelling from room to room

6. Coughing

7. Throat clearing (most easily changed)

Susan's habitual pitch was evaluated to be 196 Hz (G_1) with a basal pitch of 164 Hz (E_1). Very little pitch variation was noted. Her ceiling pitch was 262 Hz (C). No optimal pitch could be determined clinically because of her hoarseness. Maximum phonation durations were obtained on the following sounds: /a/ = 14 sec; /s/ = 21 sec; /z/ = 11 sec; s/z ratio = 1.80 (severe inefficiency). Spectrographic recordings revealed a Type IV hoarseness pattern.

Voice Profile judgments were as follows: pitch: -2 (low); laryngeal opening: $+2/-2$ (int. -3), severity of 6 (1–7 scale); resonance: 1 (normal); intensity: -2 (soft); vocal range: -2 (monotone).

The speech–language pathologist used slides to demonstrate Susan's voice and her vocal folds, then explained the pathogenesis of vocal nodules. The hierarchy of abuses was established and work begun on the systematic elimination of her abuses. It also was suggested that Susan learn to speak with a slightly higher pitch, and she was shown how to produce voice with less laryngeal tension and better tone focus.

Susan's baseline audio recording ("Rainbow Passage") was made, and she was taught to speak with a hypofunctional voice. Next, she was given the abuse counting card and instructed to count all departures from the hypofunctional voice during the next 3 days. The evaluation was done on a Friday. Susan decided not to work at the spa during the coming weekend and to call in sick for her Monday cosmetology class. An appointment was made for the following Tuesday.

That day, another recording was made of Susan speaking at a "normal" conversational level. Her data card (which she felt was not complete) indicated 35 departures from her hypofunctional voice, most of them involving yelling (calling) to her roommates. Twice she recalled using her old voice to store clerks.

The audio recording revealed a slight elevation of Susan's habitual pitch from 196 Hz (baseline) to 210 Hz ($G\#_1$). The speech–language pathologist explained that this was a good sign that perhaps some of the edema had been eliminated, causing the pitch to rise.

Within 4 weeks, Susan had systematically eliminated most of her vocal abuses, except for the talking during her cosmetology class. She felt she had no control over that factor since she had to talk with her customers and the noise level could not be eliminated. However, she was trying to decrease her amount of talking. She also was having a difficult time stopping the smoking, but had changed to a low-nicotine (tar) brand and had cut her smoking in half. Recordings continued to reveal voice quality improvement with minor exceptions.

After 2½ months of therapy, Susan was seen by her otolaryngologist, who reported that her nodules were reduced significantly, the color of her vocal folds was normal, and the swelling had been eliminated. He still could see evidence of nodules on both vocal folds, but was encouraged by her progress.

Summary: Vocal Nodules

Vocal nodules constitute a voice disorder in which organic change on the vocal folds results from function misuse. Treatment involves the identification and elimination of all forms of functional abuse/misuse. When this is done, the organicity of nodules is replaced by healthy tissues, and voice quality and vocal efficiency improve. The specifics involved in the evaluation and management of children and adults are presented in such a way that the speech–language pathologist can treat this disorder effectively.

Contact Ulcers

Another voice disorder that involves an organic change in the larynx from vocal abuse or physical trauma is the contact ulcer. Contact ulcers develop with or without ulcer granuloma. There are several suspected etiologies, including intubation trauma and vocal abuse/misuse. Brodnitz (1961) wrote that contact ulcers are rare in Europe but common in the United States, and attributed this difference to cultural factors.

Traditionally, the contact ulcer patient has been described as a male in the 40 to 60 year range who has a vocally demanding professional life, such as law, teaching, or sales. Additionally, smoking heavily and the use of a low pitch are factors. These demographic data appear to be changing. I am finding younger and more female patients involved in the pathogenesis, which is confirmed by the research of Watterson, Hansen-Magorian, and McFarlane (1990). They reported on 57 contact ulcer patients, with 21% female and 47% younger than 40 years of age. Their patients also did not manifest a higher than expected involvement in smoking and alcohol consumption. They concluded that the contact ulcer patient is similar to patients with other disorders of laryngeal hyperfunction.

Contact ulcers form at the junction of the middle and posterior aspects of the glottis at the border of the intermembranous and intercartilaginous segments where the tips of the vocal processes of the arytenoid are located (Figure 4–4). The ulceration begins at this junction and can involve the entire posterior region of the glottis, with bilateral involvement common. An abrasion in this region may result in granulation tissue development around the ulcer.

Voice Characteristics

The vocal symptoms of contact ulcers vary from person to person. Because the ulcers occur on the tips of the vocal processes of the arytenoid cartilages rather than on the vibrating muscular tissues of the vocal folds, the vocal symptoms ofter are not dramatic, particularly in the early stages of ulceration before granulation occurs. Vocal symptoms usually include an exces-

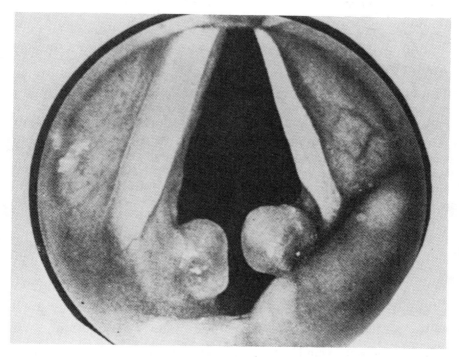

Figure 4–4 Contact Ulcer Granuloma. Reproduced with permission from *Voice Disorders: A Programmed Approach to Voice Therapy* by F. B. Wilson and M. Rice, 1977, Hingham, MA: Teaching Resources Corp. Copyright 1977 by F. B. Wilson.

sively breathy, weak voice with irregular voice onset. These symptoms increase with continued usage throughout the day.

Vocal fry (pulse register) is a common characteristic and is both a symptom and an etiological factor. Vocal fry (also called glottal fry) is difficult to describe but easy to identify once it is understood. It is best characterized as a pitch that is so low that the individual beats (pulses) of vibration can be detected. Another common voice characteristic is laryngeal tension or vocal hyperfunction (+2 on the Voice Profile, laryngeal opening parameter). Pitch breaks at the onset of phonation are common and occur because the person is unable to set the larynx properly with adequate vocal fold approximation because of the pain factor or the presence of tissue granuloma.

Clients often complain of pain during phonation and feel a sharp pain deep in the larynx, which also may extend (be referred) to the ipsilateral ear. This referred pain results from sensation carried over the internal (sensory) branch of the superior laryngeal nerve integrating with the auricular nerve (sensory) at the jugular ganglion (Maccomb & Fletcher, 1967). In summary, the typical voice profile of the adult with contact ulcers is low, breathy, and tense, characterized by vocal fry, pitch breaks, pain, and decreased durability.

As mentioned above, although contact ulcer traditionally is a disorder of the adult male, recently I have seen more adult females with this disorder. One was a female student in construction engineering who reported that, in order to avoid the critical comments from her male student associates, she tried to become "one of the guys," particularly in her speaking voice. She explained, "A sweet feminine voice just wouldn't do it." As more females enter professions previously dominated by males, the disorders associated with "male-type" professions no longer will be limited to men.

Specific Etiologies

Several specific contact ulcer etiologies have been identified, many of which include vocal abuse/misuse:

- Suffering intubation trauma
- Speaking at a habitual pitch level that is too low
- Speaking in a prolonged manner under conditions of loud noise
- Producing voice with laryngeal tissues that are inflamed and tender from excessive smoking, alcohol consumption, allergy, or upper respiratory infection
- Speaking with excessive laryngeal tension
- Initiating phonation with sudden and abrupt onset, that is, hard glottal attack (coup de glotte)
- Yelling, such as at sporting events
- Accumulating acidic secretions from the stomach and digestive tract around the arytenoid cartilages during sleep
- Presenting any of the miscellaneous forms of vocal abuse described in the section on vocal nodules

Most of these factors are clear and need no elaboration because they are described under etiologies associated with vocal nodules. However, a few additional comments are appropriate.

The vocal processes of the arytenoids can be traumatized by an endotracheal tube either directly during the introduction of the tube into the larynx during surgery or by static pressures by the tissue against the tube while in situ. Contact ulcers and granulomas from intubation are found in both females and children; these differ from the contact ulcers and granulomas that result from vocal abuse/misuse (Paparella & Shumrick, 1980).

In addition to the formation of intubation contact ulcers, Gallivan, Dawson, and Robbins (1989) reported other laryngeal trauma resulting from intubation for respiratory failure. Seventeen patients who had been intubated for a mean of 179 hours (range: 10 to 672 hours) were examined for the possibility of postintubation laryngeal damage. Only 1 patient had a normal examination. A total of 31 lesions were found related to intubation trauma, including erythema, tissue erosion, polypoid development, edema, and miscellaneous other abnormalities. One of the most interesting and common findings was that of a "keyhole" lesion which formed in the posterior larynx at the glottal level within hours after endotracheal intubation. The lesion looked like an open circle of tissue trauma similar to an old-fashioned keyhole. The authors concluded that the deleterious effects of endotracheal intubation on the tissues of the larynx and the voice have been significantly underestimated.

With regard to acidic accumulation as an etiological factor, Cody, Kern, and Pearson (1981) of the Mayo Clinic suggested that patients with heartburn and a granuloma should be referred for an esophagogram to determine whether gastroesophageal reflux during sleep causing lowered pH (increased acidity) is occurring around the posterior aspect of the larynx. Such acidity can irritate the tissue and cause tissue necrosis (ulceration).

Lumpkin, Bishop, and Katz (1989) also reported on 14 patients who had complained about voice or laryngeal disorder with concomitant dyspeptic symptomatology. These authors objectively assessed gastric reflux with pH monitoring and found that 70% of the patients experienced reflux in the hypopharynx in both upright and supine positions. Four of the 14 patients (36%) had contact ulcer/granuloma development. Whereas previous reports of reflux etiology in contact ulcer development have been essentially anecdotal reports, these authors provided objective documentation.

Although the hard glottal attack traditionally has been associated with contact ulcer etiology because of the "hammer and anvil" action that occurs between the arytenoids at the onset of phonation, Arnold (1980) disagreed. He explained that this cannot be a chief factor because contact ulcer is almost unknown in northern Germany despite the inhabitants' relatively harsh speaking style, particularly at the onset of speaking. Regardless of Arnold's opinion, A. E. Aronson (1985) and Boone and McFarlane (1988) suggested that this is an etiology factor, and I agree.

Evaluation Procedures

In contact ulcer cases, it is important that the speech–language pathologist obtain a case history to help identify background factors that require clinical attention. Using the Vocal Abuse Case History forms (Exhibits 4–2 and 4–3), the Vocal Abuse/Misuse Checklist (Exhibit 4–4), and general interviewing procedures, the speech–language pathologist should seek information about the client in the following areas:

- Nature of client's work
- Vocal characteristics associated with employment
- Noise levels in the typical speaking environment
- Onset of the vocal disorder and treatments obtained or sought
- Personality characteristics in terms of attitudes about self, lifestyle, social relations, ambitions, and achievement expectations
- Relationships with friends, family, and colleagues
- General physical and mental health factors
- Presence of reflux

The purpose is not to probe sensitive areas, but to help obtain insight into the client's personality and general behavior to determine which factors need modification.

The pitch, loudness, quality, and vocal duration parameters of phonation are evaluated next, as in the evaluation of vocal nodules. A special comment is needed, however, regarding the importance of pitch characteristics in clients with contact ulcers.

Men and women who develop contact ulcers tend, consciously or unconsciously, to speak with a lower and more authoritative voice, causing a significant vocal abuse factor. For example, if the habitual pitch level is only one or two tones from the basal, the laryngeal mechanisms are being used in a less efficient manner. This low pitch requires more vocal effort to maintain adequate loudness for speech.

More often than not, this increased effort is translated into vocal tension. Tension occurs particularly when the client uses language that involves many downward inflections, such as at the end of phrases or sentences. These downward inflection patterns place the pitch at the bottom of the range, which requires considerable effort to maintain voice. Vocal fry, heard throughout the client's voice, is particularly noticeable in these downward inflections.

The vocal processes of the arytenoid cartilages are particularly abused by these low-pitched, downward inflections since they undergo extensive medial compression from such phonation. This medial compression force is probably one of the most significant factors contributing to the pathogenesis of contact ulcers. All of this is compounded when speaking is occurring constantly in a noisy environment.

Therapy for Contact Ulcers

Since contact ulcers usually are caused by vocal abuse/misuse, it is necessary to identify all forms of that abuse and eliminate them similarly to the treatment in vocal nodules. However, there are a few differences. Since the typical client is tense and rather hard driving, it is common to find extensive muscular tension present in the laryngeal area during phonation. This also must be eliminated. The two most significant etiological factors in contact ulcers are an inappropriately low-pitched speaking voice and the hard glottal attack. These must receive careful attention.

Changing the Pitch

One of the speech–language pathologist's most challenging clinical tasks is to change an adult's pitch. Using a pitch pipe, the pathologist should blow the tone that has been found to be the client's optimal pitch, for example, B_2 (123 Hz). The person is told to hum or say /a/ at that pitch level. If the client can match the pitch pipe, and do so consistently, then the hum or vowel should be used as a starter as the individual is instructed to count, say the alphabet, or offer similar nonpropositional speech, for example, hum (B_2), 1-2-3-4-5, hum (B_2), A-B-C-D-E-F, hum (B_2), Sunday, Monday, Tuesday, Wednesday, and so forth. The speech–language pathologist must listen to ensure that the person is performing at the target pitch of the hum.

When sure the person can hit the target pitch with the help of the hum and can maintain it while counting and so forth, the speech–language pathologist directs the client to say simple phrases, such as "open the door," in a monotone. The target hum can be used intermittently if necessary to stabilize the pitch, but it should be eliminated as soon as possible. The sequence can go something like this:

Hum (B_2) Open the door.

Hum (B_2) Get the paper.

Tell the man.

Call me today.

Hum (B_2) Forget it buster, etc.

The target hum can be used periodically to ensure the proper pitch is being voiced. (Of course, the speech–language pathologist should check the pitch periodically to assure correctness.)

When the client has mastered simple phrases in a monotone using the appropriate pitch, the next step is to establish the ability to find that level without a target model and after a period of silence. To achieve this, the speech–language pathologist can discuss some topic while the client listens. Every few seconds, the speech–language pathologist stops talking and signals the client to hum the target pitch, which can be checked for accuracy with the pitch pipe. When the client is accurate in matching this pitch after an interval of not using it, the speech–language pathologist can be assured that it is stable in the client's mind.

In the next step, the client reads in a monotone at the target pitch. The speech–language pathologist can test the client's ability to maintain the new level by having the person prolong vowels in the middle of reading so the pitch can be checked for accuracy. For example, the client reads the following paragraph from a newspaper or article and, on signal, prolongs a vowel for a pitch check:

A week later, a puff of steam and ash burst forth from the mountaintop, forming a crater. Sightseers flooded theeeeee (check pitch) area, eager for a glimpse of the peee (check pitch) -ak. Steam and ash eruptions, great in magnitude, were accompanied byyyyyyy (check pitch) more earthquakes and rumbles from the mountain.

When it becomes apparent that the person can read consistently in the appropriate monotone, variation around the new optimal pitch is introduced. The client is reminded that the new target is merely the central tendency of all pitches used in speech, and the voice will go up or down around this central level to add emphasis, style, and meaning to verbal expression. Through reading and conversation, the person should practice pitch inflections around the optimal pitch under the supervision of the speech–language pathologist, who should check constantly to ensure that the optimal level remains the habitual level.

Carryover of normal pitch inflections around the new optimal level into real-life situations can be accomplished by establishing a control hierarchy. When the person has reached and learned to control pitch in the highest situations on the hierarchy, it can be assumed that the new behavior has been established clinically. The speech–language pathologist must check the stability of the new pitch periodically.

This process of changing pitch is made easier with an instrument such as the Visi-Pitch. Few clinics and training facilities accredited by the American Speech–Language–Hearing Association do not have the instrumentation necessary to change the pitch of a client. Speech–language pathologists working in the schools remain typically devoid of instrumentation and must rely on a pitch pipe or other means of pitch determination.

The speech–language pathologist using the VisiPitch or similar instrument should use the instrument's cursor to draw a line across the oscilloscope at the frequency of the client's optimal pitch (e.g., 123 Hz). This line should be stored on the oscilloscope. The client then can say /a/, count, say phrases, and later speak naturally into the microphone, and the Visi-Pitch will provide feedback that the proper pitch is being used. This instrument makes changing a client's pitch much easier. Carryover remains a challenge even with the best of instruments, and the hierarchy process described in the section on vocal nodules is recommended to achieve it.

Eliminating the Hard Glottal Attack

A hard glottal attack (coup de glotte) can be eliminated by having the person initiate voice in a manner incompatible with an abrupt onset. The client is taught to respire slightly before voicing so the vocal folds are brought into contact gently and the arytenoid cartilages are not slammed together. The best way to teach this is to have the person say an /h/ sound at the beginning of the utterance (e.g., /h/ open the door, /h/ up the stairs, /h/ kick the ground, etc.). This teaches the concept of gentle onset of voicing. For contrast with a hard attack, the individual alternates between hard and gentle onset:

Gentle	*Hard*
/h/ out	out
/h/ ask	ask
/h/ yell	yell

This contrasting step should be practiced to eliminate the hard glottal attack at each level of therapy, that is, in phrases, sentences, conversation, and so on. The speech–language pathologist should remember that the /h/ sound merely facilitates a gentle onset and should be used only to teach the concept that it is necessary to have a hard and abrupt onset.

Eliminating Muscular Tension

When extensive laryngeal tension occurs during voice production, it must be modified as part of the process of eliminating vocal abuse. This can be done by using progressive relaxation, biofeedback, or other tension elimination procedures as explained in Chapter 5, on neurogenic disorders, and Chapter 6, on psychogenic voice disorders.

Case Example of Contact Ulcers

F.F., a 42-year-old insurance salesman, was referred by a laryngologist who reported that F.F. had a contact ulcer on the left vocal process. A voice evaluation revealed a habitual pitch level of E_2 (82 Hz) and a basal pitch of D_2 (73 Hz). The optimal pitch level was found to be $G\#_2$ (104 Hz). It was obvious that F.F.'s habitual pitch was too near his basal pitch and was abusive. He spoke with considerable tension, which was apparent in his extrinsic laryngeal musculature. He manifested a loud, intense, and dynamic style of communication.

F.F. indicated that he was an emotional person, easily angered and easily upset, who became tense under those conditions. He also reported feeling considerable tension in his throat when he talked with people about emotional subjects. When speaking on the phone to a client about a topic that was upsetting, F.F. said he had a "tightness in the throat that almost chokes me." A hard onset of voicing (coup de glotte) was considered an important etiological factor.

Therapy for F.F. consisted of the following:

1. Raising his habitual pitch to $G\#_2$ (104 Hz), his optimal pitch

2. Using slides and tape recordings to introduce him to the topic of vocal abuse and its consequences

3. Identifying all forms of vocal abuse in his speech

4. Eliminating all abuses systematically, including excessive tension during phonation

At the beginning of each therapy session, the speech–language pathologist taught F.F. control over the tension in his body through relaxation training. Exhibit 4–7 is a transcript of a recording of the speech–language pathologist's instructions on one such session.

The rest of the relaxation continued in the same manner, progressing up the body until all sections had been covered. Considerable effort was directed at relaxing the neck muscles, since that area seemed to be the focus of tension.

This relaxation effort was included to some degree at the beginning of each therapy session. F.F. found it helpful in blocking out his tension. The speech–language pathologist then worked on raising F.F.'s pitch and eliminating his hard glottal attack, using the /h/ facilitator explained earlier.

After 5 weeks of therapy, F.F. was able to speak habitually at his new pitch level of $G\#_2$. He also had eliminated some of the muscular tension in difficult speaking situations and most of the tension in less difficult ones. He was aware of voicing onset and learned to avoid the hard glottal attack. As a result of the therapy, he also became aware of various forms of vocal abuse, such as yelling from room to room and shouting at sporting events, and was able to eliminate many of these factors.

Two months after he enrolled in therapy, F.F. was referred back to his laryngologist, who reported that the contact ulcer was gone. Three months

Exhibit 4–7 Relaxation Instructions at a Therapy Session

Let's begin this session by relaxing as much as possible. First, I would like you to sit in the chair in a comfortable manner. Put your feet on the floor and your hands so they are resting on your legs.

Now I want you to close your eyes and just listen to me. Follow my suggestions if you want to. Concentrate on the sound of my voice only. I will suggest that you focus your attention on various parts of your body to determine whether excessive tension is present. If it is, we will attempt to eliminate it until you are completely relaxed.

Now, first I want you to concentrate on your feet. Notice whether your toes are tight and curled at all. If they are, relax them . . . relax the foot muscles. Make them limp and relaxed. Any tension you feel in your feet must be eliminated. Now concentrate on your lower legs. Again, if you feel tension, eliminate it. Let your mind and body become totally relaxed. Your mind can control the tension you feel. (Pause of about 15 seconds.)

Now concentrate on your upper legs. If you feel tension, eliminate it. (Pause) Now concentrate on your stomach area. Let your stomach muscles be as relaxed as possible. As you breathe in air, let your stomach muscles be relaxed so your breathing is deep and full. Let each breathing cycle make you more and more relaxed. Now concentrate on your chest muscles . . . let them be as relaxed as possible. . . .

later, F.F. reported he again was experiencing vocal tension. He had seen his laryngologist and there had been no change in his larynx, but he felt the tension and wanted to get a handle on it before losing control.

When he came in for a review session, F.F. was found to be stable on pitch control and he demonstrated continued control over the hard glottal attack, but he did seem tense in his neck region by his own admission and by clinical observation. He was given more relaxation help, and it was suggested that he return for evaluations every 2 weeks until he felt he had control of the tension. F.F. has maintained his control for many years without relapse.

Medical results were reported by Bloch, Gould, and Hirano (1981) on 17 patients with contact granuloma. These 17 were treated by voice therapy without surgery. The therapy included a comprehensive case history and voice evaluation, stress reduction, relaxation help, auditory and kinesthetic feedback on voice production, pitch change, and general elimination of vocal abuse. The therapy resulted in the elimination of the granuloma in 9 patients, reduction in 4, and no change in 1 patient. Bloch et al. felt that their success rate of 71% indicates that voice therapy is a viable treatment for contact ulcer granuloma. The only failures in this study were the patients who terminated treatment early.

This study, and my experience, provide convincing evidence that voice therapy is necessary for the successful treatment of patients with contact ulcer, with or without granuloma.

Summary: Contact Ulcers

Contact ulcers occur on the posterior surface of the glottis at the junction where muscle joins the vocal processes of the arytenoids. The pathology can involve tissue necrosis or granuloma development. Vocal abuse causes the arytenoids to slam together with sufficient force, or to be pressed together with extensive medial compression, so that tissue breaks down at the point of contact.

There are several forms of vocal abuse etiology. The therapeutic procedures involve identifying the abuses and eliminating them systematically. The evaluation and management procedures are presented in such a way that the speech–language pathologist can approach these clients with greater confidence and competency.

5

Neurogenic Voice Disorders

The neurological bases of human laryngeal functions are complex yet remarkably stable in both biological and phonatory aspects. For example, the larynx functions well in its valving processes during swallowing to keep food, liquids, saliva, and other substances from entering the delicate respiratory system. However, should some foreign substance enter the larynx and stimulate the sensory end organs, it is forcefully expelled by the motor cough reflex. Thus, laryngeal sensory and motor integration of function protects the delicate tissues of the respiratory system from foreign matter.

This same laryngeal structure works well in the act of communication. It is so delicately controlled by the nervous system as to allow a great singer, for example, to set the vocal folds with the perfect amount of longitudinal tension and medial compression to vibrate at a frequency perfectly matched to the orchestra at an exact loudness level and without trial-and-error adjustments.

The central nervous system (CNS) innervation to the larynx is extensive from both left and right cortical hemispheres, the basal ganglia and cerebellum (Netter, 1983). Nerve tracts of a motor and sensory nature from these central structures, called upper motor and sensory neuron tracts, lead to the nuclei of the peripheral nervous system structures in the brainstem that directly innervate the larynx, pharynx, and other structures of the speech system. These nuclei of the peripheral nerves are considered lower motor and sensory neurons and, in the case of motor functions, lower motor neurons.

The peripheral nervous system innervation to the larynx is ipsilateral (same side), with the right and left halves of the larynx innervated by the right and left sensory and motor peripheral nerves, respectively. The bilateral control to the larynx stops at the peripheral nerves. Therefore, the right and left halves of the larynx are innervated centrally by both cortical hemispheres directed through the right and left peripheral nerves, respectively (Tucker, 1987). Because of this bilateral contribution to each peripheral nerve, under normal circumstances, laryngeal functions are completely symmetrical with regard to right and left vocal fold function.

It is essentially impossible for the normal right and left vocal folds to function out of phase with each other in adduction and abduction. Therefore, when the structures of the larynx are devoid of pathology, only a lesion or some form of disorder in the nervous system can disrupt normal symmetrical laryngeal functions. This chapter reviews abnormal neurological functions in the motor speech system, with particular emphasis on laryngeal neurological dysfunctions. First, however, a review of the normal neurological bases of laryngeal function is needed.

Innervation of Laryngeal Structures

Central Nervous System (CNS)

Motor control to the larynx is centered primarily in the inferior paracentral and postero-inferior frontal regions of the cerebral cortex. This region in the dominant hemisphere is more important than the control from the nondominant hemisphere. Tracts from these regions pass both directly to the nuclei of the peripheral nerves and indirectly through the basal ganglia before reaching the peripheral nerves.

Indirect control also is maintained by cerebellar relays from the anterior cerebellar cortex through the reticular formation and the basal ganglia that include all subcortical clusters of neurons within the brain (claustrum, amygdala, caudate nucleus, lenticular nucleus, putamen, and globus pallidus). These neuronal tracts above the peripheral nerve nuclei are called upper motor neuron tracts (Tucker, 1987). Additional central mechanisms in the brain respond to the mechanoreceptors in the larynx, which provide sensory feedback in a servosystem of laryngeal function (Kirchner, 1986; Larson, 1988).

Peripheral Nervous System (PNS)

The peripheral nerve nuclei that serve the sensory and motor functions of the larynx, as well as related structures such as the velopharynx, are located in the nucleus ambiguus of the medulla oblongata in the brainstem. The nuclei receive innervation from the CNS structures.

The peripheral nerves involved include the vagus (tenth cranial nerve) and the accessory (eleventh cranial nerve), which integrate outside the brainstem at the nodose (inferior) ganglion. From this inferior ganglion, the innervation is essentially considered to be the vagus nerve. The right vagus innervates the right side of the larynx and the left vagus the left side via the laryngeal branches. The velopharyngeal musculature is innervated by the pharyngeal nerves that exit the vagus below the nodose ganglia. The motor control of these peripheral nerves is considered lower motor neuron tracts.

Figure 5–1 shows the sensory and motor innervation of the larynx provided by the central and peripheral nervous system. The first branch off the vagus is the pharyngeal nerve, which, as mentioned, innervates the muscles of the

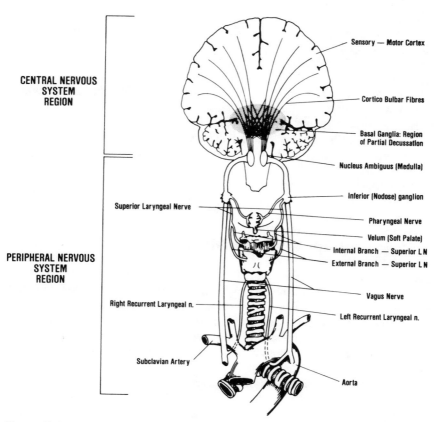

Figure 5–1 Innervation of the Larynx.

pharynx and all soft palate (velum) muscles except the tensor veli palatini, which is innervated by the motor division of the fifth cranial (trigeminal) nerve. Pharyngeal innervation is accomplished with the help of motor innervation from the ninth cranial nerve (glossopharyngeal).

Two additional branches of the vagus are important for laryngeal innervation, the superior laryngeal nerve and the recurrent laryngeal nerve. Upon exiting the vagus, the superior laryngeal nerve divides into internal and external branches. The internal branch is essentially sensory and is responsible for touch and pain innervation to the laryngeal mucosa in the ipsilateral supraglottal section of the larynx. The external branch is motor to the ipsilateral cricothyroid muscle (major pitch control muscle). Therefore, if superior laryngeal nerve innervation is normal, the sensory functions of the upper larynx (vocal folds and above) and motor control of the cricothyroid muscles are properly maintained.

The recurrent laryngeal nerve exits the vagus considerably inferior (lower) to the larynx. The left recurrent laryngeal nerve exits in the region of the aortic arch, passes underneath the arch, then ascends in a groove between the trachea and esophagus to enter the larynx. There it divides into sensory and motor components—sensory to the infraglottal mucosa for touch and pain and motor to all intrinsic laryngeal muscles except the cricothyroid (posterior cricoarytenoid, lateral cricoarytenoid, interarytenoids, and thyroarytenoids, including vocalis). The right recurrent laryngeal nerve exits the vagus slightly higher than the left, then loops under the subclavian and right common carotid arteries before ascending to the larynx.

Therefore, if the recurrent laryngeal nerve innervation is normal, the sensory functions of the lower larynx (infraglottal region) and motor functions of abduction, adduction, and vocal fold tension (vocalis contraction) are properly controlled (Tucker, 1987).

Disorders in Children and Adults

Several possible disruptions can occur along the sensory and motor tracts of the central and peripheral nervous systems to affect laryngeal function and produce a neurogenic voice disorder. Traumatic, infectious, vascular, neoplastic, chemical, or degenerative disruptions produce voice disorder. The voice symptomatology depends on the level of disruption and can occur as an isolated dysphonia or a more broadly involved disorder of the entire speech system.

The term dysarthria refers to neurogenic speech disorders that involve disruption of the respiration, phonation, resonation, and articulation speech systems to some degree. Anarthria refers to the complete stoppage of speech because of disruption in these systems. This chapter discusses the symptomatic, etiologic, evaluative, and treatment considerations of common neurogenic dysphonias, including the dysarthrias that involve dysphonia.

Vagus Nerve Lesions

Lesions can occur at any point along the vagus nerve from the nucleus in the brainstem medulla to its peripheral ending where it enters the larynx. The symptoms involved depend on the level of the lesion.

If some lesion or disease process disrupts the vagus nerve at the nucleus or any point before the pharyngeal nerve exits, the sensory and motor innervation to the pharynx and larynx are affected and a flaccid paralysis is present on the ipsilateral half of both the velum and the larynx. Velopharyngeal closure is disrupted on that side, as are vocal fold abduction, adduction, tension, and relaxation on the affected vocal fold. The paralyzed side of the velum does not lift upward and backward in velopharyngeal closure and the paralyzed vocal fold cannot adduct. The sensory aspects of laryngeal control also are lost.

The nuclei of both vagus nerves can be affected by a brainstem lesion, in which case bilateral symptoms of the pharynx and larynx are evident. A lesion outside the brainstem less commonly produces bilateral damage except in the case of widespread trauma of disease that damages both vagus trunks. The most common condition is some sort of unilateral lesion.

The speech symptoms of unilateral vagus damage above the pharyngeal nerve include hypernasal resonance on vowels, nasal air emission on pressure consonants, breathiness in the voice, reduced loudness, and lowered pitch. Diplophonia (double pitch) also is common because of the mass differences of the two vocal folds.

Nonspeech symptoms include a weakened coughing mechanism that does not have a sharp coup at the onset of the cough. Aspiration of food or liquid into the larynx is common during swallowing, causing choking and coughing. Because of reduced pharyngeal activity, swallowing is labored and slow. If a person is swallowing liquids in a bent-over position, such as at a water fountain, regurgitation of the liquid through the nose because of inadequate velopharyngeal closure often occurs.

If the lesion is in the brainstem so that the nuclei of both vagus nerves are damaged, these symptoms in speech and nonspeech areas are present in increased severity. For example, the voice usually is so breathy as to approach whispered speech. Even though both vocal folds are in an abducted position, however, there is enough closure potential during speech effort to produce a slight amount of voicing, although the overwhelming quality characteristic is severe breathiness. Loudness is compromised and the pitch of the very weak voice is near the basal level. The biological protection afforded the respiratory tract by the larynx is so severely damaged from such a bilateral lesion as to produce a life-threatening condition since all sensory and motor functions are affected.

A lesion can occur on the vagus nerve below the point of exit for the pharyngeal nerve but above the exit of the superior laryngeal nerve. In such cases, all of the laryngeal symptoms described are present, with no pharyngeal involvement. Therefore, although the voice is breathy, with reduced loudness and lowered pitch, no hypernasality or nasal air emission on consonants occurs. The vocal fold affected still is paralyzed in the abducted position from which it cannot adduct. Although rare, this same condition could occur bilaterally.

A common occurrence in neurogenic voice disorder is some condition that damages the vagus nerve below the exit of the superior laryngeal nerve, or injures only the recurrent laryngeal nerve after it exits the main trunk of the vagus. This can happen unilaterally or bilaterally. In the case of a unilateral occurrence, the ipsilateral vocal fold is paralyzed in the paramedian position from which it cannot adduct or abduct. The voice is slightly breathy, is slightly reduced in loudness and pitch, and has some possibility of diplophonia, particularly after a prolonged paralysis and subsequent atrophy of the involved vocal fold.

The most common nonspeech complaint is dyspnea (difficulty in breathing). This is particularly noticeable under conditions of extreme effort, such as running or similar activity. The dyspnea occurs because the paralyzed vocal fold is in a position near midline (paramedian) and does not abduct during inhalation. Therefore, all air must pass through the glottis, which is decreased in openness by nearly 50%. Under labored breathing, voice can be heard on inhalation, a condition called laryngeal stridor. Swallowing functions are essentially normal, and little aspiration occurs.

When the recurrent laryngeal nerve is damaged bilaterally, a much more serious condition exists. Airway obstruction is sufficient to require emergency tracheotomy in many cases. Although the voice is near normal, this is of little comfort because of the dyspnea. Bilateral recurrent laryngeal nerve damage can happen to children as well as adults. The long-term treatment consists of surgery to improve the airway (specific procedures involved are discussed later).

It is important that the speech–language pathologist understand why the vocal folds are paralyzed in varying positions, depending on the site of the lesion. As indicated earlier, a lesion that prevents innervation to the larynx from both the superior and recurrent laryngeal nerves causes the vocal fold to be paralyzed in a fairly abducted position, whereas recurrent nerve damage paralyzes the vocal fold closer to the adducted midline (paramedian) position.

The key to understanding this difference lies in the function of the external branch of the superior laryngeal nerve that provides motor control to the cricothyroid muscle. That muscle elongates the vocalis muscle to provide the longitudinal tension involved in increasing pitch. When this muscle functions properly, it pulls the vocal fold closer to midline by increasing the longitudinal tension. The following case study explains how an intact superior laryngeal nerve can influence the degree to which a paralyzed vocal fold can be moved toward midline.

Case Example of Laryngeal Nerve Paralysis

This case illustrates voice disorder resulting from unilateral lesion of the recurrent laryngeal nerve and shows that cricothyroid contractions can mask the severity of the disorder.

M.S., a 29-year-old male, was referred by a fellow employee who was a speech–language pathologist. M.S.'s main vocal concern was the voice pitch, which he felt was too high. His case history revealed that 6 years earlier he had had cancer of the thyroid gland that required surgical removal of much of the gland. During the surgery, his left recurrent laryngeal nerve had been severed, after which he reported he "hardly had a voice at all." In the ensuing years, M.S. experienced gradual improvement in the strength and quality of his voice. His only concern was that his pitch seemed too high and that he often was mistaken for a female on the telephone.

An evaluation of M.S.'s voice revealed essentially normal voice quality, indicating adequate approximation of his vocal folds at midline. However, his habitual pitch was found to be 174 Hz (F_1), which was typical of the pitch of a mature female. He also experienced pitch breaks into the falsetto range. M.S. complained of some dyspnea, as well, particularly when he ran or exercised.

Indirect laryngoscopy revealed a paralyzed left vocal fold, as expected from the case history, but with near-normal midline approximation of the vocal folds during phonation at his habitual pitch level of F_1. It was hypothesized that the midline approximation occurred because the extensive contraction of his cricothyroid muscles was sufficient to raise his pitch to the F_1 level. It was hypothesized further that, by lowering his pitch to a normal male level, the compensation mechanisms would be eliminated and the paralytic dysphonia that normally would be expected from recurrent laryngeal nerve damage would be unmasked.

Therapy during the next 3 weeks was directed at lowering his pitch from the F_1 (174 Hz) level to B_2 (123 Hz). When this had been accomplished, his voice quality became breathy and significantly reduced in loudness. Indirect laryngoscopy confirmed that a significantly altered positioning of the left vocal fold had occurred during phonation and that the fold was paralyzed in a more abducted position, producing a significant space between the folds during phonation at the B_2 level. His true paralytic dysphonia had been unmasked by eliminating the compensatory involvement of cricothyroid contraction.

M.S. then was referred to an otolaryngologist, who injected Teflon paste in three places lateral to his paralyzed vocal fold, displacing it closer to midline (Teflon laryngoplasty, discussed later). The client tolerated the procedure well, and upon recovery had an appropriately pitched voice that stabilized at a habitual pitch of C_1 (130 Hz) with normal vibration quality and loudness function (Case & Cleary, 1976).

Lesion of Superior Laryngeal Nerve

A unilateral lesion of the superior laryngeal nerve primarily affects the elongation potential of the vocal fold on that side (external branch dysfunction). A sensory disorder also is manifested in the larynx above the vocal folds on the same side (internal branch), but this does not contribute to the dysphonia. Normal adduction and abduction of the vocal folds remain, although a rotational effect on the larynx toward the normal side occurs during phonation, caused by the intact cricothyroid contraction on the uninvolved side. There also is a slight bowing of the vocal fold on the side of damage, resulting in a slight breathiness of the voice. The quality of the voice might appear slightly hoarse because of the rotational effect and the bowed paralytic vocal fold which cause asymmetrical (aperiodic) vibration of the vocal folds (Tucker, 1987).

When a bilateral lesion of the superior laryngeal nerve occurs, these same characteristics are present on both sides. The one significant difference is that the larynx does not rotate during phonation because of equal uninvolvement of the cricothyroid muscles. The anterior commissure of the larynx is masked by the overhanging epiglottis, and the vocal folds are bowed symmetrically in the middle portion of the glottis. The voice is breathy and reduced in loudness, with significantly reduced pitch variability. Increased aspiration and choking result from reduced sensory function in the upper larynx.

Bevan, Griffiths, and Morgan (1989) reported 3 cases of cricothyroid paralysis from disruption of the superior laryngeal nerve which required careful diagnoses using videostroboscopy and electromyographic analysis. Only when these objective assessment techniques were utilized was the etiology of each patient's dysphonia identified. Hartman, Daily, and Morin (1989) also reported an interesting case of coexisting superior laryngeal nerve dysfunction (unilateral) from an idiopathic inflammatory process and psychogenic dysphonia manifesting as a vocal conversion reaction. Voice therapy proved effective for alleviating the psychogenic component, and time eradicated the neuropathy. An additional concern is Reye's syndrome, a severe acute encephalopathy seen in children. J. W. Thompson, Rosenthal, and Camilon (1990) reported on 4 cases of Reye's syndrome in which superior laryngeal nerve paralysis caused absent laryngeal sensitivity. These children also had bilateral paralysis of the recurrent laryngeal nerves.

Etiologies of Vagus Nerve Lesions

Several studies on the etiologies of vocal fold paralysis of the unilateral and bilateral varieties have been reported. Tucker (1980) reviewed the selection, diagnosis, etiologic factors, and management of 390 patients with unilateral or bilateral vocal fold paralysis. This analysis shows that the most common cause of unilateral vocal fold paralysis is trauma, and that the severing of the recurrent laryngeal nerves during thyroid surgery is the major cause of bilateral abductory vocal fold paralysis.

D. D. Dedo and Dedo (1980) reported similar findings in several studies on the etiology of vocal fold paralysis, with trauma (automobile accidents, endotracheal trauma, etc.), neoplasms (tumors), infection, idiopathy (cause unknown), and vascular causes ranked in order of prevalence.

Miscellaneous causes are reported in the literature, including cases of recurrent laryngeal nerve damage following surgery of the ductus arteriosus in order to increase pulmonary blood flow in cases of right heart obstructive lesions (Seibert, Seibert, Norton, & Williams, 1981) and a large category of inflammatory causes: meningitis, polyneuritis, diphtheria, inflammatory disease of the mediastinum, thyroiditis, and neck abscesses (Tucker, 1987). Zitsch and Reilly (1987) reported vocal fold paralysis from cystic fibrosis, and Hartman et al. (1989) reported paralysis possibly secondary to herpetic infection.

Laryngeal paralysis is commonly seen in infants. Cohen, Geller, Birns, and Thompson (1982) reported on 100 cases of laryngeal paralysis involving children, based on the following factors: sex of the patient, etiology, disease onset, mother's type of pregnancy and delivery, disease-related symptoms, type of paralysis, vocal fold(s) position, need for tracheotomy, age of decannulation (removal of tracheotomy tube), preoperative diagnosis and neurological status, congenital and associated anomalies, course and progress of the disease, and statistics on recovery and resolution of the problem.

Not all of these findings can be reported here, but it is significant that central nervous system diseases occurred in 18% of the patients, birth trauma accounted for 19% of the cases, surgical and blunt trauma to the neck accounted for 11%, and 36% of the paralyses remained idiopathic with regard to etiology. A tumor (neuroblastoma) of the neck was the cause in 1 case.

Of the paralyses, 58% occurred within the first 12 hours of life. Bilateral abductor vocal fold paralysis occurred in 62% of the children studied, 45 of whom (73%) required a tracheotomy. Several neurological abnormalities, including hypotonia (floppy child), cerebral palsy, and various syndromes, were found in 33%.

The Cohen et al. (1982) article underscores the prevalence and nature of laryngeal paralysis in children. The significance of laryngeal paralysis or other abnormalities requiring prolonged tracheotomy and other forms of medical management as they relate to speech and language development was reported by Tucker, Rusnov, and Cohen (1982) and Narcy, Contencin, and Viala (1990). An excellent study on 319 children with airway obstruction including paralysis requiring tracheotomy was described by Crysdale, Feldman, and Naito (1988), who reported that the average duration of tracheotomy is almost 1 year. Of the 319 children in their study, 222 patients had tracheotomies because of airway obstruction of various etiologies.

Medical Treatment of Laryngeal Paralysis

The medical management of patients with various forms of laryngeal paralysis depends on several factors. Of primary importance is the status of the larynx in biological protection of the airway. Cannon and McLean (1982) reported on 4 patients with laryngeal paralysis who required laryngectomy because of chronic aspiration of food, liquids, and saliva into the tracheobronchial tree. An unsuccessful attempt was made to manage these patients medically with less radical procedures.

When the vocal folds are paralyzed in an abducted position and cannot close, aspiration is the primary difficulty. Although voice is weak and breathy, it is of secondary consideration. If, however, the vocal folds are paralyzed in an adducted position and cannot open, voice is not significantly dysphonic and aspiration does not occur to any unusual degree, but the patient struggles for breath (dyspnea). Medical management should be directed toward improvement of laryngeal dilatory functions. This is a well-understood rule between abduction and adduction forms of laryngeal paralysis.

Koufman (1989) reported a surgical technique for bowing of the vocal folds, involving placement of silastic implants lateral to each vocal fold plus lengthening of a central portion of the thyroid cartilage to which the vocal folds are attached by means of a tantalum shim. The combined effect of this procedure is to medially displace the bowed vocal folds and to increase their longitudinal tension by means of the shim. Koufman reported 3 cases utilizing this procedure.

Management of Abduction Paralysis

The most widely used procedure for treating bilateral vocal fold paralysis when the folds are fixed in a midline or near-midline position is arytenoidectomy. The procedure involves unilateral removal of one arytenoid cartilage, and cauterization of the muscular attachments to stimulate fibrosis and contracture and thereby provide improved dilation of the glottal space. This procedure can be either extralaryngeal, entering through the thyroid cartilage, or intralaryngeal, using suspension laryngoscopy (see Chapter 2). Both traditional and laser procedures have been reported (D. D. Dedo & Dedo, 1980; Tucker, 1987). The success of the procedure depends on whether the patient is able to breathe freely without needing a tracheotomy, has some degree of phonation, and does not aspirate food and liquid.

Kirchner (1986) described an endoscopic procedure in which lateralization of the paralyzed vocal fold occurs by microcauterizing a preassessed amount of thyroarytenoid (vocalis) muscle. Although the arytenoid cartilage is preserved, laryngeal dilation is provided with this procedure.

Nerve–Muscle Pedicle Reinnervation

A surgical procedure designed to reestablish nerve supply to the larynx is nerve anastomosis, which involves taking a pedicle of some neck strap muscle innervated by branches of the ansa cervicalis nerve and suturing it into the posterior cricoarytenoid muscle for reinnervation. The rationale for this procedure is that, during even light inhalation, there is efferent firing of the ansa cervicalis nerve and therefore, if successful, the efferent firing of the posterior cricoarytenoid could be reestablished by this means.

When the operation is successful, it can restore abduction of one vocal fold to patients with bilateral abductor paralysis. Tucker (1987) reported on the procedure and its success in many patients. Success is based on the observation of spontaneous abduction of the reinnervated vocal fold and significantly improved exercise tolerance (laryngeal abduction for high breathing demands). In successful cases, laryngeal examination revealed significant abduction of the reinnervated vocal fold.

Experimentation continues on animals, particularly dogs and cats, utilizing new procedures of laryngeal reinnervation in the hope of perfecting techniques that will be helpful to humans suffering from vocal fold paralysis (Maniglia, Dodds, Sorensen, Kumar, & Katirji, 1989).

Management of Adduction Paralysis

The most common medical management procedure for the treatment of laryngeal adductor paralysis is to inject, using a Brunings syringe, a mixture of Polytef (Teflon) and 50% glycerine-base injection into the lateral margins of the paralyzed vocal fold to displace it toward a more midline position. This is a common method, particularly when the condition of the larynx is affected unilaterally. Teflon is a chemically inert plastic material that does not absorb water, maintains its integrity over time, is not absorbed by body tissues, can be finely dispersed by syringe, and has a low tissue reactivity.

The procedure may be done by indirect or direct laryngoscopy, but D. D. Dedo and Dedo (1980) recommended the indirect approach because vocal fold tension is not altered by the laryngoscope and anesthesia. Topical anesthesia permits the patient to phonate during the procedure so that vocal quality can be used as the guide to sufficiency of the amount of Teflon injected.

The following are indications for using the Teflon laryngoplasty procedure:

- It can be done only in cases of unilateral adductor paralysis (vocal fold paralyzed in a paramedial, intermediate, or abducted position and unable to move toward midline).

- It can be done when there is bilateral bowing of the midglottal space when abduction and adduction are normal. Such bowing occurs with bilateral superior laryngeal nerve paralysis. Only one of the bowed vocal folds is injected with the Teflon–glycerine paste.

- It can be done following cordectomy, hemilaryngectomy, or blunt laryngeal trauma when there is glottal incompetency because of the removed or damaged tissue. (Cordectomy and hemilaryngectomy are described in Chapter 7.)

- It can be done when arytenoidectomy produces glottal incompetency (when the procedure is overeffective in relieving the dyspnea).

There also are several contraindications to Teflon laryngoplasty:

- It cannot be done in the majority of bilateral adductor paralyses since the procedure requires one competent vocal fold to work against the displaced (by Teflon) paralyzed vocal fold.

- It cannot be done when the vocal folds are paralyzed by CNS lesions producing generalized dysarthria and bilateral involvement.

- It cannot be done to add mass to the vocal fold for the purpose of lowering the fundamental frequency of vibration, either unilaterally or bilaterally (Zwitman & Calcaterra, 1975).

- It should not be done before 6 months after onset, except in the case of cancer-caused paralysis, since many laryngeal paralyses recover spontaneously within the first 6 months after insult (Tucker, 1987).

- It should not be done in a psychologically unstable patient (Montgomery, 1979).

- It should not be done to attempt moving an arytenoid cartilage medially. Only vocalis tissue should be moved by displacing the anterior two-thirds of the glottis without concern for eliminating a persistent posterior glottal gap. Horn and Dedo (1980) reported that several Teflon failures that were referred to them occurred because physicians had attempted to close the posterior space with Teflon.

- It should not be done for dysphonia resulting from myasthenia laryngis or hypogenesis of the vocalis muscle (Rubin, 1975).

- It should not be done for minor defects in the glottal area until vocal rehabilitation by speech pathology services has been attempted (Montgomery, 1979).

Several authors have reported on the voice improvements produced in most cases following Teflon injection in patients with laryngeal paralysis. One of the most complete single-subject studies was by Reich and Lerman (1978) on a 61-year-old male with a 24-year history of unilateral vocal fold paralysis. Following Teflon laryngoplasty, this man was evaluated for 52 weeks by a speech–language pathologist and a laryngologist. Both acoustical and perceptual data were reported. The results of the acoustical aspects indicate that, following the Teflon injection, there was a reduction of median fundamental frequency, an attenuation or elimination of certain frictional noise components, a reduction of fundamental aperiodicity for isolated but not excerpted vowels, and an increase in the energy of certain harmonic components. Many of these measures showed improvement but still were not in the normal range of acoustic measurement of normal voices (e.g., aperiodicity and perturbation). Oscillographic and spectrographic measurements provided the data.

The perceptual measurements (listener judgments) in this study revealed a reduction in perceived hoarseness and an enhancement in perceived pleasantness following the Teflon injection. The perceptual judgments were made by 20 listeners who were not informed as to when the recording was made (before injection or one of those made afterward) and used equal-appearing interval scales for hoarseness/no hoarseness, roughness/smoothness, and unpleasant/pleasant judgments.

Hammarberg, Fritzell, and Schiratzki (1984) reported excellent results of voice improvement in paralytic dysphonia on 16 patients whose voice improvement is well documented by means of acoustic data including spectrum analysis, fundamental frequency distribution analysis, waveform perturbation analysis, and perceptual judgment. An even more impressive database on Teflon laryngoplasty is provided by H. H. Dedo (1988) on patients involving 400 injections under local anesthesia. Dedo described his technique in detail and commented on the importance of the patient's being awake and able to phonate immediately after injection to determine the adequacy of the amount. The patient sat up and held his or her own tongue while the procedure was done. Dedo reported improvement in 95% of his patients using this procedure. Koufman (1988) commented that Dedo needed to provide specific data documenting the improvement in vocal parameters and expressed specific concern that Teflon should not be used to displace a vocal fold that is mobile to some degree.

A controversial analysis of vocal fold vibration patterns after Teflon injection was reported by Watterson, McFarlane, and Menicucci (1990). They used videostroboscopy to analyze the vibratory patterns of paralytic dysphonic patients with and without Teflon injection and compared them with the patterns of 3 normal subjects. Unexpected patterns of vibration were found. Patients with paralysis with uninjected folds demonstrated extensive vocal fold vibration. Such vibration was not seen in the injected vocal folds, which were essentially adynamic. The authors speculated that paralyzed vocal folds are significantly compliant because of the deinnervation and are therefore easily vibrated by aerodynamic forces. After Teflon injection, however, the paralyzed vocal folds are stiffened by the procedure and do not vibrate, even under conditions of digital manipulation or head turning, common therapy procedures. The controversial nature of this study is that no corresponding data are available regarding the vibratory patterns demonstrated stroboscopically and the acoustics of the voice. Were the voices improved or worsened by the Teflon procedure, regardless of the visual aspects of vocal fold vibration?

One postsurgical hazard occurs when excess Teflon paste is injected or there is a granuloma reaction within the injected vocal fold, causing a convex bulge across midline. Horn and Dedo (1980) reported on a surgical technique that can help correct such surgical error or abnormal tissue reaction to aid in restoring more normal function. Contrary to medical opinion that there is no way to correct a convex vocal fold after Teflon injection, those authors reported on 12 patients who were successfully treated by surgical extubation of the Teflon granuloma.

Since many patients with laryngeal paralysis are treated with Teflon injection, the speech–language pathologist must be aware of the procedure and be prepared to aid the laryngologist. It is important to document the preinjection voice with high-quality audio and, when available, videoendoscopic (including videostroboscopic) recordings, as well as to document the acoustical characteristics of the voice with a voice spectrogram. These same baseline measurements can be repeated at critical intervals following the injection to document surgical and therapeutic change. Guidelines in recording pathological voices in research as well as clinical documentation were provided by Baker (1987) and Gould (1987).

Voice therapy can help the patient stabilize pitch, quality, and loudness aspects following Teflon injection. (The specific techniques of such therapy are discussed in the final section of this chapter as they pertain to all neurogenic voice disorders.)

In some cases of vocal fold paralysis or conditions of vocal fold scarring, a protein substance of collagen has been injected. Spiegel, Sataloff, and Gould (1987) reported that collagen has two specific advantages over Teflon. First, collagen is liquid, unlike the thick Teflon paste, and therefore can be injected more accurately. Second, use of collagen in skin aberrations has shown a reduction of scar tissue in treated areas. With these advantages, collagen has been used to treat conditions of glottal insufficiency with good success (Ford & Bless, 1987). Spiegel et al. cautioned that since adverse reactions have occurred in dermatological treatments, every caution should be taken to ensure that adverse reactions in the larynx, which may compromise the airway, will not occur. They feel this can be done by using a screening skin test.

CNS/PNS Lesions and Dysarthria

To this point, the discussion has focused on lower motor neuron lesions that disrupt the innervation of the larynx and pharynx. Upper motor control of the larynx and pharynx is complex, as explained earlier, and lesions along the entire upper motor pathway can disrupt function. Upper motor neuron lesions produce spasticity of function, rather than the flaccid form of paralysis caused by lower motor neuron lesions. Upper motor neuron lesions can occur in the pyramidal tracts leading from the cortex, and when they occur bilaterally a form of spastic dysarthria results.

Pseudobulbar palsy is a syndrome caused by lesions that affect the corticobulbar tracts bilaterally. Most often, the lesions are caused by vascular disruption and are associated with arteriosclerosis, hypertension, and cardiovascular disease. Additional etiologies include congenital brain damage in cerebral palsy, neoplasms, and other degenerative diseases such as multiple sclerosis (Griffiths & Bough, 1989). A more appropriate designation probably is suprabulbar palsy. Such a condition affects motor control to structures other than the larynx, including respiration, resonation, articulation, and phonation. Thus, these upper motor neuron lesions produce a generalized dysarthria rather than a pure dysphonia. A significant nonspeech characteristic is the uncontrolled and inappropriate laughing and crying that occur frequently in these patients (Griffiths & Bough, 1989).

The speech symptoms associated with spastic dysarthria include a slowness of speaking rate, lowered pitch, reduced pitch inflections (monopitch), excessive nasal resonation on vowel sounds, and a laryngeal tension and aperiodicity during phonation that Darley, Aronson, and Brown (1975a, 1975b) have described as a harsh, strain–strangle voice quality. The speech–language pathologist thus must be aware of the dysphonic elements of this particular dysarthria, which occurs when there is suprabulbar damage to motor control centers of the CNS.

Another dysarthria with dysphonic components involves damaged cerebellar tracts, resulting in ataxic dysarthria. A distinct articulation aspect of ataxic dysarthria is that the random disruption in articulation precision and the staccato stress pattern give listeners the impression of alcohol intoxication. One client with this condition reported that his main difficulty in daily interaction with people is that he constantly is accused of being drunk; since he can drive, if he is pulled over by the police, he can count on being arrested on suspicion of driving while under the influence. Only blood tests vindicate him.

Portnoy and Aronson (1982) compared the rate and regularity of diadochokinetic syllable repetitions of /pa/, /ta/, and /ka/ in 30 normal subjects, 30 spastic dysarthric patients, and 30 ataxic dysarthric patients, and found them to be significantly different. Their data indicated that normals produce 6.4, 6.1, and 5.7 /pa/, /ta/, and /ka/ sounds per second, respectively. Spastic dysarthric patients produce 4.6, 4.2, and 3.5 sounds per second, somewhat slower than the normals. The ataxic dysarthric patients are the slowest on this task, with 3.8, 3.9, and 3.4 sounds per second.

These findings indicate that the dysarthric groups are slower than the normals; further analysis revealed that both groups are more variable in their productions. Although the ataxic dysarthric patients manifested the most variability, the researchers were surprised to find significant variability in the spastic dysarthric patients and suggested that variability may not be the discriminating factor between the spastic and ataxic dysarthric patients, as reported by Darley, Aronson, and Brown (1969a, 1969b).

Kent, Netsell, and Abbs (1979) provided further data on the acoustic characteristics of patients with dysarthria associated with cerebellar disease. They reported significant alternations of the normal timing pattern in speech, prolongation of vowel segments, and a tendency toward equalized syllable durations as discriminating factors. The more severe the dysarthria, the greater the occurrence of lengthened vowel segments. Monotone fundamental frequency and syllable-falling patterns also are common.

Dystonia

Dystonia is a term that applies to a variety of CNS dysfunctions that produce a variety of abnormal movements in the body. Generalized dystonias cause major movement functions to be abnormal, and specific dystonias affect isolated body parts. The latter are called focal dystonias. Specific focal dystonias include the eyelids (blepharospasm), mouth region (oromandibular dystonia), larynx (dystonic adductor dysphonia or spastic dysphonia), neck (spastic torticollis), and arm (writer's cramp). When two or more focal dystonias exist, the dystonia is termed segmental (Fahn, Marsden, & Calne, 1988).

Many focal and generalized dystonias significantly affect speech and voice. For example, oromandibular dystonia causes jaw and lip movements that impede motor speech production. Blitzer, Brin, Green, and Fahn (1989) treated 20 patients with this dystonia using injections of botulinum toxin (BOTOX) and reported an average of 47% improvement in various injected muscle groups (masseters, temporalis, orbicularis oris, etc.). These patients reported improvement in eating and speaking, as well as reduction of pain.

Spastic (spasmodic) torticollis is a focal dystonia that involves mainly the neck. Duane (1988), at the Mayo Clinic Rochester and the Arizona Dystonia

Institute, evaluated and treated over 1,000 cases of spasmodic torticollis. Many of these patients had voice and speech dysfunction. Case, LaPointe, and Duane (1990) reported on the voice and speech characteristics of 70 patients with idiopathic spasmodic torticollis. Compared with normals, these patients had significantly reduced levels of pitch range, /s/ and /z/ durations, phonation reaction times, and alternate movement rates for /pʌ /, /tʌ /, and /kʌ/. Apparently, the torque-like focal dystonic contractions that create the neck postural and movement abnormalities characteristic of idiopathic spasmodic torticollis create a considerable impact on the voice and speech characteristics of these patients.

Vocal tremor is heard in a variety of neurological conditions, including Parkinson's disease and essential tremor, adductor spastic dysphonia of essential tremor, and abductor spastic dysphonia of essential tremor. When the tremor involves other speech mechanisms, such as the velum, pharyngeal walls, laryngeal mechanisms, diaphragm, and tongue, a condition called palatopharyngolaryngeal myoclonus is present (A. E. Aronson, 1985). Ramig and Shipp (1987) compared acoustically the tremor of neurologically involved patients with the vibrato of singers and found more similarities than differences. The patients' tremors took the form of both frequency and intensity (amplitude) oscillations occurring at the mean rate of 6.77 Hz ($SD = 2.63$ Hz). This rate is within the range reported by A. E. Aronson (1985) of 5 to 12 Hz.

Parkinsonism

Lesions can occur in various areas of the basal ganglia to produce dysarthric and dysphonic symptoms. One such disorder is Parkinsonism. The damaged area in Parkinsonism is thought to be in the striatonigral (substantia nigra) system of the basal ganglia. One active neurotransmitter in this area is dopamine, and research has demonstrated that dopamine depletion in the striatonigral system is responsible for the neuropathological characteristics of this disorder. The deficiency of dopamine in the striatum of patients with Parkinsonism intensifies the excitatory effects of the cholinergic system within the striatum.

Therapeutic administration of drugs to enhance dopaminergic activity or anticholinergic effects has produced remarkable benefits for many persons with Parkinsonism. The most common drug is levodopa (L-dopa), which replenishes depleted amounts of dopamine in the substantia nigra. The exact etiology of Parkinsonism remains unclear, although exposure to toxins, metabolic abnormalities, infections of the slow virus types, and autoimmunity disorders are being studied (Yahr & Bergmann, 1987).

Logemann, Fisher, Boshes, and Blonsky (1978), in an analysis of articulation, laryngeal function, rate, and resonance in 200 patients with Parkinsonism, reported that 178 (89%) manifested some sort of laryngeal disorder (breathiness, roughness, hoarseness, tremulousness). Ninety (45%) showed some sort of articulation disorder, all but 1 of whom also displayed laryngeal dysfunction. Hypernasality and other resonance disorders appeared in only 20 (10%) and rate abnormality in 40 (20%). These findings are consistent with the notion that Parkinsonism often produces mixed vocal tract abnormalities of the dysarthria type.

Ramig, Scherer, Titze, and Ringel (1988) studied acoustically the voices of several groups of neurologically involved patients, including 8 patients with Parkinson's disease. Compared with a control group, these patients had greater shimmer and jitter (perturbation) values by a factor of 2, and almost one-half the harmonics-to-noise ratio. Four of the patients presented perceptible vocal tremor between 5 and 6 oscillations per second (Hz). Murdoch, Chenery, Bowler, and Ingram (1989) reported on the respiratory functions of these patients, and found essentially normal lung volumes but abnormal chest wall movements during speech. These acoustic and respiratory measures help define the perceptual characteristics that the speech–language pathologist should expect to find: breathiness, hoarseness, blurred articulation, monotonous and monoloud voice, vocal tremor, and islands of rapid or blurred speech (Griffiths & Bough, 1989).

Speech therapy for Parkinsonism has proved helpful in improving the overall communication skills of these patients. Scott and Caird (1982) demonstrated improvement in vocal prosodic control in 26 patients after only 2 to 3 weeks of voice therapy.

Amyotrophic Lateral Sclerosis

The complex and delicate nature of laryngeal function makes the larynx highly vulnerable to abnormalities resulting from numerous diseases. A common example is amyotrophic lateral sclerosis (ALS), popularly known as Lou Gehrig's disease. This progressive degenerative neuromuscular disease involves both upper and lower motor neurons of the cerebral cortex, the brainstem, and the lateral spinal tracts or the pyramidal tracts of the spinal cord, and results in both spastic and atrophic muscular symptoms. The cause of ALS is unknown, although histopathologic examination reveals widespread atrophy and loss of motor cells at all levels in the CNS.

The classical presentation of ALS is in progressive muscular atrophy of the arms, legs, and trunk muscles, with weakness, cramping, and fasciculations (tremors), leading to eventual dysfunction in swallowing, digestion, respiration, and all other motoric biological systems. The prognosis in ALS patients is poor; in most cases it is a terminal condition. Only 10% of patients survive

10 years, and death usually results from aspiration pneumonia or respiratory paralysis (Garfinkle & Kimmelman, 1982).

The generalized dysarthria of ALS involves all aspects of speech. Respiration progressively deteriorates until it is unable to sustain life. Phonation disorders parallel the respiratory deterioration, producing an aperiodic voice, sometimes tense and sometimes breathy. The vocal quality often sounds as though excessive mucus is present on the vocal folds, resulting in a wet hoarseness. This is caused by poor oral management of saliva and discharge from mucous membranes of the vocal tract. In other cases, the hoarseness is a dry type.

The pitch usually is near the basal level and monotonic. Speech phrasing is fragmented because of poor respiratory control. The intensity of the voice is soft and lacks variability, particularly in the late stages of the disease. One of the most striking features of the dysarthria involved in ALS is poor articulation, resulting from slow and inaccurate lingual and labial movements. Pressure consonants are articulated improperly, also because of velopharyngeal insufficiency that results in nasal air emission.

The relentless degeneration of ALS in terms of voice and speech characteristics has been well documented by Ramig, Scherer, Klasner, Titze, and Horii (1990), who compared the acoustic parameters of voice in a 69-year-old patient diagnosed with ALS over a 6-month period (six trials). The patient was free of vocal symptoms at the beginning of the study, but manifested significant vocal instability after 6 months of disease progression. The patient manifested increased variability in amplitude (loudness) and frequency (pitch), increased shimmer and jitter, reduced harmonics-to-noise ratio, and reduced maximum vowel duration by the time the last recording was taken. There was no significant increase in nasalization of speech over time in this patient, unlike other ALS patients. This precise form of acoustic measurement provides excellent documentation of change in progressive or degenerative diseases of the nervous system.

A. E. Aronson (1985) described ALS patients as producing a voice sound like a strain–strangle and gurgle and said that the vocal folds may adduct and abduct with less-than-normal excursions. Garfinkle and Kimmelman (1982) found that a laryngoscopic examination often revealed a pooling of saliva in the pyriform sinuses, which provided evidence for the gurgle quality that Aronson described. One of the most thorough studies of the dysarthria in ALS was provided by Hirose, Kiritani, and Sawashima (1982), who used a pellet-tracking X-ray microbeam to study articulation movements. Their findings confirmed the previously mentioned articulation patterns of ALS patients.

In the final stages of this disease, speech is essentially anarthric. Intelligence and complete awareness remain in ALS patients up to death, so their ability to maintain communication with family and friends is important since they may pass months in this condition. The speech–language pathologist must be aware of the special needs of ALS patients and be prepared to augment their communication efforts during the late stages when speech is unintelligible and anarthric.

Several communication aids are available to the speech–language pathologist for this purpose. Silverman (1989) thoroughly reviewed communication aids for persons unable to speak intelligibly regardless of the etiology involved, including the dysarthrias, apraxia, aphasia, glossectomy, laryngectomy, and mental retardation. Gestural (no instrumentation needed) and gestural-assisted (containing a readout device or display activated directly or indirectly by muscle gestures or movements) methods are described in detail.

Multiple Sclerosis

One common neurological disorder is multiple sclerosis (MS), a disease characterized by scarring or sclerosis of the white matter in various parts of the CNS. When MS develops, episodes of involvement occur and recur, interspersed with long periods of latency. Lesions can involve the cerebral cortex, the brainstem, the cerebellum, or the spinal tracts, with symptoms mirroring the site of involvement. The lesions of MS range from less than 1 mm to several centimeters, and they cause a loss of myelin on the involved neurons while the axons or dendrites remain intact (Garfinkle & Kimmelman, 1982).

There are several theories of etiology, most centering on unspecified viral infections. There also is an allergic response theory that is based on myelino-taxic substances found in the brains and cerebrospinal fluid of MS patients (Lisak, 1980).

Several clinical manifestations have been related to MS, many of which are pathognomonic to its diagnosis: ataxic gait; spastic paralysis of the legs; hyperreflexia; unilateral loss of vision; ataxic nystagmus; nystagmus of various types (central, vertical, positional, horizontal); vertigo; a tingling, heaviness, or numbness of the extremities; diplopia; bladder disturbances (incontinence); and various forms of dysarthria (Weiner & Levitt, 1978).

One of the most thorough studies of the dysarthria often associated with MS was reported by Darley, Brown, and Goldstein (1972). They said that of 168 patients with MS, 99 (59%) had speech that would be considered normal. Only 21 had speech disorders judged to be more than minimal in severity. The following specific speech deviations were found among the patients (from most frequent to least common): impaired loudness control, harshness, defective articulation, impaired emphasis, impaired pitch control, decreased vital capacity, hypernasality, inappropriate pitch level, breathiness, increased breathing rate, sudden articulation breakdown, nasal escape of air, and inadequate ventilation. Classically, patients with MS have been described as having "scanning speech," which is an equal emphasis per syllable pattern; however, Darly et al. found little evidence of that pattern (24 patients, 14%).

No cure is known for MS, but symptomatic treatment has improved quality of life by providing patients with physical therapy, audiological amplification, visual prostheses, parenteral nutrition, psychiatric support, and speech pathology services for the dysarthria. Adrenal corticosteroids and muscle relaxants often are used (Gilman et al., 1980).

Myasthenia Gravis

Myasthenia gravis is a neuromuscular disease characterized by weakened (striated) muscles, easily fatigued muscles, and prolonged latency of the return of muscle strength. Garfinkle and Kimmelman (1982) reported that several conditions or states tend to aggravate the muscular characteristics— infection, excitement, general fatigue, menstruation, and increased carbohydrate intake.

There are three major forms of myasthenia gravis: (a) neonatal, manifesting itself soon after birth by 12% of children born to mothers who have the condition; (b) congenital or juvenile, seen in children of healthy mothers usually after the age of 10 but before puberty; and (c) adult, with peak incidence occurring around the third decade of life. Muscular manifestations of myasthenia gravis include ptosis (droopy eyelids); diplopia (double vision); weakness beginning in the legs and spreading to other muscles over time; generalized fatigue; weakness in the facial muscles producing a smooth, immobile visage; dysphagia (swallowing difficulty); unnatural smile with lips elevating but not retracting; and generalized dysarthria (Carpenter, McDonald, & Howard, 1979).

Myasthenia gravis is caused by a biochemical abnormality at the junction of the motor end plates of the somatic nervous system and the muscle cells of the striated fibers. In 87% of 71 patients with myasthenia, antibodies against the development of the neurotransmitter acetylcholine were demonstrated (Lindstrom, Seybold, Lennon, Whittingham, & Duane, 1976). Although no muscular atrophy is involved, both clinically and experimentally reduced availability of acetylcholine in the myoneuronal junction appears to be the basis for the disease (Garfinkle & Kimmelman, 1982).

The dysarthria of myasthenia gravis involves all speech functions. Wolski (1967) discussed a case in which hypernasality was the presenting symptom, and A. E. Aronson (1971) described one in which a mild, breathy dysphonia was diagnosed as a psychogenic voice disorder when in fact this 20-year-old female was manifesting early myasthenia gravis. Only after the speech diagnosis manifested a marked increase in the breathiness, hypernasality, and articulation breakdown after prolonged speaking was myasthenia gravis suspected, and a referral was made back to the neurologist to establish the correct diagnosis.

A. E. Aronson (1985) described the dysarthria of myasthenia gravis as involving a breathy, hoarse voice, weak in loudness, and manifesting increased hypernasality that leads to nasal air emission on pressure consonants as speaking increases. There also are nonspeech symptoms of dysphagia, nasal regurgitation of food or liquids during swallowing, and, in severe states, inhalatory stridor and dyspnea. The voice quality often is of the wet hoarseness variety because of poor oral management of liquids and oral–nasal secretions.

Besides these symptoms, which can be observed clinically or by electromyography, there is abnormal articulation function secondary to muscle weakness of the lips, tongue, and mandibular muscles. Distortions of consonants resulting from these weakened articulation muscles are compounded by poor velopharyngeal closure for oral-breath pressure. The articulation distortions increase as speaking becomes continuous, until in severe cases it becomes unintelligible. As part of the overall medical and pharmacological management of the myasthenia gravis patient, the speech–language pathologist must be prepared to provide diagnostic and therapeutic support for the communication disorder that is a part of this disease.

Miscellaneous Central Dysarthrias

Several diseases or central conditions produce neurological abnormalities that result in some degree of dysarthric speech. They are described briefly below.

Wilson's Disease

Wilson's disease affects the body's ability to metabolize copper, causing the element to accumulate in body tissue over time until it reaches toxic levels. It first was called "progressive lenticular degeneration" because of postmortem findings showing cellular degeneration in the lenticular nuclei (putamen and globus pallidus) of the basal ganglia. It is transmitted genetically by autosomal (non–sex-linked) recessive inheritance. When copper reaches toxic levels, it causes damage to the liver, kidneys, cornea, and lenticular nuclei. Damage to the lenticular nuclei produces the neurological symptoms of dysarthria.

Berry, Darley, Aronson, and Goldstein (1974), comparing the dysarthric patterns of 20 patients before medical treatment and 10 patients before and after treatment for Wilson's disease, reported significant improvement in the overall dysarthria as a result of dietetic and pharmacological therapy. The characteristics result from a mixed dysarthria with prominent ataxic, spastic, and hypokinetic features.

Perceptual judgments reveal variation from patient to patient, depending on neurological state, but overall analysis indicates that reduced vocal stress, monopitch, monoloudness, and imprecise consonant articulation are altered most significantly in Wilson's disease patients.

Gilles de la Tourette's Syndrome

Although Gilles de la Tourette's syndrome is not common and often is not diagnosed properly, it constitutes a unique and interesting neurological disorder. The etiology is unknown, but it is thought to be some abnormality in the CNS rather than a psychological disturbance. Tourette's syndrome consists of random and uncontrolled grunting, coughing, throat clearing, whistling, and barking-type noises, accompanied by body and facial jerks and spasms. In 60% of affected patients, uncontrolled salacious and socially unacceptable obscenities are expressed, usually as isolated words in a totally unrelated sentence. The frustration of this disorder often comes from poor and improper medical treatment. Shapiro, Shapiro, Bruun, and Sweet (1978) expressed this frustration:

> Name a treatment and a Tourette patient has had it. Patients have consulted 100 physicians, spent $100,000, and received every known sedative, antianxiety, antipsychotic, stimulant, antidepressant, anticonvulsant, psychotomimetic, as well as other classes of drugs. Surgical procedures included phrenic nerve ligation, cryothalamotomy, and various types of lobotomies. Patients have been treated with megavitamins, allergic desensitization, insulin coma treatment, electroconvulsive treatment, narcosis treatment, acupuncture, and a variety of substances to correct hypoglycemic states and nutritional deficiencies. Patients have fruitlessly tried every type of psychotherapy, supportive psychotherapy, group therapy, family therapy, hypnosis, gestalt therapy, primal scream therapy, and recently, a variety of behavior therapies. One of the criteria for the diagnosis of Tourette syndrome is a fluctuating clinical course in which symptoms wax and wane. . . . These spontaneous changes are frequently misinterpreted as therapeutic effects. (pp. 5–6)

Darley et al. (1975a) provided audio samples of the dysarthria heard in Tourette's syndrome, and the speech–language pathologist would do well to become acquainted with its uniqueness by listening to these recordings. A Tourette's syndrome patient could be referred for speech management with an improper diagnosis, to which the speech–language pathologist would not want to contribute further confusion.

Kozak, Freeman, Connolly, and Riding (1989) reviewed retrospectively the medical charts of 72 patients with Tourette's syndrome to determine the otolaryngological symptomatology. In addition to the chart review, a questionnaire was mailed to 66 patients regarding ear, nose, and throat concerns. Nearly 90% of the questionnaires were returned with data that indicated that 42%

of the patients had consulted with otolaryngologists with such complaints as "sniffing and throat-clearing (likely related to the barking noises often heard)," "back of throat and nose noises," "snorting and difficulty breathing," and "noises like gulping sounds."

Cerebral Palsy

Although much has been written about cerebral palsy, a brief analysis of the dysarthria involved is appropriate. Cerebral palsy is an umbrella term for several congenital and early developing neurological disorders of the motor system. Mysak (1983) stated that brain damage between conception and 2 years of age that affects various forms and combinations of sensorimotor, perceptual, behavioral, and speech functions can be considered as part of the cerebral palsy umbrella.

Cerebral palsy manifests itself in spasticity, athetosis, ataxia, rigidity, tremor, and dystonia—separately or combined—in all degrees of severity. Hearing loss, visual abnormalities, mental retardation, emotional abnormalities, and developmental language delay can contribute to the motor dysfunction. When language is normal or near normal, the most striking speech characteristic in cerebral palsy often is some form of dysarthria. In severe cases, speech becomes anarthric so augmentation devices are appropriate, as noted earlier.

Organic Voice Tremor (Essential Tremor)

A common characteristic in geriatric populations is vocal tremor (A. E. Aronson, 1985). Although an actor or actress might use a slight voice tremor in the role of an old person, vocal tremor actually is an organic condition of unknown etiology. It is not merely an aspect of the aging process. Several specific lesion locations have been suspected, including the caudate and putamen of the basal ganglia, the cerebellum (loss of Purkinje cells), the dentate nuclei, and a triangle of substance connecting the red nucleus, dentate nucleus, and inferior olive. Organic voice tremor also is called essential or heredofamilial tremor when the hands, arms, jaw, tongue, head, or other body parts are involved and an autosomal dominant mode of inheritance can be proved (Darley et al., 1975a).

A. E. Aronson and Hartman (1981) analyzed three groups of patients with laryngeal dysfunction. One group was diagnosed as having essential (voice) tremor, a second with essential (voice) tremor but with occasional voice arrest typical of classical spastic dysphonia, and a third with spastic dysphonia (hyperadduction of true and false vocal folds during phonation, discussed later). These groups were compared on the frequency of voice tremor, among other things, and were found to be not significantly different (median tremor frequencies of 5.7, 5.0, and 5.5 Hz, respectively). Patients in all three groups also were found to have tremors in other parts of the body, other scattered neurological signs (hyperactive reflexes, asymmetric reflexes, ataxic gait, tongue fasciculations, and rigidity), and histories of life stress associated with the onset of their dysphonia. Although the research was designed to determine whether spastic dysphonia differs significantly from essential tremor, the data helped clarify the vocal characteristics of patients with organic voice (essential) tremor.

The primary characteristics of voice tremor include consistent rhythmic vibrato-like alterations in pitch and loudness, ranging from 4 to 12 oscillations per second with a frequency of oscillation around 5 or 6 Hz. As much as 5 dB of intensity variation also can be heard. The thyroid cartilage can be seen to oscillate with the voice. For a diagnosis of organic voice tremor to be made, the tremor itself should be the most prominent characteristic, although voice stoppage as heard in spastic dysphonia might occur.

Spastic (Spasmodic) Dysphonia

Perhaps no voice disorder has received the attention of the medical and speech–language pathology communities in the last few years as has the puzzling disorder of spastic (spasmodic) dysphonia. Since the first edition of this book in 1984, significant changes have occurred in the classification of this disorder, its etiological bases, the documentation of its neurological aberrations, its relationships with other neurological and psychological disorders, and its treatment methodologies.

Spastic dysphonia is a voice disorder with many characteristics that fall into the hyperfunctional category of phonation. Terms used to describe its vocal characteristics include tense, strained, overpressured, effortful, jerky, staccato, hoarse, stutter-like, spastic, laborious, and strangled. Other characteristics include hyperadduction tremor, grunts, groaning, uncontrolled pitch and loudness, facial tics, voice arrests, stoppages, and laryngospasm. It has been given a myriad of names, including aphthongia, lalophobia, mogiphonia, laryngeal stuttering, and psychophonasthenia.

A. E. Aronson (1985) and A. E. Aronson and DeSanto (1983) classified this disorder as falling into one of three general categories with subcategories in each: psychogenic adductor spastic dysphonia (adductor spastic dysphonia of conversion reaction, adductor spastic dysphonia of musculoskeletal tension reaction), neurological adductor spastic dysphonia (adductor spastic dysphonia of organic or essential tremor, adductor spastic dysphonia of dystonia), and idiopathic adductor spastic dysphonia. They described patients who fall into each of the above categories. Few other writers have categorized this disorder into as many classifications, and most have tended to generalize it into (a) a large category of patients with identifiable neurological abnormalities and (b) a small percentage of patients who fail to demonstrate neurological aberrations (Finitzo & Freeman, 1989).

In earlier literature, spastic dysphonia was considered as having a significant psychogenic basis. For example, Murphy (1964) stated that its onset

> may be sudden—following an emotional shock of some kind—or of longer duration. And, although it is usually a hyperkinetic phenomenon, hypokinetic conditions have been observed. We are probably dealing with hysteria in some cases. The disorder may be regarded psychodynamically as a somatization developed unconsciously as a defense against the recognition of unacceptable urges. (p. 71)

Almost a decade later, A. E. Aronson (1973) classified adductor spastic dysphonia as a psychogenic disorder, a form of conversion reaction, and indicated that clinicians were looking for a neurogenic component.

Few professionals today consider the majority of adductor spastic dysphonic patients as having psychogenic voice disorders. Rather, they are classified more often as having neurogenic etiology with possible psychogenic sequelae. Most professionals who work with clients having this voice disorder notice that the vocal symptoms are varied, capricious, affected by emotional states, and often absent during laughter, singing, saying "ee" in a high-pitched voice, or unusual vocal efforts. These factors give the impression that spastic dysphonia is affected significantly by psychosocial and psychodynamic factors, but such evidence does not solve the issue of etiology. A. E. Aronson and DeSanto (1983) stated that adductor spastic dysphonia can arise from one of several categories:

- Acute or chronic emotional stress that produces either heightened laryngeal musculoskeletal tension or conversion reaction

- Diseases of the CNS that produce movement disorders that either disinhibit or hyperstimulate centers responsible for laryngeal closure

- Specific neurologic syndromes that might be responsible for these laryngeal mechanisms, including essential (voice) tremor, orofacial–laryngeal dyskinesia, chorea, and spasmodic torticollis

They added that several patients they analyzed provided no identifiable cause symptomatology, resulting in a large category of idiopathic etiology.

Finitzo and Freeman (1989) studied 75 patients with either adductor or abductor spasmodic dysphonia over a 7-year period. They began their research to determine whether spasmodic dysphonia is a neurological disorder and, if so, where in the nervous system the disruptional basis or bases occur. Using auditory brainstem response, gastric and cardiac vagal nerve function studies, fiber optic analysis of vocal tract movements, electromyographic analysis, magnetic resonance imaging, brain electrical activity mapping (a combination of electroencephalographic and long-latency evoked potential assessment techniques), and positron emission tomography (PET) scanning techniques, the authors found that spasmodic dysphonia had a neurological etiology in the vast majority of their patients.

The conclusions to the above research indicate that spasmodic dysphonia is a supranuclear movement disorder that primarily, but not exclusively, affects the larynx. Over 50% of the patients manifested isolated, multifocal, or cortical lesions in the CNS, specifically in the left frontal/temporal cerebral cortex (perisylvian region), in the medial frontal cortex, or in the right posterior temporal/parietal cortex. An additional 25% of the patients presented mixed subcortical and cortical pathology. Subcortical lesions alone were found in 7% of the patients. Only 16% of the patients manifested no evidence of cortical or subcortical lesions. Thus, over 80% of these patients have documented evidence of neurological aberrations that could explain their phonatory differences. These findings are consistent with laryngeal studies of muscle function in spasmodic dysphonic patients, which would indicate that the difficulty is not in the muscle structures themselves (Ludlow & Conner, 1987; Shipp, Izdebski, Reed, & Morrissey, 1985).

In a study involving 12 spastic dysphonic patients, Aminoff, Dedo, and Izdebski (1978) found no evidence of psychiatric symptomatology. Ten males and 2 females were evaluated by a team of specialists representing neurology, psychiatry, and otolaryngology. No evidence of psychiatric or specific laryngeal pathology was found to justify the voice symptoms. However, 8 of the patients were found to have coexisting neurological disorders, including postural tremor, buccolingual dyskinesia, blepharospasm, and idiopathic torsion dystonia. Aminoff et al. concluded that spastic dysphonia should be regarded as a focal tremor of the laryngeal musculature.

Vocal Symptoms in Spastic Dysphonia

Several terms have been used to describe the vocal characteristics of spastic dysphonia. A. E. Aronson and DeSanto (1983) and A. E. Aronson (1985) identified adductor spastic dysphonia as a squeezed, hoarse, groaning, effortful, jerky, or staccato voice produced by moments of true and false vocal fold hyperadduction and laryngeal elevation.

H. H. Dedo and Izdebski (1983a) evaluated spastic dysphonic voices on dimensions of breathiness, overpressure (spasticity), tremor, and aperiodicity, and indicated that such voices contain evidence of increased overpressure, are laborious and "hostile sounding," and often are accompanied by facial grimaces. The vocal symptoms can become so severe that they produce occupational disability and social maladjustment. Depression is not uncommon among spastic dysphonic patients, because there is little relief from the disorder. They frequently resort to whispering in an effort to communicate.

Spastic dysphonia appears to be an adult disorder, and some data (A. E. Aronson & DeSanto, 1983) indicate that it is more prevalent in females (66%) than in males (33%). In that study, the average age of spastic patients surgically treated for this condition was 62, with a range from 44 to 79. These ages closely represent the age data of typical populations of spastic dysphonic patients.

Treatment of Spastic Dysphonia

One significant problem with spastic dysphonia is its resistance to treatment. Historically, because of its psychosomatic diagnostic base, patients were subjected to diverse attempts at management, including psychotherapy, voice–speech therapy, acupuncture, hypnosis, biofeedback, relaxation, respiratory therapy, electroshock therapy, meditation, tranquilizers, muscle relaxants, megavitamins, and chiropractic therapies (H. H. Dedo & Izdebski, 1983a).

I have tried a few strange and esoteric techniques without significant success. Many patients have shown improvement with traditional voice therapy and have learned to control the vocal symptoms in small units, such as monosyllabic utterances, but rarely in contextual speech. Historically, the poor prognosis is one of the most significant symptoms of this disorder and has been pathognomonic to it.

Because of the poor prognosis, an alternative treatment method has been developed by H. H. Dedo (1976). He reported on 34 patients who demonstrated significant improvement in vocal quality after Xylocaine injection into one recurrent laryngeal nerve (RLN) to produce temporary paralysis of the nerve and the vocal fold innervated by it. In these 34 patients, the RLN later was sectioned to produce permanent paralysis of the vocal fold in an attempt to eliminate the overpressure (hyperadduction) during phonation. With nerve sectioning plus postoperative voice therapy by speech–language pathologists, these patients experienced significant improvement in their voices, with half gaining near-normal voice.

It is difficult to generalize the current status of RLN sectioning for spastic dysphonia. A. E. Aronson and DeSanto (1983) reported that surgical success must be viewed in the long-term results obtained. Of 33 patients who were sectioned, 100% experienced improved voice immediately after surgery, but 3 years later 21 (64%) had failed to maintain improvement and were considered surgical failures. The voices of 10 of these 21 were considered worse than before surgery. Women patients were more likely to experience long-term failure than men, for unknown reasons.

On the other hand, H. H. Dedo and Izdebski (1983a) reported more beneficial long-term results as indicated by perceptual studies and patient self-reporting. Perceptually, 92% of patients sampled were judged to have reduced overpressure, with breathiness and voice weakness in 51%. Those with significant breathiness after surgery often were treated with Teflon injection, with improved results. Also, those who continued to have postsurgery overpressure were treated with CO_2 laser vocal fold thinning via microdirect laryngoscopy to achieve more lateralization (H. H. Dedo & Izdebski, 1983b). All patients were recommended to have voice therapy by a speech pathologist as part of the overall treatment.

If there is a solution to treating spastic dysphonia, it will come only after the passage of time, with all professionals involved continuing their efforts for objective evaluation. I have heard and judged on tape all 306 spastic dysphonic patients reported in the H. H. Dedo and Izdebski (1983a) paper and can attest that voice improvement resulted in the majority of these cases. Many cases of which I am personally aware have not been helped in the long term even after one or two subsequent CO_2 laser thinnings.

As A. E. Aronson and DeSanto (1983) stated, the differences among researchers may arise from varying research methodology (e.g., method of follow-up, types of spastic dysphonia patients selected for treatment, numbers of patients studied, criteria for success and failure, or interpretation of results).

As of this writing, RLN sectioning is being done much less by laryngologists as a result of rather discouraging long-term results. Time appears to be working unfavorably for many patients who have undergone RLN sectioning for spastic dysphonia. Because many cases have experienced only short-term improvement (e.g., H. H. Dedo & Izdebski's, 1983a, cases), I strongly advocate other treatment avenues at this time. As medical technology advances, improved techniques will continue to emerge, such as the usage of botulinum toxin, as discussed later.

Abductor Spastic (Spasmodic) Dysphonia

In 1973, A. E. Aronson described what he classified as spastic dysphonia, abductor type, which involved intermittent vocal fold abduction, resulting in spasmodic moments of unvoicing during continuing speech. He considered this phenomenon a variation on spastic dysphonia caused by an involuntary parting of the vocal folds during phonation. Patients complain that inability to maintain phonation while talking affects their loudness and intelligibility.

A. E. Aronson (1985) reaffirmed this condition and indicated that, during phonation under conditions of endoscopic inspection, a synchronous and untimely abduction of the true vocal folds produces a wide open glottal chink. Although little has been written about it, speech–language pathologists are beginning to notice this pattern of spontaneous abduction of the vocal folds at inappropriate times in speech and are reporting more cases.

It is not known whether abductor spastic dysphonia results from psychogenic or neurogenic causes, or a combination of the two. The evidence is mounting of a parallel condition to adductor spastic dysphonia; that is, the majority of cases evidence neurological aberrations with psychogenic sequelae and some cases are rather devoid of evidence supporting a neurological basis. Finitzo and Freeman (1989) provided evidence of a neurological component. One-third of their 75 patients of spastic dysphonia were classified as having abductor spastic dysphonia or a mixture of adductor and abductor, and 80% of the subject population demonstrated neurological aberrations. In any case, the speech–language pathologist must be aware of the differences involving the two forms of spastic dysphonia in order to evaluate and treat them properly.

Botulinum Toxin (BOTOX)

A growing body of literature and clinical experience indicates that injection of botulinum toxin (BOTOX) into the vocal folds of patients with adductor spastic dysphonia is an effective treatment. BOTOX is being used in a number of medical centers, and the results appear to be favorable even with repeated injections. Few sequelae are reported, other than the expected slight difficulty in swallowing for a short period of time. Injections are now being done bilaterally, and still no reported case of apnea or aspiration has occurred. The patients whom I have evaluated have demonstrated remarkable and stable vocal control essentially free of spastic voice quality for several months. Patients also report a lessening of a feeling of tightness in the throat even when the BOTOX effect is wearing off and vocal symptoms are returning. Patients also are receiving emotional support and encouragement through a national spastic dysphonia support organization (OurVoice, Managing Editor, Midge Kovacs, c/o Lenox Hill Hospital, Center for Communciation Disorders, 100 East 77th Street, New York, NY 10021), and local support groups are being formed in various cities. Speech–language pathologists, otolaryngologists, patients, and related health professionals can receive the OurVoice newsletter by writing to the above address, and thus be kept up to date on matters pertaining to adductor and abductor spastic dysphonia. Additional references regarding the use of BOTOX in the treatment of adductor spastic dysphonia include Blitzer, Brin, Fahn, and Lovelace (1988); Brin, Blitzer, Fahn, Gould, and Lovelace (1989); Gacek (1987); and R. H. Miller, Woodson, and Jankovic (1987).

Although voice therapy alone has not been successful in the majority of cases of adductor spastic dysphonia, it is an important augmentation to the medical management procedures of RLN sectioning or BOTOX injections. Patients who have been struggling with the strain–strangle effects of adductor spastic dysphonia can benefit from voice therapy directed toward teaching them not to fight and struggle with voice, but to make it a relaxed and free-flowing process. The elimination of any musculoskeletal tension might be necessary as a result of years of vocal struggle. Teaching a patient proper tone focus and less laryngeal focus would be a most important contribution. The methodology involved in these procedures will be discussed in a later section of this chapter.

Treatment for Neurogenic Voice Disorder

When a patient with neurogenic voice disorder is referred to the speech–language pathologist, independently or in combination with some medical management technique, the pathologist has several modification techniques available. If the client's symptoms include breathiness, as in the case of unilateral adductor paralysis, improved glottal approximation becomes the goal. This can be accomplished initially using the pushing technique, introduced by Froeschels, Kastein, and Weiss (1955) and explained by Boone and McFarlane (1988).

Boone and McFarlane suggested that a chair be used in a lifting process in lieu of the pushing approach to help approximate the vocal folds during phonation. Patients are instructed to lift up on the bottom of the chair as they sit on it in a futile attempt to lift themselves. This effort increases glottal adduction. During this attempt, they are instructed to produce voice by saying /a/ in a prolonged fashion. The utterances are taped for analysis to determine whether such efforts produce improved voice production. If so, the clients are instructed to repeat the task while decreasing the lifting effort and attempting to maintain the improved voice quality. Patients often can internalize the glottal closure for improved voice without needing the lifting support.

Diplophonia (double-pitched voice) is heard often in patients with laryngeal paralysis. Therapy can help eliminate diplophonia by exploring variations in pitch, loudness, and vocal effort. Isolated vocal productions of /a/ or other vowels should be recorded for analysis. When an utterance is devoid of diplophonia, the client can hear the recording and attempt to duplicate that phonation.

One clinical technique I have found helpful is to use a cassette tape endless loop (20 sec) that is played continuously during phonation efforts. When the speech–language pathologist hears an improved production, the recorder is stopped and the phonation effort is played back so the client can hear it repeatedly during simultaneous vocal effort. This helps to establish a target voice that can be expanded from the /a/ into short phrases, reading, controlled conversation, and finally functional communication. These techniques can be used with any client who has insufficient glottal approximation (breathiness) during phonation, regardless of the etiology.

When the client has hyperfunctional (musculoskeletal) tension in the voice and surrounding neck muscles, the speech–language pathologist must be prepared to help the patient eliminate the overpressure. In the case of patients with adductor spastic dysphonia, after the medical management techniques described, or any other neurologically involved patient with hyperfunctional symptoms, the following techniques should be helpful: (a) feedback, (b) relaxation, (c) yawn–sigh, and (d) tone focus.

Feedback

Clients have been helped in eliminating specific areas of body tension during phonation through visual or auditory biofeedback regarding excessive muscle contraction. Prosek, Montgomery, Walden, and Schwartz (1978) reported success with 3 of 6 patients with hyperfunctional voice disorder via biofeedback. Biofeedback methodology differs from system to system, but generally uses information from muscle or brain-wave activity as a reflection of the biophysical state of the body.

When muscle activity is being monitored, electromyography (EMG) is used. EMG electrodes are placed in surface contact with the muscle being monitored so contractions can be detected, amplified, and fed back to the client and speech–language pathologist as visual or auditory signals. When the person is made aware of the muscle contraction(s), efforts can be directed to the muscle to relax. EMG techniques also involve introducing electrodes into the muscles of the larynx to monitor contractions during phonation, but these have been used in basic research rather than clinical modification of speaking patterns.

A therapy approach using biofeedback as an adjunct to vocal management could develop as follows: The speech–language pathologist should understand the technology of operating the biofeedback instrumentation, or should work with someone who does. The client is instructed to concentrate on monitoring the signal that detects excessive contraction of the muscle(s) being analyzed. This establishes a stable baseline of biofeedback tension or contraction. The person is directed to think about relaxing activities while maintaining awareness of the signal. The purpose is to have the client use the relaxing thoughts to help eliminate the muscular tension. The signal provides the feedback necessary to indicate whether the process is working.

In gradual hierarchical steps, the client is directed to concentrate on more stressful and anxiety-provoking situations while attempting to keep the biofeedback signal at low levels. When the individual's self-projection into imagined images or situations is achieved, reality is introduced by having the person actually produce voice by humming, prolonging a sustained /a/, or performing a similar task while maintaining biofeedback control. As the task of phonating without triggering the biofeedback sensors is established, the level of difficulty is increased from phonemes to words, to phrases, to reading, and finally to conversation. At each stage, it is necessary to allow the client to adapt to the biofeedback signal for a period of time before task escalation.

The client soon should be able to determine when relaxation has been achieved without the biofeedback signal. When this has been accomplished, generalization of the control should be attempted by having the person speak in more natural settings away from the clinic under the speech–language pathologist's careful supervision. Each time the patient undertakes a speaking venture, it should be followed by a therapy time to discuss progress.

Relaxation

Jacobson (1978) proposed a method of training persons to eliminate states of tension in the body through progressive relaxation. This involves a series of muscle isolation steps to identify and eliminate tension. Jacobson wrote,

> We call the relaxation "progressive" in three respects: (1) the subject relaxes a group, for instance the muscles that bend the right arm, further and further each minute. (2) He learns one after the other to relax the principal muscle groups of his body. With each new group he simultaneously relaxes such parts as have received practice previously. (3) As he practices from day to day, according to my experience, he progresses toward a habit of repose—and tends toward a state in which quiet is automatically maintained. (p. 161)

The specific method of obtaining muscle relaxation is not as critical as focusing on the laryngeal mechanism once general body relaxation has been achieved. As Boone (1977) stated, "The clinician who chooses to use relaxation methods with particular patients should remember that these methods are usually best combined with other facilitating techniques designed especially for producing a better voice" (p. 152).

Yawn–Sigh

By teaching the client to relax and produce a long, drawn-out sigh, as in a yawn, the speech–language pathologist can hear an improved voice that can be recorded, fed back on the tape loop system, and used as a target voice. If this produces the improved target, therapy should be directed toward stabilizing it in isolation, short phrases, reading, controlled conversation, and finally functional communication.

A similar technique to eliminate laryngeal hyperfunction is to have the client produce words that start with an /h/ sound for easier onset of phonation. This can help eliminate in isolation the abrupt overpressure heard in hyperfunctional dysphonia.

Tone Focus

It is important to teach a voice-disordered client to produce voice with proper tone focus. Music teachers are excellent about teaching voice students to sing without excessive energy focus in the laryngeal area. The techniques of musical pedagogy for the singer can be helpful for the speaker. To teach proper tone focus, the speech–language pathologist should have the client take in a full breath of air using the abdominal cavity in good abdominal–diaphragmatic respiration. Repeat three or four such respirations. It is a good idea to have the client stand for this exercise, and have him or her place a hand lightly on the stomach with the thumb resting on the navel. During each inhalation cycle, notice whether stomach or abdominal distension occurs. If this distension is not occurring, work on the client's respiration until it does. Often the cue, "As you inhale, relax your stomach muscle completely" will help accomplish this end. Teach the client to exaggerate this respiratory step of inhalation.

Once the client is able to take in full breaths with major abdominal distension and only a little chest expansion, the respiratory basis for good voice production and tone focus has been established. Next, on exhalation have the client hum the /m/ sound very lightly (little intensity). Meanwhile, the client should drop the jaw as far as possible with the lips still together. The tongue should be relaxed and resting on the floor of the mouth in the mandibular cavity. During the humming, encourage the client to feel a tickling on the lips. The client should repeat this process, relaxing everything on exhalation and humming, until this lip tickling is felt. Then, encourage repetition until an increase of tickling is felt. Determine whether the client can focus on the muscles of the face to the degree that the tickling spreads from the lips to the nose and surrounding facial area. Use verbal imagery to help the client feel all the tone focus and acoustic energy in the mask of the face, and not in the neck and laryngeal area. Demonstrate this to the client with your own productions. Have him or her feel your face as you accomplish the above task of excessive vibration in the mask of the face. Have the client notice that when the above voice production is accomplished, little energy or tone focus is felt in the laryngeal area. All the effort is coming from abdominal support of respiration (and the client must be feeling lots of effort in this area) and resonant energy in the mask of the face. It is almost as if "nothing" is happening in the laryngeal area, even though that is the source of the tone. The goal is to teach the hyperfunctional client how to produce isolated tone with good respiratory support and facial tone focus.

When the above has been accomplished, move from humming to consonant–vowel (CV) productions of nasal consonants /m/ and various vowels. It is often helpful to have the client repeat the CV /mi/ several times: /mimimimimimimi/. Next, /momomomomomo/. Next, /maimaimaimaimai/. As each production occurs, ask the client to note that vibration is still felt in the mask of the face with good abdominal support and not in the larynx.

When these tasks are stabilized, move from nasal to non-nasal productions or isolated vowels. Eventually, if the client has been taught well the concept of abdominal support and resonant tone focus, generalization to larger speech units and conversation can proceed under the speech–language pathologist's direction.

Palatal Lift

When a dysarthric patient has symptoms of hypernasality and reduced oral pressure for articulation because of velopharyngeal valving difficulties, improvement is often facilitated by means of a palatal lift dental prosthesis. With the cooperation of a prosthodontist, an appliance can be constructed that will lift the velum toward the posterior pharyngeal wall sufficiently to improve resonance and oral speech pressure without significantly compromising the client's ability to breathe nasally. More information on palatal lift prostheses is provided in Chapter 8.

For further documentation of all the treatments explained above, please consult Yorkston, Beukelman, and Bell (1988) and Rosenbek and LaPointe (1985).

Case Example of Hyperfunctional Disorder

The following case study is an example of traditional therapy used with spastic dysphonia cases who have not received RLN sectioning. Although the laryngologist who referred this patient for speech–language services stated that the condition was "nonorganic," the actual diagnosis is more likely to be spastic dysphonia. In any event, the case illustrates how hyperfunctional symptoms can be treated.

J.B., a 46-year-old clergyman, referred himself for a voice evaluation because of vocal difficulty that was interfering with his ministry. He said that for several years he had found it progressively difficult to preach effectively and to deal with the problems presented by members of his congregation. He also reported having considerable difficulty with his daughter, whom he called a "free spirit." He noticed that at the beginning of the day his voice was quite clear, but as he faced problem after problem he felt it grow tighter until he was unable to speak. He recently had seen an otolaryngologist who found nothing wrong with the structures of his voice and said the disorder was nonorganic. J.B. indicated that he understood that nonorganic was a euphemism for psychologically based.

His voice examination revealed a pattern characterized by excessive tension during most phonation efforts and periodic spastic stoppages. It also was weak in loudness. Excessive contraction of muscles surrounding his neck (sternocleidomastoid, mylohyoid) and in his jaw area (masseter) supported the perception of vocal tension.

J.B.'s therapy began with a complete explanation of the larynx, how it worked, and what happened to it when used improperly, using pictures and models. The myoelastic–aerodynamic theory of phonation was explained simply. He also was shown how phonation could occur under variable amounts of tension in a continuum from hypofunctional control (breathiness), to normal phonation, to hyperfunctional control (spasticity). The purpose was to show him how much voluntary control over the voice was possible.

During the next few sessions, J.B. was given instructions on progressive relaxation and taken through the steps necessary to achieve voluntary relaxation. After he had learned to consciously relax most of the muscles of his body, including his extrinsic laryngeal ones, he was instructed to take a deep breath and let the air escape silently from his lungs in an easy, relaxed manner. After a few cycles of relaxed respiration, he was told to add a breathy sigh as he released air. This showed him that voluntary control of the tension in his voice was possible. He repeated this breathy sigh process until he was able to exhale and phonate various vowels in the same breathy manner.

As J.B. was producing these breathy utterances on vowels, the speech–language pathologist pointed out that, when phonating with this easy manner, he should not be able to feel anything happen in the larynx—all the voice vibration should be felt in the mask of the face. J.B. agreed that such was the case and said he was surprised how easy phonation could be.

At this point in therapy, negative practice (Boone & McFarlane, 1988) was introduced to show J.B. the difference between hypofunctional and hyperfunctional phonation. The ability to shift into and out of tense phonation indicated that he had achieved voluntary control over the tension level of voice. J.B. then was directed to use his new voice, which was deliberately established at a slightly breathy level, in large articulation units (i.e., monosyllabic words, any word, phrases, short sentences, connected reading, simple dialogue, and finally conversation). At each stage, negative practice was used to help him maintain the contrast of tension versus nontense, normal phonation.

When J.B. was able to converse with the speech–language pathologist about various topics with his new voice, a hierarchy was established that allowed systematic generalization to everyday communication. This involved having J.B. rank specific stressful situations while communicating on a continuum from low stress to high stress. Some of the conversation situations he ranked low in the hierarchy were speaking with his wife early in the morning and offering personal and family prayers. The highest ranking involved leading a group counseling session of young people in his church. J.B. then was instructed to attempt as well as he could to control the tension in his voice when speaking in the situations ranked low on the hierarchy and gradually move up the list. It took him 3 weeks of constant effort to approach the higher situations.

At the higher levels, he began having difficulty controlling his voice. For example, J.B. reported that at times the tension level at the counseling sessions with the young people got so high that everyone felt it. It was in these situations that control of vocal tension was rather poor. He felt he was controlling the tension better than before therapy started, but felt there was still room for improvement.

After a few more sessions in which little progress was made, he terminated formal therapy. A checkup schedule was established to help him maintain the control he had achieved. Five checkups in a 7-month period revealed only minor setbacks in J.B.'s ability to control the tension in his voice.

Summary

This chapter has reviewed normal laryngeal innervation (central and peripheral) and the many disorders that can disrupt neurological functioning in the motor speech system, with special emphasis on laryngeal aspects. Various forms of laryngeal paralysis, dysarthria, anarthria, and specific disease processes or disorder types have been analyzed. Also discussed was current literature on the etiology, epidemiology, symptomatology, and medical and nonmedical treatments of these disorders.

6

Psychogenic (Nonorganic) Voice Disorders

Although the larynx is a well-organized and stable biological structure with complex neurological control (as described in Chapter 5), its vulnerability to changes in the individual's emotional or psychological state makes it an excellent barometer of mental and psychological stability. Persons anxious and under stress often can hide the condition in every way but vocally. The pitch may go higher and the voice may acquire a slight vocal quiver or even stop suddenly in a moment of spasm, or in some other subtle way betray attempts to appear calm and in control.

Most persons have experienced the frustration of losing vocal control in an emotional situation no matter how hard they try to avoid it. For example, a major league baseball manager had been fired and a press conference called to announce his dismissal. Part way into his farewell speech, this highly verbal and seasoned man had to stop, fight his tears, and walk away. He could not control his emotional state sufficiently to speak.

Many persons have had similar experiences under even less traumatic circumstances when voice could not be produced or, if not stopped, certainly was affected negatively so that the emotional state could not be hidden or masked. Whether the emotional state is one of fear, anger, or happiness, the human voice generally communicates the condition. Indeed, it is almost impossible for individuals to mask their emotions from the voice.

Under emotion or stress, the biological functions of the larynx usually are not affected, since swallowing water or some other liquid or food does not jeopardize the integrity of the protective valving mechanisms. In an emotional state, the lungs are protected by the larynx, but the psyche is not.

All of this vocal symptomatology involving stress, fear, anger, or happiness is experienced by everyone and is normal. However, in many individuals these vocal effects are the standard, not the emotional exception. The symptoms vary from a slight but rather consistent quiver or tremor in the voice at one extreme to complete aphonia at the other. The common factor in each disorder is the absence of any physical basis that can explain the voice symptoms.

A laryngoscopic examination reveals essentially normal structures, but the voice function is abnormal. Such a person has a nonorganic or psychogenic voice disorder. This chapter details this process of functional or psychogenic loss of vocal control so the speech–language pathologist will have sufficient background to evaluate, treat, or refer the person with this disorder.

Psychogenic voice disorder occurs when vocal control over pitch, loudness, quality, or resonance is disrupted sufficiently to impede communication effectiveness rather constantly because of psychological disequilibrium. Such disequilibrium can result from unrealistic fear, anxiety, depression, anger, unresolved conflicts, personality abnormalities, psychosexual confusion, conversion reactions, interpersonal relationship disruptions, poor self-confidence, and puberty adjustment difficulties, as well as major neuroses and psychoses.

To qualify as a psychogenic, nonorganic voice disorder, (a) one of these factors or similar conditions must be present, (b) the voice must be affected fairly constantly rather than in minor episodes of extreme emotion, and (c) no physical or structural bases in the speech system (particularly the larynx) can account for the disorder.

One significant word of caution is appropriate at this point. The diagnosis of nonorganic voice disorder has been traditionally inaccurate, and many individuals so diagnosed in actuality have significant organic disease. Yang and Mu (1989) reported on 333 patients diagnosed as having functional or nonorganic dysphonia. Only 16 of these cases (4.8%) were found to have functional or nonorganic disorder after careful scrutiny (laryngoscopic, electromyographic and spectrum analysis). The majority of these patients (317, or 95.2%) had organic disease with varying degrees of laryngeal nerve paresis, usually idiopathically caused. Speech–language pathologists must be careful not to consider that a patient or client has a nonorganic or functional voice disorder until organicity has been carefully eliminated by competent medical evaluation, regardless of the similarity of vocal symptoms to psychogenic disorder.

Another consideration is that a large number of individuals consider themselves to be reticent speakers. They are shy, rather quiet, and have a general feeling that what they have to say does not need to be said and that more is to be lost than gained by talking. They are likely to have a rather flat voice, with little pitch (monotone), loudness (monoloud), and inflections to emphasize their message suprasegmentally. Generally, they would not consider themselves as having good communication skills. They might speak at a slower rate and be less fluent. Rekart and Begnal (1989) studied the acoustic characteristics of such speakers who classified themselves as reticent speakers for placement in a speech class and found many of the characteristics common to nonorganic voice disorder.

The acoustic characteristics of Rekart and Begnal's (1989) reticent speakers include differences from normal in terms of fluency and perceived pitch. The reticent speakers had greater pause durations (lower fluency) and, in the case of females, a narrower frequency range (monotone). In addition, male reticent speakers tended to have a higher pitch (F_0) than nonreticent male speakers. More research is needed in this area since many persons find themselves in employment that requires good communication skills and have difficulty matching such expectations.

Vocal Symptoms of Psychogenic Disorder

Although extensive literature compares specific voice characteristics to specific psychological states, as reviewed thoroughly by A. E. Aronson (1985), few speech–language pathologists have developed the skill necessary to differentially diagnose a particular psychological state by evaluating only the voice.

Moses (1954) stated, "Whoever diagnoses neurosis is consciously or unconsciously affected by the patient's voice" (p. 1). Moses contended that specific neurotic states can be diagnosed accurately by evaluating only vocal features (respiration, range, register, resonance, rhythm, melody, intensity, speed, accents, emphasis, pathos, mannerism, melism, exactness, pauses between words). His analysis continues to be quoted by writers on psychogenic voice disorders, although few authorities claim to have the skill necessary to utilize his system to make such diagnoses.

C. E. Williams and Stevens (1972) compared actors' simulations of various emotional states with recorded examples of voice and speech patterns of speakers under actual circumstances of emotion to determine acoustical correlations in relation to the emotional state. For example, the destruction of the German dirigible Hindenburg in 1937 was recorded by an announcer, excerpts of whose vocal patterns were compared before and during the crash by spectrograms (narrow-band). Significant differences were noted in contours of the F_0 for up and down inflection. The average F_0 was considerably higher during the crash, with a greater range of F_0 change. Some evidence of tremor and irregularities reflecting a loss of precise control of the speech musculature and breathing control were noted spectrographically.

An actor's simulation of this event revealed similar patterns, even though the actor had never heard the broadcast. The Williams and Stevens study covered the emotions of anger, fear, sorrow, and a neutral condition in a similar manner and provided spectrographic data on the acoustic patterns in these emotional states. Their data revealed how vulnerable the speech and vocal systems are to changes from psychological balance.

Physiological Speech Changes Under Stress

What happens physiologically under conditions of anger, fear, sorrow, grief, hysteria, elation, or any of the typical states of emotional change? First, it must be determined whether these emotions have different biochemical or psychophysiological bases. According to most psychophysiologists, the nervous system responds differently to rage, to fear, and to positive emotions such as joy or sexual arousal. However, the differences are not sufficient to account for the variety of emotions experienced by humans during social, sexual, competitive, and other daily interactions. Essentially, to understand changes that typically occur in the body under varying conditions of emotion, speech–language pathologists must comprehend the workings of the autonomic nervous system, particularly the limbic aspect, and the manner in which the nervous system interacts with the endocrine system.

Autonomic Nervous System

The autonomic nervous system is a functional division of the entire nervous system that has sympathetic and parasympathetic aspects. With the help of the endocrine system, it controls body homeostasis—a state of balance maintained by a certain group of biological processes. The internal environment of the body must be regulated with regard to temperature, hunger, thirst, blood pressure, oxygen content in the cells, acid–base balance, blood sugar levels, and all other metabolic functions. When some aspect of the internal environment is out of balance, a homeostatic drive occurs to achieve balance (i.e., to seek water, change temperature, etc.).

All of the cells of the body in their own specialized manner are regulated by the nervous and endocrine systems to maintain homeostasis by regulating the basic metabolic rate (BMR) of cellular function. The sympathetic and parasympathetic divisions of the autonomic nervous system are responsible for either increasing (sympathetic) or decreasing (parasympathetic) the BMR by stimulating the endocrine system to maintain homeostasis.

For example, the thyroid gland, under stimulation of the autonomic nervous system, is the master controller of the BMR by means of thyroxine secretions. The thyroid is stimulated to increase thyroxine secretion under the direction of the anterior lobe of the pituitary gland, which secretes thyrotropin (or thyroid-stimulating hormone, TSH). TSH directly stimulates the thyroid. This is one example of the complex interaction between the nervous system and the endocrine glands in maintaining homeostasis (Gilman, Goodman, & Gilman, 1980; Netter, 1983).

Limbic System

The section of the brain thought to be responsible for regulating emotion is the limbic system. This is a set of forebrain structures that form a border around midline structures in the brain, thus the term limbic (from the Latin *limbus*, meaning border). The system includes the hypothalamus, the hippocampus, the amygdala, the olfactory bulbs, parts of the thalamus, and the cingulate gyrus of the cerebral cortex (Kalat, 1981; Netter, 1983).

Through direct stimulation to animal and human brains, as well as through postmortem studies, sections of the limbic system have been found to be directly related to many emotional aspects of pleasure and displeasure. For example, electrical stimulation to the septum, hippocampus, and cingulate gyrus of rats produces penile erection, self-grooming, and related pleasurable responses. Damage or stimulation to certain nuclei in the amygdala produces increased aggressiveness in animals and humans, whereas damage or stimulation to other nuclei of the same structure causes tameness and passive behavior (L. R. Aronson & Cooper, 1979). Thus, it can be seen that humans' emotional status is dependent on the regulation of many nervous system and endocrine interactions.

Exactly what happens to the human body when some environmental (internal or external) change occurs to upset homeostasis, and how does that change relate to speech and voice processes? Only a partial answer can be provided here as a foundation to generally understanding psychogenic voice disorders, but some sources mentioned in this chapter provide additional information on the psychophysiological processes of emotion.

From Basic Level to Excitation

Basically, when a person is resting and not digesting food, the metabolic rate is at its basic level. Heart rate is normal, blood pressure is normal, cellular metabolism rate is normal, respiration cycles of inhalation and exhalation are steady and regular, and the person generally is experiencing a sensation of calmness. Should an environmental change generate an emotional response, however, several changes occur to offset homeostasis and physiological balance.

In the case of a stress signal causing fear, rage, or anger, for example, the sympathetic nervous system acts to prepare the person in the classic "flight-

or-fight'' reaction. The nervous system stimulates the adrenal gland to secrete epinephrine and norepinephrine. Epinephrine raises blood pressure by cardio-acceleration, and norepinephrine does so by vascular constriction of the blood vessels leading to the skin and viscera. Epinephrine output by the adrenal medulla also elicits adrenocorticotrophic hormone (ACTH) output from the anterior pituitary gland that increases carbohydrate metabolism and nervous excitability. Respiration cycles increase to provide more oxygen for cellular metabolism, blood sugar levels rise, a feeling of ''butterflies'' in the stomach is created because of blood drainage from it, arteries of the digestive system contract and somatic muscle arteries expand to divert blood where it is needed, bronchial tubes to the lungs dilate to accommodate increased respiration, pupils of the eyes dilate, sweating increases to cool the body, stomach and intestine muscles stop digestion, and mucous membranes that line the body cavities such as the mouth and throat dry significantly. The degree of these effects depends on the significance of the emotional stimulus (Netter, 1983).

Many of these reactions are part of the well-known phenomenon of ''stage fright,'' but to a lesser degree than in the ''flight-or-fight'' sympathetic nervous system–endocrine reaction. Persons who are to perform or speak before audiences often experience a lack of control over body functions and experience increased sweating, rapid heartbeat, flushing of the skin, dryness of the mouth and throat, and a general feeling of anxiety and nervousness. It does little good to say, ''Be still my heart!'' When about to speak or sing, persons might focus particularly on how dry the mouth and throat are since such dryness affects the phonation and articulation processes significantly.

An individual who has trouble speaking because of these reactions is having a psychogenic speech–voice manifestation. However, such a psychogenic disorder, notwithstanding its reality and effect on the communication process, is not considered a communication disorder in the clinical sense.

Most speakers who have had stage fright, upon the conclusion of the speaking event and after the parasympathetic nervous system has countered the effects of the sympathetic nervous system and brought the body back to homeostasis, tend to say, ''Let me do it again; I could do so much better now.''

Case Examples of Psychogenic Voice Disorder

The following example illustrates how an emotional experience can affect the voice beyond the duration of the triggering experience. R.T. was an 18-year-old female who was referred because of a severe voice disorder. She had been held up while working late one night as an attendant at a gasoline station. The robber held a knife to her throat and told her to empty the cash register. After she complied, he took the money, but before leaving he ran the knife across R.T.'s throat. She was taken to the hospital and examined for possible laryngeal damage. Only a superficial cut of external tissue was found; there was no laryngeal damage. Laryngoscopic examination revealed normal form and function of her vocal folds. However, R.T. could produce only a weak and breathy voice even 3 weeks after the incident. She was essentially aphonic. This is an example of true psychogenic aphonia. (The resolution of her situation is discussed in the aphonia case example later in this chapter.)

Another example is a child who had his tonsils and adenoids surgically removed. Upon awakening from the anesthesia, the physician told him not to talk for a few days or else he could "hurt his throat real bad." This boy was very conscientious and would not make a sound. He gestured and pointed to his throat as though to say, "I can't talk." After a few days, his physician told him he could start talking, but the boy could not make a voice. Encouragement from his physician and parents did not seem to help. Luckily, after a few days this boy spontaneously began to use his voice and is functioning normally today. Similar examples are reported by Boone (1966) involving a child after surgery and an adult after prolonged illness that required therapy to restore voice.

A final example involves an elderly woman who was seen after 3 years of aphonia. Hospital records revealed that 3 years before the examination, she had undergone thyroid surgery for tumor removal. After the surgery, she lost her voice completely. While reading the hospital record as part of the voice evaluation, the speech–language pathologist noticed that the patient continually coughed strongly and was constantly clearing her throat with a phonated grunt. The hospital records indicated that her laryngology examination showed normally functioning vocal folds in every respect.

When asked to speak, the woman moved her lips as though attempting to speak, but no sound emerged. During the evaluation, the pathologist pressed on her neck in the general area of the larynx, asked her to cough, and said, "Oh, yes, I can see what the trouble is, you cannot bring your vocal folds together to produce voice. Let me help you and I think your voice will be fine." In the next few minutes, the woman produced many examples of normal voice in words and short phrases, but no functional communication was established even after an hour of intense effort.

The next day in therapy she was unable to produce any voice at all. The speech–language pathologist also noticed she was holding her breath for several seconds, then quickly breathing to catch up, then holding her breath again. Her daughter said this was new behavior which, as far as she knew, her mother had not done before. The pathologist soon learned that this woman was on welfare because of her voice disorder and had been for 3 years. The psychological mechanisms underlying her aphonia then were clear, as were the reasons why the woman was resisting reestablishment of her voice; she seemed to be afraid of losing the welfare payments if she regained her voice.

These examples illustrate the relationships between the mind and the voice. (Details of therapeutic management of such cases are provided in the therapy section of this chapter.)

Specific psychogenic voice disorders should be examined in terms of symptoms, etiology, evaluation, and treatment considerations. Many psychological or psychiatric disorders can and do affect communication processes, many of which have a specific effect on the voice. The American Psychiatric Association (1987) classifies mental disorders according to the categories (including subcategories) listed in Exhibit 6–1. Many of these categories have little to do with communication, and others have direct relationship. Some of the disorders also involve communication dysfunctions that are not treated as a separate aspect of the disorder since improved status in the condition is paralleled by improved communication skill. This chapter deals only with psychogenic disorders that have communication (particularly voice) disorders that are treated as separate aspects of the conditions.

Aphonia (Conversion)

A conversion aphonia can involve one of the somatoform disorders listed in Exhibit 6–1. Essentially, somatoform disorders are those in which symptoms suggesting physical etiology occur for which no identifiable organicity can be demonstrated, no physiological basis is inferred, and symptoms are linked through positive evidence or strong presumption to psychological disturbance or conflict.

The essential features of somatoform disorders are that the patient often seeks medical care from many physicians, sometimes simultaneously, and presents a complicated medical history in which numerous diagnoses of possible conditions have been made. Somatoform disorders can involve any of the organ systems, but typically are pseudoneurological (blindness, deafness, paralysis), gastrointestinal (abdominal pain), female reproductive (painful menstruation), psychosexual (sexual indifference), or cardiopulmonary (dizziness).

In any event, the physical symptom serves to reduce or eliminate anxiety from some sort of unresolved conflict. In the patient with conversion aphonia, the striking symptom is the absence of phonation during attempts to communicate. The patient often uses only a whispered voice in a functional turnoff of phonation, producing only articulated air. Some patients with the same psychogenic etiology are classified as conversion dysphonic since a slight amount of voicing can be heard in speech attempts, but the striking feature is a breathy voice, weak in intensity. The conversion at times is so effective in reducing the anxiety that caused it that the patient displays an attitude of unusual calmness considering the severity of the symptomatology, a phenomenon called *la belle indifference.*

The question often is asked as to why in the conversion aphonic or dysphonic patient the physical symptom occurs in the voice rather than some other organ system. There is no clear answer, but at least two characteristics

Exhibit 6–1 Classification of Mental Disorders

- Mental retardation (all degrees from mild, moderate, severe, to profound)
- Attention deficit disorder (with or without hyperactivity associated)
- Conduct disorder (undersocialized, aggressive or nonaggressive, socialized aggressive or nonaggressive, etc.)
- Anxiety disorders of childhood or adolescence (separation, avoidant, or overanxious disorder)
- Other disorders of infancy, childhood, or adolescence (schizoid disorder, elective mutism, identify disorder, etc.)
- Eating disorders (anorexia nervosa, etc.)
- Stereotyped movement disorders (chronic motor tic disorder, Tourette's syndrome, etc.)
- Other disorders with physical manifestations (stuttering, functional enuresis, sleepwalking, etc.)
- Pervasive developmental disorders (infantile autism)
- Specific developmental disorders (developmental reading, arithmetic, language, articulation, and mixed disorder)
- Organic mental disorders (primary degenerative dementia, senile onset, with delirium, delusion, depression, or uncomplicated)
- Substance-induced organic mental disorders (alcohol, barbiturate, sedative, hypnotic, opioid, cocaine, amphetamine, hallucinogen, phencyclidine (PCP), cannabis, tobacco, caffeine, etc.)
- Substance use disorders (see above substances such as alcohol, tobacco, cocaine, amphetamine, etc.)
- Schizophrenic disorders (catatonic, paranoid, undifferentiated, etc.)
- Paranoid disorders (paranoia, acute paranoid disorder, atypical paranoid disorder, etc.)
- Psychotic disorders not elsewhere classified (schizophreniform disorder, brief reactive psychosis, schizoaffective disorder, etc.)
- Neurotic disorders [these are included in Affective, Anxiety, Somatoform, Dissociative, and Psychosexual categories—the next five listed—no separate category for neurosis is advocated by the American Psychiatric Association]
- Affective disorders (with or without psychotic features, melancholia, with mania, with depression, cyclothymic disorder, dysthymic disorder, etc.)
- Anxiety disorders—phobic disorders or phobic neuroses (agoraphobia or fear of being alone in a large space, with or without panic reactions, social phobia, and all other phobic categories)
- Somatoform disorders (conversion disorder or hysterical neurosis, conversion neurosis, psychogenic pain disorder, hypochondriasis, etc.)
- Dissociative disorders—or hysterical neuroses of the dissociative type (psychogenic amnesia, psychogenic fugue, multiple personality, etc.)
- Psychosexual disorders—gender identify disorders (transsexualism, asexual, homosexual, etc.)
- Psychosexual disorders—paraphilias (fetishism, transvestism, zoophilia, pedophilia, exhibitionism, voyeurism, sexual masochism or sadism, etc.)
- Psychosexual dysfunctions (inhibited sexual desire, inhibited sexual excitement, inhibited orgasm, premature ejaculation, etc.)
- Factitious disorders (false disorder with no apparent goal as compared with malingering disorders in which patient fakes a disorder to gain or avoid some consequence)

Exhibit 6–1 continued

- Impulse control (kleptomania, pyromania, isolated or intermittent explosive disorder, etc.)
- Adjustment disorder (with depressed mood, with anxious mood, with mixed emotional features, with work, with withdrawal, etc.)
- Conditions not attributable to a mental disorder that are a focus of attention or treatment (malingering, adult antisocial behavior, academic problem, occupational problem, phase of life problem, marital problem, parent-child problem, other specified family circumstance, noncompliance with medical treatment, childhood or adolescent antisocial behavior, bereavement, and other interpersonal problems)
- Personality disorders (paranoid, schizoid, schizotypal, histrionic, narcissistic, antisocial, borderline, avoidant, dependent, compulsive, passive-aggressive, and atypical or mixed personality)

Note. Adapted from *The Diagnostic and Statistical Manual of Mental Disorders* (3rd ed. rev.) by the American Psychiatric Association, 1988, Washington, DC: Author. Copyright 1988 by the American Psychiatric Association.

in the case history of the typical conversion aphonic patient provide some clarification:

1. There usually is evidence of a breakdown in communication between the patient and some other person of importance, such as a spouse, parent, child, or person of authority. The loss of voice seems to serve the function of eliminating the burden of attempting to continue, maintain, or reestablish the communication that has become so psychologically painful to the patient.

2. There often is evidence that at the time of onset of the aphonia, or just prior to it, the patient experienced actual loss of voice from a cold, upper respiratory infection, episode of laryngitis, or similar condition.

The relationship between this actual dysphonia and the conversion aphonia can be explained in part in the following dialogue between a speech–language pathologist and a patient with conversion aphonia:

SLP: When did you first lose your voice?

PT: (Using a whisper voice) During May of this year, I caught a bad cold and became very hoarse. This cold lasted for several days and then I started to feel better, my nose stopped running, and I no longer had aches and pains, but my voice never improved. It kept getting worse and worse until I couldn't make any sound at all . . . like this today.

I saw my doctor and he gave me some pills . . . decongestants, I think, but that didn't help at all. They just made me sleepy and I felt worse, so I stopped taking them. I don't know, maybe I shouldn't have stopped. But my voice has been like this all the time since.

As the interview continued, the patient reported that at the time this cold was developing she was experiencing extreme interpersonal difficulty with her mother. It seems her mother had been unusually protective and demanding of high moral values and behavior, embarrassing her in front of boyfriends by asking them of their physical intentions, and in general accusing her of being "loose" with sex.

The patient learned, at about the same time her cold developed, that throughout these dating years her mother had been a prostitute. She said, "I could not understand how my mother could demand such moral perfection from me and be living a life of a prostitute at the same time. I can never forgive her for that." She confronted her mother with her inconsistencies, arguments developed, and communication broke down. It was easy to deduce that the development of her cold and actual hoarseness became a means of avoiding these verbal conflicts, resulting in her conversion aphonia once the cold was over.

Conversions can take the form of conversion aphonia (no voice but articulated air stream), conversion muteness (no attempt to produce voice or articulate, or perhaps the lips are moved as though attempting to speak without exhaling), or conversion dysphonia (some voice but abnormal quality, pitch, or loudness function).

Conversions have been reported in the literature as being caused by strong suggestions not to talk after surgery (Boone, 1966), adjusting to divorced parents, adjusting to the death of a loved one, difficulty accepting being involved in an extramarital affair, difficulty adjusting to the role of being a tough policeman, and difficulty accepting the fact that an only daughter is annoying (A. E. Aronson, 1985). These are only a sampling of the many etiologies that have produced conversion aphonia, muteness, or dysphonia.

One case of a 40-year-old female who developed a significantly high-pitched voice (320 Hz) was labeled as hysterical conversion dysphonia. Voice therapy (symptomatic) using a modification of the pushing approach (Boone & McFarlane, 1988) was successful in lowering this client's voice to a normal habitual pitch level of 213 Hz. Although the American Psychiatric Association (1988) regards hysterical neurosis as another term for conversion disorder, A. E. Aronson (1985) considers the two as separate entities and provides criteria for the differences between them.

It is clear, therefore, that conversion aphonias or dysphonias can have varying vocal symptomatology in pitch, resonance, and hyperfunctional laryngeal valving. The most common form, however, is hypofunctional laryngeal valving. Loudness can be affected by psychological states so that the person speaks in a very soft voice. Some adults present abnormal pitch inflections. All of these voice dimensions can interact in subtle ways to produce a complex of symptoms of underlying psychological disorder.

One unique characteristic of many forms of psychogenic voice disorder in the conversion area is the variability of voice symptomatology in the same patient. Within the same voice sample, the trained speech–language pathologist often can detect vocal hyperfunction, vocal hypofunction manifested as breathiness, and even instances of normal vocal fold vibration. These symptoms occur randomly during a communication utterance and can be so unusual that no organic condition could affect the larynx and vocal system in such an extreme and variable manner.

Excessive muscular tension in the extrinsic and intrinsic laryngeal structures is present even when the primary vocal symptom involves hypofunctional voice (breathiness or aphonia). Tension can be detected in the masseter, sternocleidomastoid, and mylohyoid muscles. Most other strap muscles manifest similar tension, but, because they are easier to palpate, it is easier to identify the tension. The hyoid bone and thyroid cartilage often rise excessively during phonation attempts. The speech–language pathologist should not be confused by these seemingly incompatible symptoms.

Laryngoscopic examination of the laryngeal structures may reveal slight swelling or reddening (edema or erythema) of the vocal folds, giving the impression that there is an organic or structural basis for the voice disorder. It should become apparent, however, that the severity and extreme variability of vocal symptoms is inconsistent with the slight organic factors. The edema or erythema most likely results from the general tension associated with psychogenic voice disorder and can be considered as a slight vocal abuse factor. In any case, this abuse factor is not sufficient to explain the presence of the voice disorder.

Another unique characteristic in conversion aphonia or conversion muteness is the presence of phonation during coughing, laughing, or throat clearing and its absence during speech. Typically, the person with this sort of voice disorder does not seem to realize that the sound produced by the vocal folds during coughing, laughing, or throat clearing uses the same mechanism as in speech phonation. The following dialogue demonstrates the typical manifestation of this phenomenon in conversion aphonia:

SLP: What happened to your bank job while you were confined to the state hospital?

PT: Well, they kept me on the payroll. (Patient was whispering only)

SLP: For 3 months, even though you started working there only 1 week before you went to the hospital?

PT: (Whispering) Yes, they have been very good to me.

SLP: I'm impressed with that bank. I think I will switch banks!

PT: (Patient laughs loudly with phonation, then again whispers) I don't know why, but they seem to want me back.

SLP: When I open my new savings account with that bank, I will tell them why I am switching.

PT: (Patient laughs again with phonation and gives no indication she has just produced voice, then again whispers) Thanks, that might help them keep me forever.

Evaluation Procedures

Before proceeding with an evaluation and management of a patient with some form of psychogenic voice disorder, the speech–language pathologist should be sure the client is evaluated medically by an otolaryngologist or other physician. Organic conditions of a neurogenic nature (Chapter 5) produce voice symptoms similar to psychogenic voice disorders, so medical referral is necessary to diagnose the etiology properly.

A. E. Aronson (1985) reported a case diagnosed as having "functional aphonia" that actually was based on myasthenia gravis, a myoneuronal junctional disease that produces a generalized dysarthria (see Chapter 5). Only after case-history examination and endurance speech testing was the vocal deterioration noted, prompting the neurological testing that determined the actual etiology.

When a medical examination has eliminated organicity as the basis for the voice disorder, the speech–language pathologist should begin the evaluation by taking a thorough case history (Chapter 3). Questions should explore background and general aspects of life-style to identify possible interpersonal or environmental sources of stress and conflict. In a general and nonthreatening manner, the speech–language pathologist should discuss with the client such areas as family and marital relationships, employment stress factors, attitudes about self-worth and self-acceptance, financial concerns, and general life-style considerations.

Many of these areas are private, emotionally laden, difficult to express, embarrassing to the client, and in general highly sensitive. It is not necessary to probe deeply into the individual's private life ("Tell me all about your sex life," etc.), as that would be inappropriate for voice symptom management. Rather than probing, a general atmosphere of communication encouragement and acceptance is appropriate.

The speech–language pathologist should begin something like this:

It has been found that persons with voice patterns similar to yours are experiencing conflicts and stresses that might be affecting the voice. Is anything happening in your life that might be important for us to understand? What about your family life? Your marriage? Job? Financial concerns? These or any other areas? What do you think?

An encouraging attitude from the speech–language pathologist can stimulate communication about these areas. The client at first may deny any such conflicts, but time and rapport in an encouraging atmosphere usually provide the forum for the person to start talking about these sensitive concerns.

Why should the speech–language pathologist ask about such areas? Is he or she playing psychiatrist or psychologist? Should he or she not deal merely with vocal symptoms and leave the psychology to the psychologist or psychiatrist? These are significant and legitimate questions. The answer lies in the fact that the speech–language pathologist often is the first professional to see a person with a psychogenic voice disorder. If that is so, it is important to determine the psychological status of the client in a general sense to determine when referral for psychological or psychiatric services is necessary. The speech–language pathologist may be the only professional who asks such questions in an attempt to determine the nature of the dysphonia. Rollin (1987) has written extensively on the psychological aspects of communication disorder including dysphonia, and has provided excellent guidance to the speech–language pathologist on dealing with this aspect of the job.

Speech–language pathologists often treat clients with psychogenic voice disorder by direct referral from a laryngologist who sees these patients, determines that the voice disorder is not organic, assumes it is functional or psychogenic, and refers for voice therapy. It then is necessary for the speech–language pathologists to determine how critical the psychological or psychiatric symptoms are. Can symptomatic voice therapy remove the dysphonia before psychological or psychiatric referral? Or must the patients be seen immediately by another professional and referred back later for symptomatic voice therapy?

Such a determination can be made only after the speech–language pathologist has heard the clients discuss their background. The more background he or she has in psychology, the more comfortable he or she will be in determining the psychological status of clients. Nevertheless, that determination must be made.

In my experience, therapy to eliminate abnormal symptomatology in psychogenic voice cases usually is effective only with patterns that are extremely distinguishable from the patient's emotional or psychological status. The patient who has dysphonia only when crying or having an emotional confrontation with some other person is unlikely to be helped by symptomatic voice therapy. Such a client would benefit more by immediate referral for psychological and psychiatric services.

By the end of the evaluation period, it should be clear whether the significant aspects of the client's voice disorder are nonorganic or psychogenic. Medical evaluation should have produced a diagnosis of functional or psychogenic dysphonia, and the speech–language pathologist should expand on that diagnosis with an analysis of the vocal symptoms. Therapy then can begin to remediate the dysphonia.

The therapy procedures recommended in this chapter involve removal of vocal symptoms found to be abnormal in the evaluation, without much attention to underlying psychological or psychiatric dysfunction. If the therapy is successful, the person will continue to have stress, interpersonal relationship difficulties, coping difficulties, or emotional disorder, but with a better voice. Such a therapeutic process has been labeled symptomatic voice therapy (Boone & McFarlane, 1988) since only symptoms are removed, not causes.

Therapy Procedures

The prognosis for removing abnormal symptoms in conversion aphonia or dysphonia depends on several factors. One of the most important is the time between the onset of vocal symptoms and the initiation of therapy to remove them. The sooner the speech–language pathologist is consulted after the voice disorder begins, the better the prognosis for improvement. However, several months or even years may elapse before the client seeks help. Under such conditions, it is more difficult to eliminate the abnormal symptoms. The passage of time seems to stabilize the need for the symptoms.

Another prognostic factor is the severity of the symptoms. The more extreme they are, whether hypofunctional or hyperfunctional, the better the prognosis for improvement, particularly when managed soon after onset. Aphonia, whispering, or extreme tension all are easier to modify than slight vocal quivering or tremor that is psychogenic and not neurologically based.

Symptomatic voice therapy with an adult or child with newly developed and extreme patterns of voice production, such as in aphonia, can be managed in a direct and straightforward manner. One of the most effective facilitators is to use a simple coughing pattern of voice initiation.

Adults with psychogenic aphonia, as mentioned earlier, often do not realize that the sound heard in a cough involves the same valving and vibration principles as true phonation. The sound of the cough is the sound of vibrating vocal folds. When asked to cough, the aphonic client produces "voice" without realizing it. By extending the cough phonation into normal vowel production, normal phonation is facilitated.

Once the person can cough and prolong it into a vowel, the speech–language pathologist can suggest that the cough be dropped while holding onto the vowel. The individual may have trouble doing that without dropping the cough phonation. If that is the case, the speech–language pathologist should suggest that the client think of beginning to cough without actually doing so. The person should feel the "set" of a cough without actually coughing, then prolong the set into a normal vowel.

A suggestion to grunt as though lifting something heavy can produce the same valving action of the vocal folds as is heard in coughing or normal phonation. This form of voicing then can be prolonged into a vowel in the same manner as the coughing method. The client also can be asked to demonstrate a forceful hum.

Coughing, grunting, and humming all are techniques of distraction. The client suddenly is producing voice without being aware of it. Whichever technique is used, it is important that the speech–language pathologist move the client quickly through steps leading to normal voice usage in communication:

1. Coughing or similar technique

2. Prolongation into a normal vowel with the cough

3. Production of all vowels

4. Monosyllabic words

5. Any word

6. Simple phrases

7. Oral reading

8. Simple conversation

9. Conversation about anything and with anyone in the clinic setting

10. Generalization to everyday communication

Because a number of suggestions or techniques are workable, I have a word of caution regarding how to proceed. Before trying any particular technique, such as coughing or grunting, the speech–language pathologist should make a general statement such as, "You have not lost your voice. You have merely lost the ability to make it work. We are going to try a variety of things to help you regain this ability. Let's see how they work. Let's begin by having you . . ." With such an approach, the speech–language pathologist is not setting the stage for one powerful technique: "I command you to be healed." A general statement permits one technique to be attempted; if it fails, another can be tried without discouraging the client.

Once the client can communicate with voice in the therapy session, it is important to move as quickly as possible into conversation by following the steps listed. When the aphonia has been of rather short duration, the client often can move quickly into a conversation mode without the aphonia. The speech–language pathologist should accept such rapid change and say something such as, "There, you have your voice back! You have done the right thing(s) to get it going again, and you do not need to worry that you will ever lose it again."

The speech–language pathologist should continue the conversation mode until convinced of vocal stability, then make an appointment for a checkup in a few days. Telephone contact between appointments is helpful to ensure client voice stability away from the clinic. When rapid and successful change occurs, the speech–language pathologist should remember that only the symptom of psychological disturbance has been removed, not the disturbance itself.

It is a good idea to refer the client to a psychologist or psychiatrist to help with unresolved conflicts and adjustments, if such a relationship has not previously been established. In any case, the speech–language pathologist can have confidence that the aphonia is neither likely to return nor to be replaced with some other symptom. Symptoms have been known to recur, but the common clinical finding is that they do not.

Case Example of Aphonia Treatment

The following example illustrates the therapy approach recommended for conversion aphonia. It is the case introduced earlier of R.T., the 18-year-old female victim of a gas station robbery.

R.T. was referred because of a recently developed severe aphonia. After the holdup, as mentioned earlier, the robber cut R.T.'s throat superficially. Laryngoscopic inspection revealed an intact larynx in terms of neuromusculature. However, from then until her evaluation 3 weeks later, she had been "unable" to produce voice; she could only whisper.

At her evaluation, the speech–language pathologist decided that no long case history about her emotional status was necessary since it seemed rather obvious that she suffered a conversion aphonia from a specific incident. General questioning of the mother indicated that R.T. had been a well-adjusted person before the robbery, with no evidence of voice disorder. It was decided to initiate symptomatic voice therapy immediately.

The speech–language pathologist instructed R.T. to cough. She gave a loud and abrupt cough. She then was told to cough again and prolong it into a vowel /a/, which the speech–language pathologist demonstrated. R.T. accomplished this without difficulty. Several other vowels were attempted in this same manner, and the cough was eliminated without difficulty.

Next, she was asked to repeat several words from a list, then to count from 1 to 20. Following the counting, she was asked to name the days of the week, months of the year, and items that could be purchased in a department store; to describe how to scramble eggs; and finally to tell what her plans were for the next few days. She explained in a clear and strong voice ("This is my normal voice") that she was planning a wedding and that she was glad to have her voice back before her wedding day.

After a few minutes of conversation about the wedding plans, the speech–language pathologist was convinced that R.T.'s voice was entirely normal and no further therapy would be needed. An appointment was made for her to return in 3 days for a checkup to ensure stability. The speech–language pathologist also mentioned that she might experience some horror memory from the holdup and that it might be helpful to see a psychologist or psychiatrist, even though her voice had returned, to help her cope and adjust. She was not sure how she felt about that suggestion but said she would consider it. When the time came for her next appointment, her mother called to say that because of the wedding pressures, R.T. did not want to come for the checkup and that her voice was entirely normal. The case of R.T. clearly represents successful voice therapy for conversion aphonia.

Therapy for Conversion Dysphonia

Many forms of conversion dysphonia, and even some aphonia cases, are not managed as easily as was R.T. For example, when considerable time has passed between the development of the voice disorder and the initiation of therapy, the prognosis for quick improvement is diminished. When the client has had the voice symptoms for several months or even years, it is as though they become an integral part of everyday coping strategies. The voice pattern seems to become part of the client's communication personality and, as a result, is more resistant to easy modification.

This should not discourage the speech–language pathologist because such resistance to easy change is more typical of the everyday clinical experiences in communication disorder. Quick and easy solutions are the exception rather than the clinical rule in any therapy of communication disorders, so why should voice therapy be different?

With patients who have experienced significant, long-term psychogenic change, a simple cough, hum, or grunt technique will not produce voice. Change will come only when the client learns how to produce voice; how factors such as tension, pitch, loudness, and quality can be regulated; and how stress affects them. The client must become informed and aware that although personality, emotion, and voice are highly intertwined, considerable conscious control can be exerted over the vocal system, even in emotional states. This control will not develop easily, but with careful instruction and therapeutic direction, vocal stability can be achieved by those who really seek such improvement.

Several techniques have been reported in the literature as clinically effective in achieving control over long-term psychogenic voice disorders. Most of these are directed at reducing the hyperfunctional aspects of voice production. When tension exists and the voice manifests it, it is not enough to suggest that if the person could relax when talking the voice would improve. Rather, the individual must be taken through systematic stages of control over the muscles involved in the hyperfunctional basis of phonation. The following sections describe techniques that have been used to accomplish this control.

Progressive Relaxation

Jacobson (1978) proposed a method of training clients to learn to contrast states of tension in the body with its elimination through progressive relaxation.

The specific method of obtaining muscle relaxation in the person with psychogenic voice disorder, however, is not as critical as focusing on the laryngeal mechanism once general body relaxation has been achieved. In Chapter 4, in a case of contact ulcers, part of the therapy involved directions for achieving relaxation by means of progressive control. This is a specific example of how progressive relaxation therapy can be integrated with voice disorder of any form when excessive muscular tension is present.

Clinical Hypnosis

Hypnosis is a common technique in psychiatry and psychology and is being used more often in all aspects of clinical medicine and dentistry. Hypnosis can be defined as a state of suggestibility characterized by attentive, receptive focal concentration with diminished peripheral awareness. All forms of hypnosis, in the true sense of what actually happens in hypnotic induction, are self-hypnosis since the client allows the induction process to occur. This intense concentration can be used to achieve specific goals that are suggested by the therapist and accepted by the client (Spiegel & Spiegel, 1980).

Horsley (1982) analyzed the successful treatment of a 46-year-old professional woman with psychogenic dysphonia who had received traditional voice therapy from a speech pathologist for more than 3 months without significant improvement. Horsley used a progressive relaxation form of hypnotic induction coupled with mental placidity. The client was instructed during hypnosis to exercise control over physical and emotional tension through daily sessions of self-hypnosis designed to improve her feelings of self-worth and self-confidence. Notable improvement occurred within the first week of hypnotherapy and was maintained throughout 16 months of follow-up evaluation. Her voice characteristics reflecting improvement were evaluated by a team of five speech pathologists who rated recordings of her voice.

Clinical hypnosis is being used successfully in the treatment of many symptom-oriented disorders, including smoking, anxiety reduction, phobia elimination, and pain reduction. To this list must be added the treatment of psychogenic voice disorder. It is not a method devoid of problems and myths, and many cautions on its use have been communicated to professionals (Kendall & Norton-Ford, 1982; Spiegel & Spiegel, 1980). In the hands of a well-trained professional, however, clinical hypnosis can be an effective tool in the treatment of many forms of voice disorder, particularly the conversion aphonias and dysphonias.

Biofeedback

Clients have been helped in eliminating specific areas of body tension by receiving information of excessive muscle contraction fed back through visual or auditory means, as explained in Chapter 5.

Digital Manipulation of Phonation

Although it is difficult for the typical person with a hyperfunctional voice disorder to understand, normal phonation should be an easy process. The speech–language pathologist should demonstrate that the larynx does not work efficiently under tension, but does its best when little or no effort is involved. Easy, relaxed phonation should result in the client's feeling vibration not much in the larynx but in the resonance chambers above it.

Most of the vocal energy during phonation should be felt in the oral and nasal cavities, referred to by music teachers as the mask of the face. This balance of resonance in the mask of the face can be demonstrated by having the client feel the vibrations in the speech–language pathologist's face during normal phonation. The client should place one finger lightly on the side of the pathologist's nose, another finger on the face around the lips, and another lightly on the side of the larynx around the thyroid laminae.

As the speech–language pathologist phonates an /m/ sound, the client should be able to detect a balance of vibration in all three areas, with most of the sound concentration felt in the mask of the face around the lips. The client then can phonate an /m/ sound and feel the results in the same manner. The person also should experience a tingling sensation generally throughout that area and around the lips. If this is felt, chances are excellent that the larynx is being vibrated efficiently without excessive tension.

The speech–language pathologist should point out how phonation in this manner seems devoid of effortful vibration in the larynx. I strongly recommend this as an effective method of monitoring normal phonation in clients with hyperfunctional voice disorders.

Vocal Abuse as a Psychogenic Disorder

Several writers have classified dysphonia resulting from vocal abuse (vocal nodules, contact ulcers, acute laryngitis from abuse, etc.) as a form of psychogenic voice disorder. A. E. Aronson (1985) indicated that since clients who develop vocal nodules and contact ulcers tend to fit the same typical personality profile (highly vocal and intense in verbal interactions, hard driving, perfectionistic, loud speakers, etc.), they should be classified as having psychogenic voice disorders.

Koufman and Blalock (1982) agreed with the classification of dysphonias from vocal abuse as functional in nature, but separated them from the hysterical aphonia/dysphonia and true psychogenic category. Although I recognize the psychogenic component in many cases, I consider these disorders separately from traditional psychogenic voice disorder (Chapter 4).

Puberphonia (Mutational Falsetto)

One of the most easily corrected psychogenic voice disorders is puberphonia, also called mutational falsetto. During puberty, the typical male experiences major body transformations as a result of hormonal changes that produce growth spurts and the development of secondary sex characteristics. Failure to adjust the voice to reflect these changes is the basis for puberphonia. Chapter 1, in the section on age and sex differences in F_0, refers to the specifics of laryngeal change during pubescence. The growth changes in the larynx during this time essentially parallel general body development. Kahane (1982) and Zemlin (1988) discussed these changes in terms of (a) vocal fold length, (b) vocal fold mass or thickness, and (c) cartilage and tissue weight. The interaction between the changes reflected in pubescence, which is the biological change, and adolescence, which is the psychological change, constitutes the basis for the development of psychogenic voice disorder at that age.

The process of biological growth is a gradual one, beginning around age 11 for girls and 12 for boys. In girls, breast and pubic hair development and height increase all begin about 12. Their growth spurt peaks about 12.5, and by age 16 the average girl has reached adult height. Menarche (menstruation) in girls generally begins around the peak growth spurt of 12.5 (United States), but often does not start until 16. In boys, the testes begin to grow at about age 11.5 and are adult size by 16. Penis growth begins about 12 and usually stops about 15. The growth spurt for height and general body size in boys begins about age 12 and peaks as a spurt at about 14. By 17, the typical male has achieved adult height (Offer, 1980). There may be significant variations in individual differences since these figures reflect averages.

Most adult hormonal levels are achieved by the age of 16 for both sexes. The interaction between the hypothalamus of the CNS and the pituitary, thyroid, ovaries, and testes of the endocrine system in producing the hormonal bases of puberty, associated growth, and secondary sex characteristic development is complex and cannot be treated in significant detail here. However, full details can be found in Offer (1980). Generally, the factors are as shown in Exhibit 6–2. As noted, this exhibit offers only a partial indication of the functions. For a more complete description of each hormone and its physiological effect (as well as pharmacological constitution), see Gilman et al. (1980).

With an understanding of the complex growth (body and larynx) and hormonal changes associated with puberty, one can better understand the effect of abnormalities in biology or psychological pressures of adolescence. With regard to puberphonia, the psychological pressures of adolescence seem to have more of an effect on the genesis of the disorder than do the biological changes of puberty.

During puberty, the typical male experiences major body changes due to growth and hormone factors. The larynx similarly changes rapidly. Voice quality and pitch change significantly, often in a matter of a few months. The pitch of a young man's voice manifests the most significant and noticeable vocal change. As a result of rather sudden increases in vocal fold length and mass, the typical young male's pitch will drop about one octave, or eight whole tones. The voice also becomes more resonant and acquires a richer and fuller quality. Essentially, in a few short months, the boy's voice becomes a man's.

In some instances, the transition from boy to man is not easy. Not only is it difficult to handle increased responsibility in life, but the rapid body changes can be confusing and difficult to understand. When a boy has difficulty in making these adjustments, puberphonia or mutational falsetto can develop.

S. L. Kaplan (1982) described mutational falsetto as the psychological failure of the adolescent's voice to descend or maintain its descent to a normal adult pitch at puberty. Instead, the adolescent (usually male) raises his voice above its prepubertal pitch and consistently speaks in a falsetto or near-falsetto voice. Untreated, according to Kaplan, the symptom may be lifelong. Kaplan contrasted mutational falsetto voice with what he calls persistent pubertal voice, which involves symptoms beyond voice that suggest the possibility of an endocrinologic disorder manifesting itself as delayed puberty. My experience indicates that this voice disorder of puberty and adolescence can have the following characteristics:

1. A pitch level that is typical of the prepuberty voice that is maintained after the boy has essentially completed the biological changes of puberty

2. A pitch level that is excessively higher (usually falsetto) than that of the typical prepuberty voice after the biological changes of puberty have occurred

Exhibit 6–2 Factors in Sexual Maturation

Organ[a]	Hormone Secreted	Hormone Function (Partial)
Hypothalamus (part of CNS)	TRF (Thyrotropin-releasing factor)	Causes pituitary to release TSH (thyrotropic hormone or thyroid-stimulating hormone)
	LRF (luteinizing hormone-releasing factor)	Causes pituitary to release LH (luteinizing hormone)
Pituitary gland (endocrine)	TSH	Stimulates thyroid gland
	LH	In female: causes ovary to produce progesterone In male: causes testes to produce testosterone
	FHS (follicle-stimulating hormone)	In female: causes ovary to produce estrogen In male: causes testes to produce sperm
	Oxytocin	Affects mammary glands and uterus
	ACTH (adrenocorticotrophic hormone)	Stimulates adrenal gland to secrete steroid hormones
	STH (somatotrophic or "growth" hormone)	Promotes muscle and bone growth and metabolic processes (utilization of glucose for fuel)
Thyroid gland	Thyroxine and triiodothyronine	Increases metabolic rate; promotes growth, bone development, sex gland maturation, maturation of nervous system
Ovary glands	Estrogens, including estradiol	Affects female secondary sexual characteristics, including breast development, female sex drive, ovulation
	Progesterone	Maintains pregnancy
	Androgens (small amounts)	Not clearly understood in females
Testes	Androgens including testosterone	Affects male secondary sexual characteristics, including penis size, pubic hair, body hair, sex drive, sperm production
	Estrogens (small amounts)	Not clearly understood in males

[a] Only the organs and glands pertaining to the topic of this chapter are included here.

Note. Based on *Biological Psychology* by J. W. Kalat, 1981, Belmont, CA: Wadsworth Publishing Co.

3. A pitch level that is typical of the prepuberty voice when the biological changes of puberty have not occurred at an age at which they normally would be completed

4. A voice that is unusually high for a mature male but is compatible with the size of the laryngeal structures while incompatible with body size

The first three of these disorders are functional, the last is structural, and all have psychogenic components. In all cases, the pitch and overall quality are the dramatic characteristics of dysphonia.

Pitch and Maturation

The most common form of puberphonia occurs when a boy goes through the biological changes of puberty and experiences body and laryngeal growth changes but does not allow the pitch of the voice to descend to its adult level. This functional voice disorder results when a boy is not able to make the vocal transition to manhood. The perceptual effect is a boy's voice in a man's body. The actual development of this disorder is not understood clearly other than from the perspective of clinical experience. Several cases I have seen provide the profile described below.

The boy who develops puberphonia usually is shy and somewhat insecure in personal relationships. Case history data from parents and clients verify this point. I think that most boys experience some embarrassment about the rapidly changing voice during puberty, although this seems to be a momentary concern for most. During this period, pitch breaks and other voice adjustment problems occur, but they seem to have a significant effect only on the boy who has a poor self-image or who is shy and insecure.

For example, should a pitch break occur around a friend or group of peers, teasing may result. Nobody enjoys being teased, but the boy who has a poor self-concept and is not secure in peer relationships can be devastated psychologically by it. The boy is likely to become concerned about a recurrence. It is almost as though he becomes so worried about a pitch break that it is on his mind each time he begins to talk, especially if he is in a socially difficult situation, such as with a girl or around peers. The boy may think such thoughts as, "I wonder if my voice will squeak or break if I talk to her. I hope it doesn't happen here."

This concern about pitch stability before speaking sets the stage for the development of puberphonia. To obtain pitch function and ensure that breaks will be unlikely to occur, the boy may attempt to keep his pitch at the level he has always used (i.e., his prepuberty level). It is not long before his old pitch becomes stabilized and the puberphonic dysphonia has been established.

The following sections describe typical voice characteristics of the male who has developed puberphonia.

Pitch Factors

Few data are available regarding the pitch of individuals with puberphonia. Although Welch, Sergeant, and MacCurtain (1988) presented data on vocal and laryngeal characteristics of male falsetto singers (countertenor or male alto), the only pitch data specific to puberphonia have been presented by Case (1987). Pitch levels of 7 cases of puberphonia were recorded before and after therapy on high quality instrumentation (Nakamichi 550 Dual-Tracer Stereo Recorder). All subjects were male (mean age 16.8, range 14 to 18 years) and indicated (self-report or parental report) that essential completion of physical puberty and secondary sex changes had occurred. All therapy was accomplished in one session, an average time of 1 ½ hours. Although checkups were scheduled and maintained, no relapse was found.

The audio recordings of pre- and post-therapy speech samples were analyzed using the Micro Speech Laboratory (MSL) speech and signal analyzer, which digitized the sample at 10 KHz/sec. This sampling provided a mean F_0 every 25 msec.

Figure 6–1 provides the results for the 7 subjects. Fundamental frequency is represented along the ordinate (y-axis) and the subjects are represented along the abscissa (x-axis). Individual subject means (before and after therapy) are provided, as well as group means.

The group mean before therapy was 250.4 Hz. These data indicate that the pre-therapy mean was well above the mean acceptable F_0 for 16-year-old males (150 Hz, acceptable range 125 to 180 Hz; D. K. Wilson, 1987) and even above the acceptable level for 16-year-old females (215 Hz, range 180 to 255 Hz; D. K. Wilson, 1987). In other words, these male subjects had a mean pitch level at the upper end of what Wilson described as acceptable for normal females. The highest mean for subject J.O. was 377 Hz, which is not acceptable for a person of any age or sex.

The group mean after therapy was 126.9 Hz. As a group, these subjects were well within normal limits of pitch and even at the lower end of the range of normal expectations as reported by Wilson. The lowest subject mean was 105 Hz, which is even lower than the expected mean of 18-year-old subjects.

Except for the breaks, the habitual pitch level of the boy with puberphonia is often monotonic and devoid of natural inflections. Diplophonia (double pitch) is common. However, the unnaturally high voice is the striking characteristic of this disorder. Sex confusion over the phone is common; when the boy answers the phone and the caller asks, "Hello, is your husband home?" fuel is added to the psychogenic factor. Under the Wilson Voice Profile system described in Chapter 3, the typical perceptual judgment for the puberphonic client is +2 or +3 (pitch).

Quality Factors. The voice of the puberphonic speaker usually is of normal quality in terms of laryngeal vibration and resonance. Hoarseness is rare.

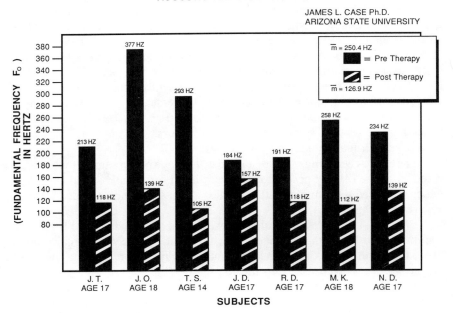

PUBERPHONIA: BEFORE AND AFTER THERAPY
ACOUSTIC ANALYSIS OF PITCH

JAMES L. CASE Ph.D.
ARIZONA STATE UNIVERSITY

Figure 6–1 Vocal Pitch in Puberphonia.

Slight tension is heard at times, but is a minor concern and probably results from the speaker's use of a pitch level that is not optimal, so that increased effort is necessary to maintain voice continuity. Using the Wilson Voice Profile, the typical laryngeal opening judgment is 1 (normal) or +2 (tension).

Loudness Factor.   The boy has essentially normal loudness ability in conversation but sometimes complains of not being able to yell. This is related to using a pitch level that is not compatible for the larynx under optimal conditions, and thus limits its projection potential. It also is related in many cases to a shy personality that is nearly incompatible with yelling in social situations.

Resonance Factor.   Puberphonia does not produce any significant alteration in vocal resonance. Hyponasality or hypernasality in the vocal signal probably results from an independent factor (see Chapter 8). Therefore, resonance is expected to be normal.

Management Procedures in Puberphonia

Developing a Case History

Developing a case history is fairly straightforward. The speech–language pathologist asks when the pitch disorder first occurred, when the onset of puberty was, what was happening socially during the puberty change, whether there were instances of speaking avoidance because of embarrassment about pitch breaks, and whether any conscious attempt was made to keep pitch at a high level. Generally, it is necessary to gain perspective only about the relationship between puberty and the current state of the voice. A. E. Aronson (1985) suggested exploring such additional factors as delayed maturation of the laryngeal structures because of endocrine imbalance, severe hearing loss that makes pitch monitoring difficult, neurological disease during adolescence change, and general debilitating illness during puberty.

From this information, the speech–language pathologist can determine whether medical referral is necessary. If any question exists after such a case history as to the possibility of a physical basis for the pitch disorder, it is important to obtain current medical information by appropriate referral.

Voice Evaluation

The voice characteristics of the puberphonic youth are rated first on pitch, quality, and loudness. This is important in obtaining a measurement of the habitual pitch level using procedures outlined earlier. The speech–language pathologist then records a 5-min conversation during which the student reads a short paragraph. Any instances of low-pitched voice should be noted.

In most cases, after a case history and voice evaluation have been completed, it should be apparent that puberphonia is the basis for the disorder. It is particularly helpful to have medical information on the youth, either before or shortly after the evaluation, indicating that the laryngeal structures are normal for voice production.

Stimulation Techniques

Once puberphonia is established as the basis for the pitch disorder, the speech–language pathologist should explain to the youth the likely relationship between the onset of puberty and the voice problem. The professional then describes either or both of the following techniques that will be used in an attempt to find the boy's true pitch:

1. *Cough:* A human cough creates a sound that is a result of air vibrating the closed vocal folds. It is a rough form of phonation using the same mechanisms as in normal voice production. Because coughing, compared with normal phonation, is a biological act, it is not subject to the emotions associated with phonation in human communication. Therefore, the youth coughs, and the sound usually reflects the condition of the vocal folds in a natural state. The pitch of the cough roughly approximates the optimal pitch of the voice. A cough can facilitate the use of the optimal pitch.

2. *Digital Manipulation:* Gentle pushing on the thyroid cartilage of the larynx during phonation suddenly relaxes the vocal folds and the pitch drops approximately one whole tone. The technique is to have the young man relax and say "ah" as the speech–language pathologist pushes gently on the thyroid cartilage. The pitch goes down and, when the dropped tone is heard, the youth is instructed to hold onto it as the pressure on the thyroid cartilage is released. The process is repeated as the student lowers his pitch in whole-tone steps. When the pupil has a pitch that is optimal for his age, the speech–language pathologist stabilizes and shapes it into conversation using techniques explained below.

A Case Example of Puberphonia

This example illustrates how evaluation and treatment procedures for puberphonia can be handled. R.D., a 15-year-old male, was referred by an otolaryngologist because of persistent diplophonia (double-pitched voice) and an inappropriately high-pitched tone. He also had been treated by another physician, who had diagnosed R.D. as having contact ulcers on his vocal folds.

His case history revealed nothing of significance about his pitch disorder other than the fact that his "voice did not change when it was supposed to." It seemed apparent that, because recent examinations by otolaryngologists indicated normal laryngeal structures and the case history was devoid of significance other than the delayed voice change at puberty, R.D. was a true puberphonic. The following recording of the speech–language pathologist's explanation to the youth is an example of voice management of this disorder.

> Let me explain what has happened to your voice. During the years of puberty change, as your body was growing and changing, you probably experienced some frustration handling the pitch of your voice. This frustration led you to keep the pitch of your voice with which you were most familiar rather than let it change. We are going to try some techniques to help you find your best pitch. It may be easy; it may be hard. Let's find out.

First, I want you to cough like this. (Speech–language pathologist demonstrates cough.) Did you notice that the sound of your cough was low . . . much lower than your speaking voice. That is because your vocal folds were vibrating at a pitch that was natural for them.

Now, try it again. (R.D. coughs at D#$_1$.) Good, try it again . . . and again. Now cough and prolong the cough into an "ah" sound like this. (Speech–language pathologist demonstrates.) (R.D. coughs, followed by an "ah" at the same pitch level.) Good. Notice your pitch stayed low with both the cough and the "ah." Do it again . . . and again.

Now, I want you to "think" of a cough without actually coughing and say "ah" at that pitch. (R.D. does it.) Good. Do it again. Now say "ah" like you have been, then go into an "o" sound like this. (Speech–language pathologist demonstrates.) (R.D. does it.) Good. Now you can say any sound at that pitch level. Say the following sounds after me. (R.D. repeats 10 different vowel sounds after model.)

Now count to 20 at the low pitch level. (R.D. does it with two slight breaks into a higher pitch.) Now say the ABCs at that pitch. (R.D. does it.) Now tell me your address and phone number. Good. Now I want you to read this list of sentences using your new pitch level. If you get confused as to where your pitch should be, just cough gently or think of a cough and speak at the cough level.

In a few minutes, using a biological state of the larynx to facilitate normal phonation at an optimal pitch level, R.D. learned to control his pitch and left the therapy session with a new voice. As he became comfortable with his new pitch, he relaxed and his voice lowered to an optimal and habitual pitch of A$_2$ (approximately 110 Hz). During the first session, he was able to read orally, converse with the speech–language pathologist about school, then chat for 20 min with his sister who had accompanied him. This conversation was monitored by the speech–language pathologist to determine that the youth maintained his new pitch level.

As he left the clinic, R.D. was instructed to use his new pitch in any situation in which he felt comfortable. Called a few hours later by the speech–language pathologist, the youth reported he had no difficulty using his new pitch in all speaking situations, including those with close friends. He mentioned that several persons had commented on his new voice, but he dismissed these by saying he had a cold. Four days later, R.D. returned to the clinic and was recorded in conversation. All aspects of his voice were judged normal, including pitch, quality, and loudness. He was using his voice in all speaking situations and felt comfortable with it.

Special Considerations in Puberphonia

Although puberphonia is a functional voice disorder and easy to remediate when done properly, a few cautions need to be stated. As the speech–language pathologist begins to change the student's voice, care should be taken not to indicate to a client that if one specific technique is used, the proper pitch level will occur (i.e., cough and the proper pitch will emerge). Rather, the speech–language pathologist should indicate that several methods will be attempted to help the student find his new pitch and that one of them should work. Then, if failure occurs on the first technique, the youth will not become discouraged easily. All the eggs have not been placed in one basket, so a new technique can be attempted easily.

When a youth hears his new low-pitched voice, he often will comment that he does not like it. This is understandable because he has never heard himself speaking low. Since he does not like it because he is not used to it, he may be somewhat reluctant to try it with others, assuming that they will not like it either. The speech–language pathologist should tell him he soon will be used to it and that others will like it immediately. He should test his new voice with strangers, such as store clerks, and he will notice no negative reactions to his pitch. Such experiences will help him develop confidence in the normal nature of his new pitch.

Care also should be taken not to lower the youth's voice too much; rather, the speech–language pathologist should seek an optimal pitch level about three or four tones from the basal. This new level will allow all downward inflections in the young man's voice without approaching the basal, which would produce tension. Even when the pitch still seems somewhat high after lowering it, it should be kept in mind that, as the student matures into adulthood, his voice will become deeper in pitch and richer in resonance.

When the student expresses concern about using his new pitch around persons other than the speech–language pathologist, it may be necessary to carefully control the process of generalization from the clinic or school therapy to other situations. This can be done through ranking all speaking situations in task difficulty. This is called hierarchy analysis of typical speaking situations (Boone & McFarlane, 1988) and is done by assigning the student to speak with his new voice first in situations low on the task hierarchy before moving onto the more stressful levels.

It is important that the change of pitch from puberphonic to normal occur quickly compared with typical school communication disorder therapy durations of weeks and months. Within 2 or 3 days, the change should be complete. Even in settings such as the school, where youths may be seen by the speech–language pathologist only a few minutes a week, it is important to change their schedules to accommodate intense therapy. The speech–language pathologist must be assertive in expecting the student to use the new pitch in situations that may be rather uncomfortable at first. The youth should be told that any discomfort he experiences will be momentary and that people soon will not even notice the change.

Working with youths who have puberphonia can be most satisfying to the speech–language pathologist, who is accustomed to only slight change in communication performance even under prolonged therapy. To hear a boy, in a few hours or days, significantly change a voice pattern that has caused so much concern and embarrassment can compensate for more frustrating therapy efforts.

Literature Review in Puberphonia

In addition to the factors discussed, A. E. Aronson (1985) identified several etiologies to mutational falsetto (puberphonia):

- Delayed maturation in endocrine disorders that retard laryngeal development, perpetuating a high-pitched voice which then becomes difficult to abandon because of longer than normal persistence into adolescence, even after the larynx has attained normal size.

- Severe hearing loss, preventing the individual from perceiving his or her voice during adolescent voice change.

- Weakness or incoordination of the vocal folds or of respiration during puberty because of neurologic disease.

- General debilitating illness during puberty, which not only may delay overall growth during puberty, but because of the physical restrictions of being bedfast, may reduce the range of respiratory excursions and consequently tidal air volumes, preventing the development of adequate infraglottal air pressure.

A. E. Aronson also indicated that several patients have been seen as adults (50s and 60s), often for the first time, in an attempt to change their voices. The prognosis for changing even these adults' voices generally is excellent using the methods outlined.

S. L. Kaplan (1982) presented a unique case of mutational falsetto that appears different from the typical profile. In this case, a 15-year-old male who had been speaking in a falsetto for 2 years was treated for the dysphonia by psychotherapy. This boy was able to demonstrate to the psychotherapist that he was capable of speaking in a lower voice but failed to understand why his parents were so concerned that he did not speak using it. He persisted in speaking in a falsetto. After two sessions of psychotherapy directed toward helping the client understand his motivations for using the falsetto, the boy began speaking in his low voice. Therapy was terminated after five sessions with the boy using the low voice consistently; a 6-month follow-up revealed the pitch was maintained at the low level.

Six months after the follow-up, the boy began to develop symptoms of behavior deterioration in school and social coping, with auditory hallucinations that people were calling him a homosexual and telling him to physically assault classmates. He was diagnosed as developing a psychotic disorder and was admitted to an inpatient psychiatric unit with a diagnosis of schizophreniform disorder. On the night of admission, he physically assaulted staff members because he felt his display of physical prowess would communicate to the voices (hallucinations) that he was a man. He was treated with high-dose phenothiazine medication and was released after 2 months. Although this case appears unique and is the first reported in the literature in which mutational falsetto preceded schizophrenia, it certainly must alert professionals who treat this disorder to monitor the psychological or psychiatric status of these clients during and subsequent to voice therapy.

Hartman and Aronson (1983) reported an interesting case of psychogenic aphonia that masked itself as mutational falsetto. A 14-year-old boy experienced aphonia because of laryngeal inflammation that persisted as a psychogenic aphonia after the inflammation subsided. The psychogenic aphonia became superimposed on the unstable pitch of adolescent voice change. The details of treatment in that case are consistent with the procedures outlined above.

Organic Mutational Falsetto

In some cases of voice disorder, for organic reasons the larynx fails to develop to its adult size and the voice remains at prepuberty pitch, quality, and resonance. Endocrine imbalance must be suspected in such cases, and the only reasonable treatment is medical. When the voice, larynx size, status of pubescence, and general development of secondary sex characteristics are delayed, such endocrine imbalance must be considered as an etiology and must be evaluated by an endocrinologist or other physician.

The ancient custom of castration of male adolescents and adults for a variety of reasons provides evidence of the effect of endocrine imbalance on the voice. For example, castration was done to produce eunuchs as slaves in brothels, harems, and the courts of royalty; for religious excommunication; for revenge on prisoners of war; and to produce a certain singing quality in early religious music. St. Paul wrote, "Let your women keep silence in the church" (I Corinthians 14:34); therefore, women could not be used in church choirs. Much has been written about the famous castrato voice but an excellent reference is Brodnitz (1975).

Transsexual Voice Disorder

The term unisexual describes cultural, sociological, and personal phenomena that are not clearly dimorphistic with regard to sexual identification. Whether it is in dress, vocations, avocations, hairstyles, jewelry, or a variety of other elements, the unisex concept more and more applies to today's society.

The developing embryo has clearly defined unisexual potential until the endocrine system makes its mark and the infant becomes sexually defined. Examples of the hermaphrodite, who is intermediate between normal male and female in anatomy, or with genes of one sex and anatomy of another, are common abnormalities (Kalat, 1981). No behavior is clearly recognizable as male or female during the first year of life.

With all of this sexual confusion, it is a wonder more people do not experience difficulty with gender identity. Brodnitz (1975) indicated that voice professionals are seeing increased numbers of individuals with puberphonia or other forms of gender identity difficulty. One such disorder being seen more commonly now by speech–language pathologists is the transsexual, particularly male-to-female. Most authors writing on transsexualism apply the term to anyone who claims to belong to the wrong sex and who wishes to change to the opposite sex. Such persons seek sex changes through surgery or hormone therapy to make their bodies appear and function as members of the opposite sex.

Stoller (1980) provided a thorough description of the literature dealing with the etiology of transsexualism, so only voice characteristics and treatment considerations of transsexualism are presented here.

A male who wishes transsexual change to female can do so in appearance through cross-dressing, hormonal treatment (estrogen), and electrolysis to remove body hair. Surgical alteration of the penis to form a vagina has been done successfully in some cases, but is approached with caution because of its nonreversibility and common surgical complications (bowel perforations, repeated bouts of cystitis, sloughing of grafts, and closure of the artificial vagina). Extensive psychiatric treatment is recommended so that such persons can confront directly the negative side of their wish to change sex. That can enable them to rediscover the dimensions of residual masculinity and commitment to their male bodies, decide against radical surgery, and approach the issue more conservatively. Often, they decide they can live more comfortably as they are (Stoller, 1980).

When the male does change sex (surgically or medically) and wants to appear female, the voice and communication style often are the troublesome aspects. Increased testosterone lowers the female voice in the female transsexual who wishes to become male. Although increased estrogen for the male-to-female transsexual increases breast size, it does not decrease the laryngeal size and cause it to produce a higher pitched voice naturally (Laing, 1989).

Surgical alteration of the larynx has proved successful in providing a higher pitch for the male-to-female transsexual. Donald (1982) reported on a surgical alteration of the larynx to provide shorter vocal folds and therefore a higher fundamental frequency of vibration. By means of laryngofissure, the anterior one-third of each vocal fold on 3 transsexual patients was surgically denuded and approximated to the opposite vocal fold to form an anterior web. This process resulted in pitch elevation in all 3 cases by surgically shortening the vocal folds.

Additional surgical techniques to raise vocal pitch have been reported by Isshiki, Taira, and Tanabe (1983) and Gould and Lawrence (1984). Isshiki et al. used techniques which include cricothyroid approximation to stretch the vocal folds, longitudinal incision of the vocal folds to increase the stiffness by scarring, and decreasing the vocal fold mass by intrachordal injection of steroid or partial evaporation of the vocal fold by CO_2 laser. They reported data on 14 patients (13 females diagnosed with androphonia; 1 male-to-female transsexual) whose pitches were raised successfully without significant negative consequence. Differences were noted from technique to technique, and Isshiki et al. reported the cricothyroid approximation technique to be safest.

Isshiki et al. (1983) also reported on a surgical procedure to lower vocal pitch when voice therapy (3 to 6 month trial period) has been unsuccessful in lowering it. This surgery is done under a local anesthesia, with some sedative administered to allow the patient to phonate upon request during the surgery. The technique is designed to shorten the anteroposterior length of the thyroid cartilage, which decreases the longitudinal tension of the vocal folds and thus lowers the pitch. Several variations of the basic procedure, called Thyroplasty Type III, were reported on 9 patients (all male, diagnoses of mutational voice disorder or vocal fold atrophy). Greater success was reported with those patients whose etiology was mutational voice disorder than with those whose vocal folds were scarred or atrophic.

When surgery is not done or is not successful in raising the pitch of the male-to-female transsexual, the services of a speech–language pathologist may be needed to accomplish this goal.

One case illustrates the male transsexual's concern for voice. C.E. was referred to the Arizona State University Speech and Hearing Clinic for an evaluation of voice. C.E. was a male-to-female transsexual who wanted to present herself more successfully as a female. On her application for an evaluation, she did not communicate that she was a transsexual, but merely indicated she was female by sex and had a glandular condition. She wrote,

> I have a glandular condition similar to the problem that a bearded lady in a circus side show had (the gonads are producing more than the normal amount of androgen (male sex hormones)). Under normal circumstances ovaries produce both estrogen and androgen but proportionately less androgen than the female sex hormone (estrogen). My androgen levels are disproportionate, causing among other things a deeper voice than I should have. I need speech training to "feminize" my very masculine sounding voice.

Later this person reported that she was indeed a transsexual who wanted help in a more female presentation.

It is important to remember that raising the pitch alone will not be sufficient to communicate female sexual gender. Key (1975) and Laing (1989) identified the many differences that distinguish the sexes in communication style, including raised pitch in the female, increased use of modal constructions (can, will, may, shall, must), and intonation patterns of pitch, stress, and duration of phoneme production that appear more feminine. There also are female body language factors that have gender communicative effect and also must be considered as part of the treatment.

A study that quantified the concerns expressed by Key (1975) reported on intonation and fundamental frequency patterns in male-to-female transsexuals. V. I. Wolfe, Ratusnik, Smith, and Northrop (1990) evaluated 20 transsexuals to determine frequency and intonation patterns that would be judged as female or male. Of the 20 experimental subjects, 9 were judged as female and 11 as male. Those judged as female had significantly higher pitches (mean F_0 172 Hz, range 155.5 to 195 Hz). Those judged as male had lower pitches (mean F_0 118 Hz, range 97.2 to 145 Hz). Transsexuals rated as male also had more significant and extensive downward inflections of the voice. Those subjects rated as female had a higher percentage of upward inflections than male-rated subjects. V. I. Wolfe et al. also found that patterns of intonation were related to the gender identity of these transsexual subjects. This is an excellent reference for any speech–language pathologist working with persons who are seeking help in gender transformation.

Bralley, Bull, Gore, and Edgerton (1978) presented a case of a 49-year-old male-to-female transsexual who was administered voice therapy following surgery. She also received hormone therapy for 18 months, including Premarin (estrogens) taken orally or by injection. These produced no marked change in voice quality or pitch level. Her initial pitch level was 145 Hz (D_1) and she had approximately two octaves of pitch range (100 to 425 Hz). During therapy, her pitch was raised to a habitual level of 165 Hz (E_1), and she was instructed to increase the range of pitch inflection used in conversational speech.

Samples of voice at baseline and during treatment were included with other male and female voices and randomly presented to 15 judges who rated each sample on a scale of 1 to 7 (1 for *very masculine* and 7 for *very feminine*). The baseline mean judgment for the client was 3.7 (for the females 5.9, and the males 2.0). The treatment judgments for the client increased to 4.7 and 4.6, indicating that therapy helped increase the probability of a more feminine voice judgment. Bralley et al. reported that the client's voice more nearly resembled the feminine after treatment than before but still was clearly discernible from the voice of a typical female.

In helping a transsexual to raise or lower the pitch, the therapy must be complemented with work on the overall communication pattern. Objective assessment of the effect of clinical change must be documented in a manner similar to the Bralley et al. (1978) procedure. However, I think that because communication in most cases involves visual aspects as well, both audio *and* video recordings should be used in any study. I have used video recordings of transsexual patients in classes, presenting the patient for some other reason to determine whether the naive class members are suspicious as to the sexual identity of the client. Should the class member not comment of the gender of the client, a rather successful voice treatment has been obtained.

Stage Fright

Many persons experience in daily life or in formal performance the physiological changes associated with stage fright. The physiology behind these body reactions to "performance," whether in speaking or singing, were previously discussed in this chapter. It is very disconcerting to even the experienced professional when anxiety prior to speaking or performance causes physiological changes that affect vocal and speech control. Shakespeare was correct when he said, "All the world's a stage, and all the men and women merely players. They have their exits and their entrances . . ." (*As You Like It*). It is perhaps the natural state to experience anxiety (stage fright) when one is about to enter one of these stages and speak in an unusual situation with strangers or before large groups. Most persons merely struggle through it, often with voice quivering, with tension apparant in a slightly higher tone, and perhaps with thoughts somewhat cluttered. When the anxiety becomes so significant that performance might be compromised, however, physicians have procedures that might be helpful.

Beta blockers are used widely by performers and athletes to modify objectionable feelings of anxiety or stress prior to performance, particularly those related to muscle tremor or heart palpitations. Some performers, particularly those with extreme anxiety, might benefit from medically supervised low-dosage usage of Beta blockers. This is somewhat supported in the literature (Brantigan, Brantigan, & Joseph, 1982). However, Gates and Montalbo (1987) and Colton and Casper (1990) presented evidence that questions the positive benefits of Beta blockers, at least on musical performance. A physician can help a performer decide whether such drug treatment would be helpful. The usage of synthetic saliva (e.g., Salivart) might also be helpful to modify the dryness in the mouth which often accompanies stage fright or speech anxiety.

The Speech–Language Pathologist and the Psychology of Voice

As this chapter has indicated, the voice is intricately intertwined with the psyche. When aphonia or dysphonia occur because of psychological or psychiatric disintegration, the speech–language pathologist can be effective in restoring improving voice as part of the overall therapy team. Many speech–language pathologists have extensive training in psychology, are comfortable with the psychogenic bases of communication disorders, and have no difficulty knowing when to treat and when to refer. Other speech–language pathologists may not have the slightest idea when symptomatic voice therapy is appropriate and when it is not.

Certainly, it is wise to refer for psychological or psychiatric consultation whenever in doubt about the appropriateness of treatment for psychogenic voice disorder. When dealing with such clients, it is important to consider that, whether intended or not, symptomatic voice therapy is treating both the voice and the psyche. One of the most significant analyses of voice and psychological considerations was written by Brodnitz (1981):

> The success of vocal rehabilitation depends to a large degree on the search for emotional dynamics that have produced the disorder of the voice. Just to act as a kind of "vocal gymnastics teacher" who puts the patient through vocal routines, manipulates pitch, and corrects faulty breathing, is to treat the symptoms of a disorder instead of its etiology. Of course, such attempts to normalize vocal production have their place in voice therapy, but they have to be supplemented by a deeper understanding of psychological dynamics. A quiet hour of probing into the background of vocal difficulties, covering such essential facts as family situations, professional problems, and emotional conflicts will go far in obtaining a proper perspective for the understanding of dysfunction of the voice and for the handling of vocal rehabilitation. (p. 24)

Brodnitz ended by describing Rembrandt's *Christ Preaching* in which Jesus is preaching to 25 or more people, and not one of the listeners is looking directly at Him. Rather, each is in a state of attention, contemplation, and reflection in an attempt to understand what is being said. They are receiving the message entirely through their ears.

All speech–language pathologists can learn from this example, particularly when working with psychogenic voice-disordered clients. They must tune in to the messages the patients are communicating and attempt to understand their significance. Only then can speech–language pathologists be effective in knowing when to treat, when to refer, and what effect their management procedures are likely to have on clients with psychogenic voice disorders. It is evident to the reader that little information has been given in this chapter about instrumentation. Instruments other than audio or video equipment have little value to the speech–language pathologist working with a patient with psychogenic voice disorder. I contend that advances in technology will never make the human senses extinct, and this is never more evident than in the area of psychogenic voice disorder, its evaluation and treatment.

Summary

This chapter has covered the many interrelationships between voice and psyche. Several forms of psychogenic voice disorder have been described, including conversion aphonia and dysphonia, vocal abuse, mutational falsetto (puberphonia), transsexual voice disorder, and stage fright. Voice characteristics and treatment considerations have been analyzed. The interactions between the nervous system and the endocrine systems in the pathogenesis of psychogenic voice disorder have been presented in general terms. With this background, the speech–language pathologist should understand the nature of psychogenic voice disorder and treatment considerations.

7

Alaryngeal Phonation Therapy

Each year since around 1887, when the first laryngectomy was reportedly performed (Duguay, 1989), thousands of persons throughout the world have lost to surgery their vital organ of voice—the larynx—because of cancer or trauma. In the case of cancer, the patient's larynx must be sacrificed surgically to stop the spread of malignant cells in the hope of saving the person's life. In the case of trauma, the larynx is removed surgically because it has suffered damage that has incapacitated laryngeal valving mechanisms necessary to protect the respiratory tract from aspiration of food, liquids, or saliva. Regardless of why the larynx must be removed, life for the person involved is altered significantly: psychologically, sociologically, economically, often in employment, and particularly in communication. One whose larynx is removed surgically becomes a laryngectomized person. The term laryngectomee is used to identify such individuals, but the trend is to use the designation laryngectomized person. Laryngectomy is the surgical procedure involved.

Laryngectomized persons have many adjustments to make in life after surgery, often in all of the areas just identified. The speech–language pathologist working with such an individual must understand the overall significance of laryngeal amputation on the client and family members, particularly as to the impact on communication. Only then can the speech–language pathologist function competently in the rehabilitation process of restoring communication. This chapter provides perspective to the speech–language pathologist on the overall impact of laryngectomy, with particular emphasis on alaryngeal communication training.

The Nature of Cancer in the Larynx

Cancer of the larynx can begin in any location of intrinsic or extrinsic laryngeal tissue. Laryngeal tumors are classified as being supraglottal (above the vocal folds but in the larynx), glottal (on the vocal folds), and subglottal (below the vocal folds but still in the laryngeal region). The supraglottal zone involves the epiglottal region, including the valleculae, the aryepiglottal folds, the arytenoid cartilages, the ventricular folds, and the ventricular cavity. Glottal tumors arise on the vocal folds and on the anterior commissure for posterior aspect. Transglottal tumors appear both above and below the ventricle. Subglottal tumors are rare and arise more commonly from the lower margins of the vocal folds.

The location of the tumor is called the primary site. Any cancer that spreads from a primary to a secondary site is an indication of metastasis, which means the disease has transferred from one organ or part to another not directly connected with it. In the case of laryngeal cancer, metastasis occurs through the cervical lymphatic node system.

Exhibit 7–1 presents the American Joint Committee for Cancer's (1983) TNM classification of laryngeal cancers according to location of tumor (T) (supraglottis, glottis, subglottis), nodal (N) involvement, evidence of metastasis (M), and staging. With this classification system, physicians can determine the effectiveness of various treatments in terms of survival and recurrence.

Etiology of Laryngeal Cancer

Several factors have been identified as being etiologically related to the pathogenesis of laryngeal cancer. Smoking and excessive alcohol consumption are significantly correlated with its development, particularly in supraglottal and glottal cancers. Heavy alcohol intake has been shown to significantly increase the risk of laryngeal cancer as long as smoking is also present. When no tobacco usage is present, alcohol intake does not appear to increase the risk of laryngeal cancer (W. Lawson, Biller, & Suen, 1989).

Additional factors include exposure to organic amines and polycyclic hydrocarbons, herpes simplex infections, chronic infections, irradiation, air pollution, and leukoplakia or keratosis on the vocal folds. However, direct evidence of a relationship in an etiological sense is lacking in these factors (Myers & Suen, 1989; Ogura & Thawley, 1980). Case (1982b) reported a clinical example of the relationship between vocal abuse (nodules) and the development of laryngeal cancer without establishing or implying an etiological relationship.

Types of Laryngeal Cancer

The most common form of laryngeal cancer is squamous cell carcinoma. As indicated in Chapter 1, the true vocal folds have a covering of stratified

Exhibit 7–1 TNM Classification for Laryngeal Cancer

	Staging
Primary Tumor (T)	
T_x	Tumor that cannot be assessed by rules
T_0	No evidence of primary tumor
Supraglottis	
TIS	Carcinoma in situ
T_1	Tumor confined to region of origin with normal mobility
T_2	Tumor involving adjacent supraglottic site(s) or glottis without fixation
T_3	Tumor limited to larynx with fixation and/or extension to involve postcricoid area, medial wall of pyriform sinus, or preepiglottic space
T_4	Massive tumor extending beyond the larynx to involve oropharynx, soft tissues of neck, or destruction of thyroid cartilage
Glottis	
TIS	Carcinoma in situ
T_1	Tumor confined to vocal cord(s) with normal mobility (including involvement of anterior or posterior commissures)
T_2	Supraglottic and/or subglottic extension of tumor with normal or impaired cord mobility
T_3	Tumor confined to the larynx with cord fixation
T_4	Massive tumor with thyroid cartilage and/or extension beyond the confines of the larynx
Subglottis	
TIS	Carcinoma in situ
T_1	Tumor confined to the subglottic region
T_2	Tumor extension to vocal cords with normal or impaired cord mobility
T_3	Tumor confined to the larynx with cord fixation
T_4	Massive tumor with cartilage destruction or extension beyond the confines of the larynx, or both
Nodal Involvement (N)	
N_x	Nodes cannot be assessed
N_0	No clinically positive nodes
N_1	Single clinically positive homolateral node less than 3 cm in diameter
N_2	Single clinically positive homolateral node 3 to 6 cm in diameter or multiple clinically positive homolateral nodes, none over 6 cm in diameter
N_{2a}	Single clinically positive homolateral node, 3 to 6 cm in diameter
N_{2b}	Multiple clinically positive homolateral nodes, none over 6 cm in diameter
N_3	Massive homolateral node(s), bilateral nodes, or contralateral node(s)

Exhibit 7–1 continued

N_{3a}		Clinically positive homolateral nodes, none over 6 cm in diameter
N_{3b}		Bilateral clinically positive nodes (in this situation, each side of the neck should be staged separately; that is, N_{3b}: right, N_{2a}: left, N_1)
N_{3c}		Contralateral clinically positive node(s) only
Distant Metastasis (M)		
M_x		Not assessed
M_0		No (known) distant metastasis
M_1		Distant metastasis present

Stage Grouping

Stage I	$T_1 \ N_0 \ M_0$
Stage II	$T_2 \ N_0 \ M_0$
Stage III	$T_3 \ N_0 \ M_0$
	T_1 or T_2 or T_3, N_1, M_0
Stage IV	T_4, N_0 or N_1, M_0
	Any T, N_2 or N_3, M_0
	Any T, any N, M_1

Residual Tumor (R)	
R_0	No residual tumor
R_1	Microscopic residual tumor
R_2	Microscopic residual tumor

Source: Reprinted with permission from *American Joint Committee for Cancer Staging and End-Results Reporting: Manual for Stages of Cancer* (pp. 38–39), 1983, Philadelphia: J. B. Lippincott.

squamous epithelium. In carcinoma in situ, the epithelium of the vocal folds is replaced by a full thickness of cells with malignant cytologic features that can be detected by microscopic analysis. In the carcinoma in situ classification, there is no invasion of these malignant cells beyond the squamous epithelium.

When these cells develop beyond the epithelium, the carcinoma becomes invasive into the underlying muscle and other tissues of the larynx. Simple squamous cell carcinoma (in situ or invasive) represents the uncontrolled growth of squamous cells. Laryngeal carcinoma often is preceded by laryngeal keratosis (also called hyperkeratosis, squamous cell hyperplasia, or epithelial hyperplasia) (Crissman, 1982).

Other forms of laryngeal cancer include tumors that arise in the cartilages of the larynx (called chondrocarcinoma), as reported by Neel and Unni (1982), and of the glandular tissue (adenocarcinoma) (Ogura & Thawley, 1980). Sarcomas and chondrosarcomas are tumors of the connective tissues of the body, such as the bone and cartilage (Hicks, Walker, & Moor, 1982; Myers & Suen, 1989).

Epidemiological Considerations

Many studies to isolate factors of age, sex, and geographic location as they pertain to laryngeal cancer were summarized by Ogura and Thawley (1980). Basically, 85% of laryngeal cancers occur in the fifth, sixth, and seventh decades of life. However, Newman and Byers (1982) identified 33 patients with squamous carcinoma in the larynx who were under age 35 (mean 29 years, range 5 to 34 years). Lawson et al. (1989) provided extensive incidence, epidemiology, and etiological data on laryngeal cancer and indicated that laryngeal cancer is increasing among males.

Laryngeal cancer comprises 2 to 5% of all malignancies diagnosed annually in the United States. A slight increase in the prevalence has been noted since about 1960 (Myers & Suen, 1989).

Symptoms of Laryngeal Cancer

As indicated, laryngeal cancer can arise in the supraglottal, glottal, or subglottal regions and its symptoms depend on its location. Fortunately, cancers in the glottal region present an almost immediate symptom of hoarseness, one of the danger signals identified by the American Cancer Society. As Ogura and Thawley (1980) stated, "Any patient who is hoarse longer than two weeks should receive a careful inspection of the larynx" (p. 2518) since hoarseness can be caused by irregularities of the vocal cords, narrowing of the glottal chink, invasion of the vocalis muscle, fixation of the cricoarytenoid joint, or neural invasion.

Dyspnea (difficulty in breathing) and stridor (voice heard on inhalation) are late-appearing symptoms caused by bulky tumors or vocal fold fixation. When the patient responds to early hoarseness symptoms and seeks medical attention that leads to prompt diagnosis and treatment, the prognosis for survival is excellent.

In supraglottal cancers, the first symptom is dysphagia (difficulty in swallowing), followed by weight loss, halitosis, neck swelling, bloody discharge, and pain. Many times, the pain associated with laryngeal tumors is referred to the ipsilateral ear via the sensory portions of the tenth cranial nerve (vagus). In subglottal tumors, the most common symptoms are pain and dyspnea.

Treatment of Laryngeal Cancer

The treatment of laryngeal cancer involves radiation, surgery, or combinations of those procedures. The treatment of choice depends on the bias of the physician, based on experience and research data. The most conservative treatment for specific laryngeal cancers is radiation only, and for T_1 and T_2 lesions (Exhibit 7–1) the cure rate is from 85 to 96% by irradiation. In such cases, the basic voice is preserved to some degree and the airway remains oral and nasal; tracheostoma is avoided.

Several researchers have reported on the success and complications of various partial forms of laryngectomy. Bocca, Pignataro, and Oldini (1983) showed a 75% success rate after 30 years of supraglottal laryngectomy. Difficulty in aspiration often is a complication in such cases. Flores, Wood, Levine, Koegel, and Tucker (1982) discussed surgical techniques that can maximize the potential of successful deglutition following this procedure.

Dickens, Cassisi, Million, and Bova (1983) indicated that, except in a few specific cases, surgery may not be the treatment of choice for T_1 and T_2 lesions; instead, radiation therapy alone for 139 patients provided results that were at least equal to surgically treated cases but with better voice quality. Biller and Lawson (1981) discussed the vertical partial laryngectomy, and Hicks et al. (1982) described a conservative approach to management of chondrosarcoma of the larynx.

For T_3 and T_4 lesions, many surgeons resort to total laryngectomy. Pearson, Woods, and Hartman (1980), however, found success with extended hemilaryngectomy for T_3 glottal cancers. DeSanto, Pearson, and Olsen (1989) reported data on 28 patients with supraglottal cancer, 8 with cancer of the pharynx, and 3 with other nonglottal upper aerodigestive system cancers. Near-total laryngectomies were performed. In the 28 patients with supraglottal cancer and near-total laryngectomy, 18 were successfully rehabilitated with lung-powered speech and no aspiration. All 11 patients with pharyngeal, tongue, or invasive thyroid cancer were able to speak without aspiration. These authors reported success in the majority of these cancer patients by means of conservative near-total laryngectomy without loss of voice or significantly altered respiration. (See also the following references for conservative laryngeal surgery in cancer: Hirano, Kurita, & Matsuoka, 1987; Wenig, Stegnjajic, & Abramson, 1989.)

The specifics involved in total laryngectomy are well described in the literature (DeWeese & Saunders, 1982; Myers & Suen, 1989; Ogura & Thawley, 1980) and need not be repeated in detail here. The speech–language pathologist should understand the basic anatomical and physiological changes involved in this procedure (Figure 7–1).

The general procedure for total laryngectomy has changed little since early times (Myers & Suen, 1989). Basically, in a total laryngectomy, the larynx—including all cartilages, intrinsic muscles and membranes, and the

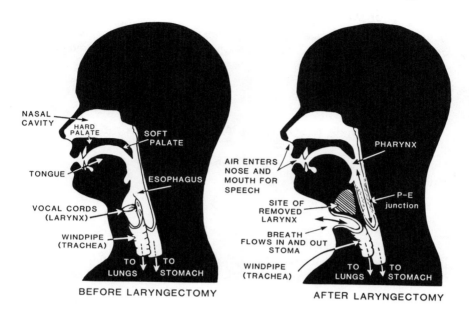

NASAL CAVITY
HARD PALATE
SOFT PALATE
TONGUE
ESOPHAGUS
VOCAL CORDS (LARYNX)
WINDPIPE (TRACHEA)
TO LUNGS
TO STOMACH

PHARYNX
AIR ENTERS NOSE AND MOUTH FOR SPEECH
SITE OF REMOVED LARYNX
P–E junction
BREATH FLOWS IN AND OUT STOMA
WINDPIPE (TRACHEA)
TO LUNGS
TO STOMACH

BEFORE LARYNGECTOMY

AFTER LARYNGECTOMY

Figure 7–1 Profile Before and After Laryngectomy. Reprinted with permission from *Clinical Management of Speech Disorders* (p. 212) by D. E. Mowrer and J. L. Case, 1982, Austin, TX: PRO-ED. Copyright 1982 by PRO-ED.

hyoid bone—is removed. The upper tracheal rings usually are sacrificed, and the exposed trachea is brought forward and provided with external attachment in the neck region just above the sternal notch. This external opening is called the tracheostoma, or stoma, and is the orifice for all respiration following the surgery. The stoma creates a permanent change for all patients as they become neck breathers for the remainder of their lives. Total laryngectomy often involves unilateral or bilateral radical neck dissection of strap muscles when there is evidence of metastatic disease; however, this is not without controversy. DeSanto, Holt, Beahrs, and O'Fallon (1982) reported no significant differences in cancer recurrence at 2 years between patients who were treated with radiation alone and those who had neck dissection.

The primary role of the speech–language pathologist in working with laryngectomized persons is to facilitate alaryngeal communication. Extrinsic and intrinsic alaryngeal sources of voice are available to help in this process. Extrinsic sources of phonation include all devices used external to the body to generate a pseudolaryngeal sound. These include the battery-driven electrolarynx (many types) or the air-driven pneumatolarynx (several sources) that utilizes air from the stoma to activate a reed to produce voice. Intrinsic sources of alaryngeal phonation include generation of voice by tissue vibration in the buccal cavity, in the pharyngeal cavity, at the junction of the pharynx and the esophagus (P-E junction), or by means of some surgically constructed shunt that connects the trachea to the esophagus to vibrate tissue and produce sound.

Extrinsic Methods of Alaryngeal Phonation

The following are the commonly used extrinsic methods of producing alaryngeal phonation.

Cooper–Rand Electronic Speech Aid

Figure 7–2 shows the Cooper–Rand electrolarynx. It is an intraoral device that consists of a battery-powered pulse generator and battery case that is approximately 3″ × 4″ and fits into a shirt pocket. This pulse generator and battery case are connected by a heavy-gauge wire to a hand-held tone generator that produces the alaryngeal voice. Connected to this tone generator is a plastic tube that fits into the oral cavity. The tone produced is channeled

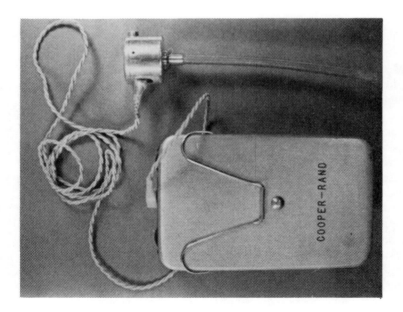

Figure 7–2 Cooper–Rand Electronic Speech Aid.

into the oral cavity for articulation and resonance purposes. Two dials on the top of the pulse generator control loudness and pitch. The speech–language pathologist must keep in mind that the two-pronged connector on the cord must be plugged into the hand-held transducer in only one direction; plugging in reverse results in a significant impedance mismatch and a noticeable reduction in loudness.

Many patients using the Cooper–Rand have difficulty at first coordinating the voicing with articulation. The placement of the tubing becomes a mild obstruction to the rapid movements of articulation until practice provides proper positioning. Once the individual becomes used to articulating with tubing in the oral cavity, good intelligibility is obtained. The lingual-velar consonants /k/ and /g/ are not produced well because the tubing placement is not far enough back into the oral cavity to facilitate the stop portion of these consonants. Context usually is sufficient to produce intelligible speech even in the absence of these consonants.

A primary advantage of the Cooper–Rand is that it is an intraoral device. Since a laryngectomy in most cases does not involve the oral cavity, the client can use the device immediately after the operation. Other extrinsic devices held against the neck are not as comfortable to use at that time because of soreness and tissue healing. The Cooper–Rand is an excellent alternative to writing during the first few days of postsurgical rehabilitation and is used by clients as a primary means of alaryngeal phonation.

Tokyo Artificial Larynx

The Tokyo artificial larynx is a pneumatic device that is driven by air from the stoma during respiration (exhalation). This is a rather simple sound source for the laryngectomized person, who merely places the mouthpiece end of the device against the stoma so air can be blown through it to vibrate a rubber reed. The other end of the device is placed into the oral cavity so the sound generated by the vibrating reed can be resonated and articulated into human speech sounds. The Toyko artificial larynx thus is also an intraoral device similar to the Cooper–Rand, but it is driven by air rather than by a battery.

Weinberg and Riekena (1973), in a study of a single subject using the Tokyo, presented data on its acoustic and perceptual characteristics. They reported 95% intelligibility with this subject, whom they cautioned might be extraordinary in ability. Since the Tokyo requires no batteries and has no mechanical moving parts, it is a simple and inexpensive option for alaryngeal phonation. The only parts that must be replaced are the stretched rubber membrane and rubber band that constitute the vibration source. The tension of the rubber membrane coupled with variation of breath pressure provides pitch variability.

Several modifications of the Tokyo have made it more convenient in many respects. One involves putting a soft rubber cover over the stoma mouthpiece to make it more comfortable to use against the delicate tissue. Another modification involves a hole at the top of the housing through which the client can breathe without taking the Tokyo away from the stoma. By placing the thumb or finger over the hole, air is shunted against the rubber membrane to produce voice.

Other similar pneumatic artificial larynges include the Osaka (Yamamura) artificial larynx, the Van Humen artificial larynx, and the Neher 5000 artificial larynx. These have been described in detail by Salmon and Goldstein (1978).

Western Electric 5C

The most widely used electrolarynx for placement against the neck is the Western Electric 5C (Figure 7–3). The client holds the device in one hand and puts its vibrating head in contact with the neck, controlling both the placement and the pressure exerted. The vibration generated by this device is transmitted into the vocal tract through the neck, and the sound then is articulated into human speech. Neck placement is most important to avoid sound spillage that is not directed into the vocal tract. Internal pitch adjustments are possible by adjusting a set screw while activating the instrument.

Zwitman and Disinger (1975) reported an experimental modification of the Western Electric electrolarynx to make it into a mouth-type electrolarynx.

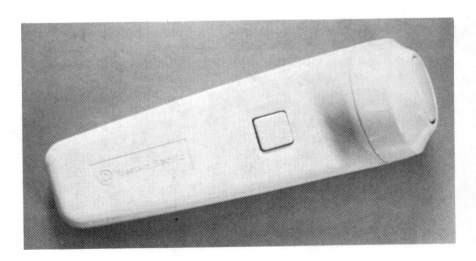

Figure 7–3 Western Electric 5C Electrolarynx.

It then functions essentially the same as the Cooper–Rand electrolarynx, against which it was compared in this study. Intelligibility data on the two instruments indicate no clear superiority for either, and both proved to be functional means of communication. The specific details of this and other modifications have been described by Salmon and Goldstein (1978).

Another study comparing the Western Electric electrolarynx with esophageal speakers was reported by Kalb and Carpenter (1981). This was discussed in a later section comparing esophageal speech with various artificial devices.

Servox Speech Aid

The Servox Speech Aid (Figure 7–4) and the Aurex Neovox (Figure 7–5) are similar instruments. Each uses a rechargeable battery system and has an adaptable intraoral extension. The Servox is a German instrument that has perhaps the best overall quality of all the neck-type electrolarynges. The sound is produced when a piston strikes a fixed diaphragm at a high velocity. The quality of the tone can be adjusted slightly. Pitch and loudness control also are adjustable but not in a variable manner during speech. These are expensive electronic devices, but the overall quality makes them worth the price. A similar electrolarynx to the Servox and Aurex is the Romet, as shown in Figure 7–4.

Several other artificial tone–generating devices for alaryngeal communication are available (Salmon & Goldstein, 1978). Centers for training laryngectomized persons to use the device are located across the country.

Intrinsic Methods of Alaryngeal Phonation

Buccal Speech

Although discussions on buccal speech are not common in the literature or in the clinical practice of most speech–language pathologists, it is a form of alaryngeal phonation and must be recognized and understood by persons working with laryngectomized individuals. Basically, buccal phonation involves producing a pseudovoice by pushing air through a constriction between the facial cheeks, lateral dental arch, and possibly tongue in the buccal cavity area of the oral cavity. The sound produced in this manner is then resonated and articulated into human speech, as is the case in any form of alaryngeal phonation.

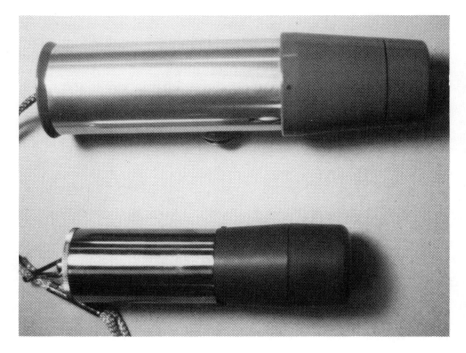

Figure 7–4 Servox and Smaller Romet Electrolarynges.

Buccal phonation in a laryngectomized individual should be discouraged, and an alternate form of alaryngeal phonation provided. Duguay (personal communication, 1984) feels that few laryngectomized individuals use buccal phonation.

Pharyngeal Speech

Pharyngeal speech involves pseudophonation that is similar to the buccal method, except that the locus of vibration is more posterior in the oral–pharyngeal cavity. It is produced by forcing air through a constriction between the back of the tongue and the posterior pharyngeal wall. It is easy to accomplish, and clients often generate this sound early in the therapy process when trying to achieve esophageal speech. It also is rather unintelligible, but less so than buccal speech; the likely reason for this is that the tongue is involved in both phonation and articulation in pharyngeal phonation.

Case (1981) presented a study of a 49-year-old male who was laryngectomized as a result of cancer of the upper esophagus. His surgery was rather

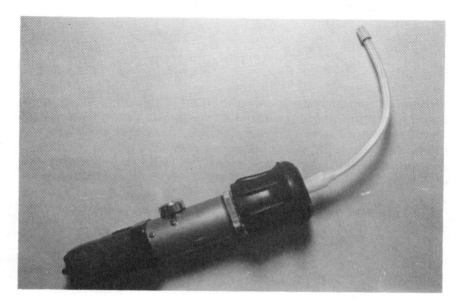

Figure 7–5 Aurex Neovox with M-550 Adapter.

atypical in that both his upper esophagus and larynx were removed. This required reconstruction of a pseudoesophagus by displacing stomach tissue upward to connect it to his pharynx.

Before learning esophageal (pseudo) phonation, this man developed excellent pharyngeal speech. Although the vibration source was not studied by radiography, it was thought to be the back of the tongue against the posterior pharyngeal wall. His fundamental frequency was 85 Hz and his speaking rate was 90 words per minute. His intelligibility was rated at 85% on the Rainbow Passage. In therapy, this man later learned superior pseudoesophageal phonation.

His pharyngeal speech served him well and was understood by most everyone except when talking on the phone. As an executive for a large national company, he frequently had to make long-distance calls. Because of his unintelligibility, many times the answering party would hang up on him, thinking it was a prank call. This frustration prompted him to attempt to learn another form of phonation.

Pharyngeal and buccal phonation must be recognized by the speech–language pathologist as undesirable and should not be reinforced when they occur. Once a client begins generating voice at a pharyngeal or buccal locus, it is difficult to correct, so it is better to avoid it at the outset.

When a client does learn pharyngeal speech, the speech–language pathologist should attempt to change the locus of vibration to the esophagus.

Torgerson and Martin (1976) described a case study in which this alteration occurred.

Esophageal Speech

Most laryngectomized persons attempt to learn to speak again using the upper musculature of the esophagus as a vibrating site for alaryngeal phonation. This is called esophageal phonation or speech. To produce esophageal phonation, the client moves air, which is present in the hypopharyngeal space above the esophagus, into the upper esophagus below its constrictive opening, then reverses the process so air is forced out of the esophagus under pressure. This causes the tissue of the upper esophagus to vibrate to produce alaryngeal phonation. The sound is then resonated and articulated into human speech in the vocal tract by the structures of articulation.

Esophageal Sound Mechanisms

To the laryngectomized person, producing speech by esophageal phonation is a simple process of using air to vibrate the tissues of the upper esophagus to produce sound, which is then formed into human speech. To the scientist or clinician, this simple process becomes extremely complex and is the subject of much debate in laboratory studies.

Hundreds of articles have been written in an attempt to isolate the mechanisms involved in (a) air intake, (b) air reservoir (neolung), (c) air expulsion, and (d) nature of the vibrator. The following sections highlight those areas of investigation to provide the speech–language pathologist with the knowledge necessary to help laryngectomized persons learn to speak again.

Methods of Air Intake

The schematic profile of the laryngectomized person (Figure 7–1) makes clear that surgical changes result in a trilevel configuration that is critical to understanding esophageal phonation: (a) the pharynx (lower aspect called the hypopharynx), (b) the P-E junction, and (c) the esophagus leading to the stomach.

Air intake for esophageal phonation involves somehow moving the air that is present in the hypopharynx through the P-E junction into the upper esophagus so that it then can be forced back through the junction to vibrate its tissues to produce sound. Two methods of accomplishing this air intake have been identified: injection and inhalation.

Injection

The primary investigation of methods of air intake, including injection, was done by Damsté (1958). The injection method is divided into two forms, one occurring before the initiation of speech (glossopress) and the other simultaneously with speech (consonant injection).

Glossopress

The glossopress (also called glossopharyngeal press) method involves using the tongue (glosso) as a pumping mechanism for pushing or pressing (injecting) air into the esophagus. Although Diedrich and Youngstrom (1966) distinguished between a glossopress and a glossopharyngeal press, they are regarded here as a single process, described as a glossopress.

In this method, the laryngectomized person usually closes the lips and always closes the velopharyngeal mechanism to trap the air present in the oral and pharyngeal cavities, then uses the tongue to press or pump the air into the esophagus. The tongue essentially sweeps or squeezes the air along the hard and soft palates and then along the pharynx in a progressive wave to force the air back down into the esophagus. As air is pushed through the P-E junction, a "klunking" sound can be heard as evidence that the esophagus has been loaded with air and is ready to be used to vibrate tissue to produce sound.

Because these processes are similar to tongue movements involved in swallowing, speech–language pathologists have used the terms "half-swallow" or "swallow air" or "the beginning stage of swallow" in teaching clients. The use of such terms or phrases should be discouraged for several reasons.

It is counterproductive for the laryngectomized person to associate this injection process in any way with swallowing, because the latter involves complex neuromuscular processes designed to move substances into the stomach. The air in esophageal phonation must not go into the stomach, and if the patient is attempting to duplicate in any fashion the process of swallowing when loading the esophagus with air, there is a great probability that air will be taken into the stomach.

Swallowing also involves a significant lag between occurrences, making it difficult for the movements involved to be repeated quickly as is needed in esophageal phonation. This can be self-illustrated by dry swallowing, then as quickly as possible attempting to swallow again, then again, then again. It soon becomes apparent that several seconds pass between swallows. This latency is counter to efficient esophageal loading for alaryngeal phonation.

Salmon (1979) suggested that the speech–language pathologist should avoid comparing esophageal injection to swallowing, even semantically. She recommended that the speech–language pathologist order the client not to swallow.

Perhaps such a strong statement can help the laryngectomized person learn to inject air without needing to equate it with deglutition.

Consonant Injection

The second method of injecting air into the esophagus for alaryngeal phonation occurs simultaneously with consonant production. Inherent in the voicing of many consonants, particularly stops and fricatives, is intraoral breath pressure that builds behind the place of articulation. This breath pressure can be used to force or inject air into the esophagus during the articulation of the sound. The quick movement of air into and out of the esophagus provides tissue vibration for voice. Thus, esophageal voice is produced rather simultaneously with the articulation of the consonant.

To attempt voicing with this consonant injection method, the client is instructed to articulate sounds such as /pa/, /ta/, /ka/, /sta/, /tʃa/, and /θa/. If the process works, esophageal voice is heard on the vowel sound following the consonant. The greater the air pressure on the consonant, the greater the probability that air will enter the esophagus. This method is effective for producing words that begin with the high-pressure consonants: *pie, tie, kite, stop, scotch, scratch, skips, paper,* and so on.

A word such as *toothpaste* has sufficient pressure consonants to load the esophagus for all the vowel sounds, and the client can say the word without much effort by merely articulating it as though a larynx existed. This also is true of such phrases as "pick it up" or "pass the salt." Unfortunately, most languages have many words and phrases that begin with vowels or low-pressure consonants such as "I am here" or "roll your eyes." Consonant injection is not effective as a method of esophageal loading for such phrases, and other methods must be attempted.

Inhalation

The injection methods described (glossopress and consonant) involve action of the tongue that increases the air pressure above the P-E junction to force air into the esophagus. The inhalation method is the opposite: The person is instructed to inhale air into the esophagus simultaneously with the inhalation cycle of breathing air into the stoma. Just as negative pressure in the lungs draws air into them during inhalation, a similar negative pressure occurs in the esophagus, drawing air that is present in the hypopharynx into the esophagus.

This inhalation method loads the esophagus with air to be used in producing esophageal vibration. Only the method of loading the esophagus is different. In the inhalation method, the tongue is passive and in a relaxed position in the oral cavity. The oral and nasal cavities are open so air is free to move into the esophagus as negative pressure increases, which draws air in.

The normal relaxed (at rest) esophagus has a mean negative pressure of −4 to −7 mm Hg (mercury) below atmospheric pressure and may drop to as much as −15 mm Hg (Dey & Kirchner, 1961). During loading of the esophagus by inhalation, the negative pressure in the esophagus drops to −15 to −20 mm Hg. If the tonicity of the P-E junction is sufficiently relaxed, this drop in negative pressure is sufficient to draw air into the esophagus in a pressure-equalizing process. The more relaxed or devoid of tension the P-E junction, the more efficiently air is drawn into it during inhalation.

This inhalation method loads the esophagus, a step that then must be followed by a reversal of the process to force the air out of the P-E junction under positive pressure. By this means, the tissues vibrate and produce alaryngeal phonation. Another study of this increase in positive pressure in the esophagus (Dey & Kirchner, 1961) found around 25 mm Hg to be sufficient to force the air out of the esophagus to vibrate the tissues.

Air Reservoir (Neolung)

One reason why esophageal speech is less efficient than normal laryngeal speech as a means of communication is that the air reservoir for driving the vibrator is reduced significantly. In normal phonation with a larynx, the lung capacity is enormous—2,000 to 4,000 cc (Zemlin, 1988). The air capacity of the esophagus as a neolung to support alaryngeal phonation generally is around 80 cc, which Salmon (1979) stated is equal to about 5 tablespoons. Little wonder that the adult with a normal larynx can sustain phonation for as many as 30 sec but the laryngectomized person does well to hold it for 2 sec.

Nature of the Vibrator

Diedrich and Youngstrom (1966) provided information on the nature of the tissue that vibrates and thus forms the neoglottis in typical esophageal phonation. This tissue is referred to here as the P-E junction. However, it is clear that the vibrator is more than simply a junction between two anatomical divisions of the gastrointestinal tract.

Diedrich and Youngstrom, looking at the nature of the pharyngoesophageal junction, analyzed 27 laryngectomized patients (23 males) with cineradiography and still radiograms. They indicated that the level of the P-E junction was variable and located between cervical (C) vertebrae 3 through 7, with most around C_5 to C_{5-6}. They summarized the findings of several studies, and reported general agreement that the P-E junction lies between C_4 and C_6.

Diedrich and Youngstrom also reported tremendous individual differences in the morphology of the P-E junction in both intersubject and intrasubject comparisons. They described the morphology of the junction as involving constriction of tissue on the dorsal or ventral side of the pharyngoesophageal lumen, usually in some combination form. It must be kept in mind, however, that these observations of the shape of the P-E junction were observed two-dimensionally from a lateral radiographic image. Three-dimensional perspective in endoscopic examination from a superior aspect might reveal even more varied patterns of morphology.

The length of the P-E junction responsible for alaryngeal phonation is as varied in intersubject and intrasubject comparisons as is the morphology. Diedrich and Youngstrom found a range between 18 and 23 mm for different vowel phonemes. They also reported a mean P-E junction length of 21 mm when measured by cinefluorograms and 29 mm from spot films; however, during actual phonation, the length of the junction was at least 5 mm of contact tissue and as long as 15 mm. These length factors were not found to be significantly related in any way to proficiency of alaryngeal phonation.

Perceptual and Acoustic Characteristics

After studying the nature of mechanisms responsible for the production of phonation involved in alaryngeal speech, it is important to investigate the characteristics of the sound produced by these mechanisms and the way they affect communication. The characteristics involve pitch, loudness, voice quality, speaking rate, and intelligibility of esophageal speech.

Pitch

The pitch or frequency of esophageal phonation has been studied thoroughly, as reviewed by Weinberg (1980). These studies in the early 1960s and early 1970s revealed the same typical information regarding esophageal fundamental frequency: The average fundamental for male laryngectomized persons is about 65 Hz, with a range of about four semitones.

The primary factors that determine fundamental frequency of esophageal vibration are tissue tonicity and vibrating mass, which differ slightly from person to person. Weinberg and Bennett (1971) reported data that distinguish male from female esophageal speakers. Naive listeners were able to distinguish the sex of the speakers 98% of the time for males and 80% for females.

Data presented in semitone form for statistical comparison showed female esophageal speakers averaged seven semitones higher voice fundamental frequency (F_0) than males. The F_0 for 15 female speakers ranged from 33 to

200 Hz. Strangely, the lowest fundamental among 15 females and 18 males was produced by a female (33 Hz), but it should be kept in mind that 8 of the 15 females had F_0s exceeding the upper limit of the range of males.

Loudness

Loudness is the perceptual correlate of intensity. It stands to reason that esophageal speakers should have reduced loudness potential since their air support and airflow amounts are significantly less than those of normal speakers. In my clinical experience, reduced loudness that makes communication difficult in noisy places is one of the most distressing aspects of esophageal speech. Laryngectomized persons often complain of having difficulty being heard in restaurants, in traffic, in automobiles while driving, or even in a room with a television turned on.

Snidecor and Isshiki (1965) reported that esophageal speakers have less ability to generate a loud sound. They found that a superior esophageal speaker could produce a spontaneous /a/ at 85 dB, compared with 95 dB by normal speakers. The normal speaker made smooth loudness changes ranging up to 45 dB, whereas the esophageal speaker could manage only about 20 dB. It should be noted that an ability to sustain an /a/ sound at 85 dB does not reflect an ability of the typical or even superior speaker to speak continuously at even close to those loudness levels. Therefore, it is misleading to assume that a superior esophageal speaker should be able to communicate functionally at those levels.

Increased loudness of the esophageal voice can be produced, but usually at the expense of other dimensions, such as quality and durability. I think that increases in loudness should be managed clinically only after functional communication has been established and the speaker essentially has automatized the processes involved in esophageal phonation. Then loudness increases can be attempted for specific communication needs without significant sacrifice of control in other relevant dimensions. Cooper–Rand manufactures a small pocket amplifier which helps increase the loudness of esophageal speakers (see Figure 7–6).

Voice Quality (Periodicity)

The voice quality of esophageal speech is described as perceptually raspy or hoarse. The variability in morphology of the P-E junction is responsible for the aperiodicity of vibration and vocal roughness heard. Of course, voice quality varies from person to person; there is considerable intrasubject variation as well.

One laryngectomized person with whom I worked put it best when he said, "You know, most people have good days and bad days. With regard

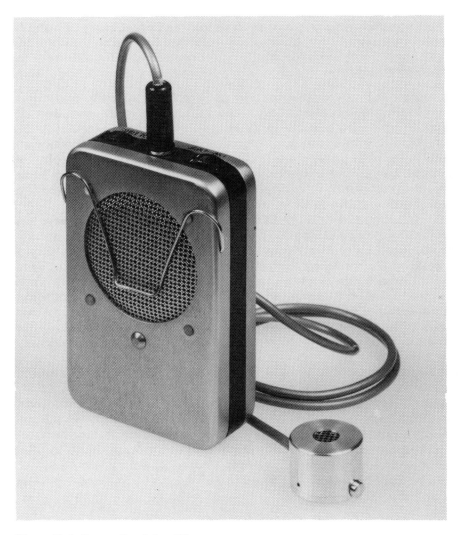

Figure 7–6 Cooper–Rand Amplifier.

to my voice quality, I have good minutes and bad minutes.'' Another laryn-gectomized male said, ''My voice quality is so bad, when someone who doesn't know me expresses concern about my bad cold, I feel I have been given a wonderful compliment.'' One female client expressed concern to her hus-band that she would never be able to sing. He said, ''Hell, Betty, you never could sing, so why the concern?'' All of these statements are testimony to the vocal quality that is typical of esophageal speech.

In a study on voice quality of esophageal speakers, Smith, Weinberg, Feth, and Horii (1978) tested earlier research findings which indicated that listener perception of the severity of vocal roughness was related to the degree or magnitude of spectral noise in the acoustic signal and that a strong, positive relationship existed between the magnitude of cycle-to-cycle frequency variation (jitter) and the degree of perceived roughness. Their findings indicated that jitter values of esophageal speakers were significantly greater than those of normal laryngeal speakers or persons with vocal/laryngeal pathologies.

When trained listeners were asked to rate the severity of vocal roughness, they were able to do so reliably, and the esophageal speakers manifested varying degrees of vocal roughness. However, mean fundamental frequency, mean jitter, or jitter ratios were not useful predictors of the perceived severity of vocal roughness. Therefore, it is not clear as to what physical variables form the basis for the perception of vocal roughness in esophageal speakers, other than assumed vibration aperiodicity.

Speaking Rate

The esophageal voice speaking rate is slower than others because the process of loading the esophagus, then squeezing the air out to produce voice, involves significant delays in the number of words spoken per minute. The scientist or research clinician studies speaking rate in terms of words spoken per minute. However, words spoken per minute do not convey the problem as clearly as did another laryngectomized person with whom I have worked: "By the time I tell my wife to go to hell, she has already died and gone there!"

Snidecor and Isshiki (1965) in a study of 6 excellent male esophageal speakers, reported that, compared with a normal speaking rate of 166 words per minute (50th percentile of Darley, 1940), these subjects were considerably slower in most cases. Five of the 6 had a rate of 80 to 128 words per minute, all below normal rates. One spoke 153 words per minute—within normal limits for the normal speaker—but this individual was an exception. The goal for esophageal speech probably should be around 100 words per minute for adequate functional rate of speaking.

Intelligibility

Regardless of speaking rate, pitch, loudness, and overall voice quality factors, if a laryngectomized person's speech is not intelligible, communication is thwarted and no other factors are important. Like the traveler in a foreign country unable to speak the language there, the laryngectomized person can order filet of sole and end up with chicken soup if the speech is unintelligible.

For this reason, several researchers have focused on the intelligibility of esophageal speech (Hoops & Noll, 1969; Shipp, 1967). Their findings seem to indicate that esophageal speakers are significantly less intelligible than normal speakers and vary more from individual to individual than do normals.

Many of these studies focused more on acceptability than on direct measurements of intelligibility, but in either case effectiveness of communication was being analyzed. Factors found that significantly influenced intelligibility and acceptability included aperiodicity of the vocal signal (which is really a measure of quality), amount of respiration (stoma) noise during speech, amount of silence, vowel durations, rate of speech, and consonant error factors. This last factor refers to difficulty in distinguishing between voiced and voiceless cognates such as /p/ and /b/, /t/ and /d/, /k/ and /g/, and /s/ and /z/.

Recognizing that intelligibility is influenced significantly by contextual and visual cues, Hubbard and Kushner (1980) investigated esophageal speakers in terms of intelligibility ratings obtained via three modes of stimulus presentation: visual, auditory, and auditory–visual combined. Normal speaker controls were used for comparison. These researchers reported no difference between the intelligibility of the normals and the esophageal speakers in visual mode alone (8% and 5%, respectively, both low). However, there were differences in the auditory and auditory–visual modes combined, with the esophageal speakers 88% intelligible in the auditory alone and 92% in the combined mode, a statistically significant improvement. The normal speakers were completely intelligible in both modes.

These data indicated that visual augmentation is helpful in improving intelligibility ratings of esophageal speakers. However, a vital point is that this study was done in a quiet environment (18 dB ASL), an ambient environment that does not approximate natural speaking situations. In more natural environments with higher ambient noise levels, esophageal speakers would be expected to have much lower intelligibility ratings.

One interesting adjustment that esophageal speakers seem to make in providing cues for improved intelligibility is to increase the duration of their vowel sounds, particularly in consonant–vowel (CV) contexts in which the consonant is voiceless (Christensen & Weinberg, 1976). This finding led to an investigation as to whether esophageal speakers systematically varied voice onset time (VOT) to distinguish prevocalic stops (voiceless) /p, t, k/ from the vocalic cognates /b, d, g/, and whether variance was dictated by place of articulation (Christensen, Weinberg, & Alfonso, 1978).

These researchers found that average VOTs associated with the production of prevocalic voiceless stops of esophageal speakers are significantly shorter than those of normal speakers, and that esophageal speakers increase VOT as a function of moving place of articulation from labial /p/ to velar /k/.

These results indicated that esophageal speakers are sensitive to the need for cognate distinction. Therefore, they attempt phonologically to modify articulation/phonation dimensions to accomplish these differences by varying VOT and increasing vowel duration in specific phonological contexts.

Esophageal Versus Artificial Larynx Phonation

Two studies compared esophageal speech and artificial larynx speech in terms of intelligibility and other measures of preference. Kalb and Carpenter (1981) discerned significantly lower intelligibility scores for subjects who use only esophageal speech (78.5%), those who use only artificial larynx speech (61.8%), and those who use both methods (67.3% for esophageal sample and 70.7% for artificial larynx sample) when compared with normal speakers (98.4%).

Green and Hults (1982) compared several factors, including intelligibility, in Tokyo pneumatic aid speech, Servox electrolarynx speech, and poor esophageal speech. Speech produced by the Tokyo aid was preferred by the majority of judges involved, although the visual aspect of Tokyo production was least preferred. The poor esophageal speaker was rated least preferred. As to intelligibility, the judges preferred both the Tokyo and the Servox over the esophageal. This information is helpful in terms of providing the speech–language pathologists data to show that alternate forms of communication such as the Tokyo or Servox are preferred and are more intelligible than poorly produced esophageal speech.

Rehabilitation of Laryngectomized Persons

The rehabilitation of a laryngectomized person requires the efforts of many people. A medical team is responsible for the physical care of the patient before, during, and after the surgery. Other laryngectomized persons in social clubs organized under the auspices of the International Association of Laryngectomees, a branch of the American Cancer Society, are helpful. Friends and family can offer such valuable support that successful rehabilitation is almost impossible without them. Psychologists and psychiatrists usually are available for counseling service. Finally, the speech–language pathologist is the primary professional responsible for communication rehabilitation. Each of these persons, professionals as well as loved ones, must function as a team working toward the successful adjustment and rehabilitation of the laryngectomized individual.

Presurgery Visit by the Speech–Language Pathologist

The role of the speech–language pathologist in the rehabilitation process often begins before the surgery. Many physicians request that the speech–language pathologist visit the patient, perhaps accompanied by a trained laryngectomized person who can provide a model of successful general and communication adjustment. Regardless of whether this individual is included, the visit must be planned carefully if it is to contribute successfully to the psychological well being of the patient and family members.

The presurgery visit should start with advance notice to the client so that family members can be present if the patient desires. This visit usually occurs a day or two before the surgery when the patient is in the hospital for testing. The speech–language pathologist should realize that the patient is often in a state of shock, anxiety, and confusion about the surgery and its implications for the future, even when the physician has spent time explaining in detail the procedures and likely results. In this visit, the speech–language pathologist should discuss briefly the changes that will exist after surgery, particularly from a phonation point of view. The following dialogue is taken from a tape recording of a presurgery visit by a speech–language pathologist the day before patient R.A. had a total laryngectomy:

SLP: I know Dr. R. has gone over the specifics of the surgery but I wanted to review the implications of what the surgery will mean from a communication point of view. This diagram (see Figure 7–1 or similar diagram) shows the before-and-after surgery changes. The main point is that your larynx will be removed. Your larynx is important for two reasons: First, it is a valve that protects your airway to the lungs (trachea) from food, liquid, saliva, and so on. Second, when air is forced through the valve during exhalation, the air vibrates the tissues of the valve and sound is produced. The tissues that vibrate are the vocal folds in the larynx. The sound of the vibration is what is known as the voice. You can feel the vibration of the larynx when you are talking by touching here. (Demonstration.)

R.A.:   I think I understand about that.

SLP: Good. Now, since the larynx must be removed, the protective valve will be gone and the tissue that produces voice will also be gone. To protect your airway, the operation will include bringing your trachea forward and attaching it to an opening in your neck. You will breathe through this opening in your neck for the rest of your life. It is called stoma. Do you understand that?

R.A.:   Yes, I knew that.

SLP: So after your surgery you will breathe through the stoma and air will no longer go up through your mouth and nose, and you will no longer have a voice. You will not even be able to effectively whisper since whispering requires air movement. (Demonstration.) And that is why I am here: To help you regain the ability to communicate, to help you find new ways of producing voice. Any questions so far?

R.A.: Dr. R. said I should be able to talk within a few weeks after surgery, is that right?

SLP: My plan is to begin working with you as soon as possible. Dr. R. will have to tell me when you are ready. Then, when he gives me the green light, we will work as hard as possible to get you talking again. We have many options available to help you with communication. Some can be used immediately after your surgery. Some will be faster than others, and I want to go over some of those options now. First, many devices have been invented and are available to laryngectomized persons. Some of these devices are very effective in giving the laryngectomized person almost immediate communication. Let me demonstrate some of these. (The next few minutes were spent in demonstrating the Cooper–Rand, Aurex Neovox, Tokyo, and Western Electric 5C.)

R.A.: Do you sell these?

SLP: No, but I can tell you where you can get one, and loaners are available until you can get your own, should you decide to do that. Most laryngectomized persons try to learn what is called esophageal speech, even when they are using one of these devices. What this involves is taking air that is always present in your mouth and throat down into your esophagus right here. (Shows diagram.) This air is then pushed gently up past this constriction and these tissues in the constriction are vibrated, very much like your vocal folds in the larynx are vibrated. This vibration produces a new sound, a new voice, and this sound is then resonated and articulated into the sounds of human speech. Because the esophagus is vibrating, it is called esophageal speech.

R.A.: You swallow air and I heard someone say it is belched up, is that right?

SLP: Not quite. You won't swallow the air because that would take it into the stomach, and we don't want it to go down that far; just a little ways into the esophagus. Then it is brought back up to vibrate the tissue. There are many ways to get the air into the esophagus without swallowing it, and I will help you learn them when the time is right to begin. I want to play some tapes of people who have been laryngectomized who speak with esophageal speech. Some of these people are very good and others are more typical. Then later, after surgery, I will visit you again with a man who has been laryngectomized and speaks with esophageal voice. I think you will find his visit quite helpful. (Tapes are played and discussed.) I will leave these pamphlets (American Cancer Society) and this book with you. You and your family can look the material over. Here is my card with phone numbers. If you or any members of your family have questions, please call. Good luck on your surgery tomorrow. Dr. R. is an excellent surgeon and you could not be in better hands. I'll be in touch.

This is a typical example of how a presurgery visit can be handled. It is short, involves demonstrations and materials, involves the patient as well as family members, and is encouraging about the future of communication. It provides information but not in great detail. It offers an opportunity for the patient to ask questions. Most importantly, it establishes the professional relationship necessary for good communication rehabilitation. It must be remembered, however, that it should not occur until the physician has asked for it.

The Artificial Larynx Controversy

The artificial larynx is not without controversy in the rehabilitation of laryngectomees. Many laryngologists and laryngectomized persons have strong negative attitudes about the use of artificial devices for communication, as reported by Case and Holen (1976) and Salmon and Goldstein (1978). Reasons for this attitude vary, but generally the objections are the artificial nature of the sound generated and the fact that the use of the devices prevents the learning of esophageal speech. It is evident from the literature and clinical experience, however, that many laryngectomized persons do not learn functional and intelligible esophageal speech (Diedrich & Youngstrom, 1966). A physician with a strong bias against the use of artificial devices can have such a strong influence on patients that they develop the same attitude.

This attitude is unfortunate because many persons fail to develop esophageal speech for a number of reasons. These individuals then have to turn to what is described as a crutch or a backup system because they could not learn the "best" method. A more reasonable attitude should be for all persons working with a laryngectomized person to have an open mind about all forms of alaryngeal phonation, expose the patient to each of them, and allow the individual to choose the form of communication after the surgery. The decision belongs to the patient, not to the physician, not to the speech-language pathologist, and not to another laryngectomized individual who might be in a position to offer advice.

Because some laryngectomized persons fail to develop esophageal speech, making alternate forms of communication necessary, Gates and Hearne (1982) developed criteria for predicting the successful acquisition of esophageal speech. The interaction of factors of site of lesion, preoperative phonation duration, postoperative physical performance status, postoperative dysphagia, and postoperative radiation therapy correctly predicted the acquisition of esophageal speech in 83% of cases in their study and also predicted failure to acquire esophageal speech in 93% of cases. Such information may prove helpful to physicians and speech–language pathologists in selecting patients for alternative forms of postlaryngectomy speech rehabilitation, making it even more important that an open mind be maintained with regard to the use of artificial devices.

The speech–language pathologist often provides specific instructions on the use of an electrolarynx before surgery. The Cooper–Rand or some modification of another type of device that involves intraoral sound generation is demonstrated and given to the patient to practice speaking. Then, a few days after surgery, when the patient is out of intensive care and feeling stronger, the electrolarynx can be used in communication. Neither a neck device such as the Western Electric or Servox nor a pneumatic device is likely to be appropriate soon after surgery. If an intraoral device is introduced, the speech–language pathologist should visit the patient a few days after surgery to determine whether it is being used. Therapy can be given at that time to facilitate its use for immediate postsurgical communication.

A speech–language pathologist who visits the patient should note in the hospital record the essentials of the call, that is, whether an electrolarynx has been presented, questions answered, and any specific instructions given about communication of which the medical staff should be aware. This also informs the physician that contact has been made. (See Miller & Groher, 1990, on laryngectomee visitation.)

Formal Alaryngeal Therapy

The speech–language pathologist usually begins formal and regular therapeutic visits when the physician indicates the patient is ready. Diedrich and Youngstrom (1966) reported therapy begins 2 to 4 months after surgery, but the actual time may vary; in recent years, it usually is much sooner—10 days to 2 weeks. The time to initiate therapy depends on many factors, such as recovery progress, whether radiation is to occur before therapy, and physician attitudes, but the speech–language pathologist should not begin until medical referral for therapy has occurred.

The initial therapy efforts should be directed at facilitating communication with artificial devices as well as with esophageal speech, assuming the patient has chosen these options. If the patient has been given an electrolarynx such as the Cooper–Rand before surgery and wishes to continue using it, the speech–language pathologist should evaluate the effectiveness of mouth placement, as well as articulation accuracy and intelligibility. If another device is desired, the speech–language pathologist should help the patient learn to use it.

When a neck device is chosen, the speech–language pathologist should provide direction, with the following recommendations:

- The nondominant hand should be used to hold the device against the neck. This frees the dominant hand for writing, holding another object, gesturing while talking, or shaking hands.

- The placement on the neck is critical for proper transmission of sound into the vocal tract. The speech–language pathologist should direct trial-and-error placement until the optimal spot is found.

- The patient should be able to place the device against the neck accurately without significant latency. This requires practice in moving the device to and from the neck in rapid sequence. This should be practiced before a mirror to help coordinate the process.

- The patient should be instructed in coordinating the activation of the electrolaryngeal tone with speech articulation. Users commonly turn the device on too early or too late for proper sequence with articulation. Patients also have a tendency to keep the device vibrating during speech pauses, resulting in an unarticulated buzz. Learning to turn the device on and off quickly and in concert with articulation is important and requires considerable practice.

- The patient should be encouraged to articulate with care and precision to distinguish between voiced and voiceless sounds (e.g., /t/ vs. /d/ and /s/ vs. /z/).

- Practice on the telephone with the device is important. The patient must have confidence in the ability to communicate using the device for emergency, social, and business calls.

- The electrolarynx should be set at a low intensity level for most communication situations. It is disconcerting to the patient using a device in public when everyone can hear what is being said. When the patient is in a noisy place, the loudness setting can be increased.

Accomplishing these steps will take more than one therapy session. Some part of each of the first few sessions should be directed at achieving excellence in the use of the artificial larynx.

During the first session, the patient also should be introduced to esophageal speech. The speech–language pathologist should determine how technical the instructions should be. Most patients do not understand complex instructions regarding the anatomical and physiological bases of esophageal voice, so a behavioral approach is recommended. The speech–language pathologist instructs the patient to do things that invoke esophageal voice without concern for whether the individual understands what is happening.

A. E. Aronson (1985), Boone and McFarlane (1988), Colton and Casper (1990), and my clinical experience indicate that a simple, rather direct approach is better during the first few sessions. It is better to tell the patient to say

"/ta/" and determine whether esophageal voice occurs than to say something such as, "I would like you to put your tongue behind your upper teeth, build up some pressure, hold the pressure a little while until it has a chance to move down into your esophagus, then, when the air goes into your esophagus, bring it back up and that will cause the tissues to vibrate. That vibration will be your new voice and with it you can say /ta/." While the speech–language pathologist was giving these complex instructions (which more than likely would not be understood), the patient could have practiced several /ta/ sounds.

With this concept of simplicity in mind, the following format for teaching a patient to produce esophageal voice is recommended. These steps are based on the work of many professionals already referenced, as well as my clinical experience. The order of the following steps is not critical, but each procedure should be attempted until esophageal voice is elicited.

Esophageal Voice Production

Step 1: Burp and Belch. The speech–language pathologist asks whether the patient has experienced a burp or belch since the surgery. If the answer is yes, the patient is asked whether this can be produced again. If the patient can do so, the speech–language pathologist asks for several repetitions. Next, the patient continues belching but with the mouth shaped for an /o/ sound. The speech–language pathologist should demonstrate the process. The mouth then is shaped for an /a/, then a /u/, and so on, until all the following vowels have been attempted: /i/, /ɪ/, /e/, /ɛ/, /æ/, /a/, /o/, /ʊ/, /u/, /ʌ/, and /ɚ/. Some vowels will be easier to produce than others. The patient should practice until each can be said intelligibly. Such quick belching generally does not involve air from the stomach.

Step 2: Consonant Injection. If the method in Step 1 is not successful in stimulating esophageal voice, elicitation with a consonant injection can be attempted. The patient is instructed to say /ta/, /pa/, /ka/, /sta/, /tʃa/, /dʒa/, and all other stop and fricative consonants followed by a vowel that is produced with the tongue low in the mouth, such as /a/.

By having the patient attempt all of the consonants, the speech–language pathologist can determine whether one is a better esophageal loader than another. If a specific one is, the patient should practice that consonant in combination with all of the vowels. For example, if the /t/ sound is found to stimulate a high incidence of esophageal voice when followed by an /i/ vowel, the patient should say the /t/ consonant with all the vowels: /ti/, /tɪ/, /te/, /tɛ/, /tæ/, /ta/, /to/, /tʊ/, /tu/, /tʌ/, and /tɚ/. It may be necessary to provide key words for each vowel such as /ti/ as in *tea*. This drill can be practiced many times. The same process then can be attempted with another consonant until all stops and fricatives have been tried.

Step 3: Inhalation.   If the first two steps have not facilitated esophageal voice, the inhalation method (explained earlier under "Methods of Air Intake") can be attempted. The patient is told to relax the throat muscles as much as possible, open the mouth as though about to yawn, then quickly inhale air into the stoma and attempt to sniff air into the nose at the same time. The speech–language pathologist should demonstrate this rather than describe it orally. If it works, as air is drawn into the stoma, it also will be drawn into the esophagus.

The patient then is instructed to say /a/. If sound is heard on the /a/, the process should be repeated until consistent voice is demonstrated. The patient then can shape the mouth for other vowel sounds as the esophagus is loaded by this inhalation method. Consonants can be added to the vowels to form simple words such as *pie, tie, kick, I,* and *above.* In the inhalation method, it does not matter whether the words begin with a consonant or a vowel.

Step 4: Glossopress or Glossopharyngeal Press.   If all these steps fail to stimulate esophageal voice, the speech–language pathologist can attempt to elicit it with a glossopress or glossopharyngeal press method, explained earlier. Essentially, these methods involve using the tongue to press or inject air into the esophagus in a piston-like fashion. The patient is told to put the tongue tip on the roof of the mouth just behind the incisor teeth, then pump it against the palate or pharynx to squeeze air into the esophagus. The movements in either of these methods are similar to the beginning stage of swallowing, except that air rather than food or liquid is being moved. As explained earlier, however, the use of the term swallow should be avoided.

As air is moved into the esophagus with these pressing methods, a slight noise (klunk) can be heard. This is the signal for the patient to push the air out of the esophagus to generate the voice sound. The voice then is shaped into sounds and words in a manner described in Steps 1, 2, and 3. The sequence is:

inject . . . say "/a/"; inject . . . say "/i/"; inject . . . say "/o/."

Later, after continued practice, the sequence is:

inject . . . say "above"; inject . . . say "drink it"; etc.

With this method of loading the esophagus, the patient can say sounds or words in any CV or VC combination.

The end result of these steps is that the patient learns to produce esophageal voice and speech. It is quite possible that the individual will learn to take air into the esophagus in a manner that does not exactly parallel any of those described. However voice is accomplished, if the patient can duplicate the process, and there are no negative aspects in the judgment of the speech–

language pathologist, it should be reinforced. It also is quite possible that after the patient begins to put sounds and words together into functional speech, combinations of methods can be used to load the esophagus with air. There is no problem with this, and it is more typical than atypical. Combinations are likely to occur without the patient's awareness as a consequence of the dynamic movements involved in alaryngeal voice and articulation processes.

Alaryngeal Phrasing

Once alaryngeal voice is produced and used in monosyllabic words, the next task is to teach simple phrases. It is the speech–language pathologist's responsibility to select phrases that are rather easy to acquire early in training. Examples of such phrases, as well as other helpful information, have been published by Lauder (1985). The speech–language pathologist also can have the patient practice words that are easy to say, such as *pack, tack, stack*, and *pick*, and put them into phrases such as "pack it, tack it, stack it" or "pack it up, tack it up, stack it up." The patient should articulate these phrases quickly. It is quite probable that esophageal voice, limited as it may be in this early stage, is sufficient to support the entire phrase.

Once a patient consistently and reliably produces esophageal voice and puts it into easy phrases, steady progress into functional communication occurs. It is important for the speech–language pathologist to keep the patient functioning at a high percentage of success (80% or better) as task difficulty is increased. For example, if a patient is reading a list of phrases, and 80% are intelligible, it is not necessary to be concerned about the 20% that are causing difficulty. The patient should pass over them after a single attempt. Often, on some future reading of the list, the difficult ones will be spoken clearly. It is counterproductive to become hung up on difficult tasks.

In addition to consistency and reliability of voice production, it is most important to work for esophageal speech that is intelligible. Strangers should listen as the patient speaks lists of words or phrases to determine whether the speech is intelligible. The speech–language pathologist often becomes too familiar with the practice lists to remain a good judge of intelligibility. It is of some help if the speech–language pathologist turns away from the patient as lists are read to determine whether they are intelligible without the conscious or unconscious help of lip reading. If a patient can be intelligible without the listener's having the benefit of lip reading, the speech–language pathologist can be sure progress is being made toward functional alaryngeal speech.

Esophageal Speech Phrasing

Early in the esophageal speech training of laryngectomized persons, it becomes obvious that careful attention to phrasing is necessary. The patient soon learns that the capability has not yet been developed to produce sufficient voice to complete some long phrases, so the esophagus must be loaded with air again in order to continue. This loading process should be done at breaks that are natural to the flow of the utterance and must be practiced repeatedly. Long phrases can be marked at suggested places:

Open the door/and bring/the book to me./

Stay awhile/but please/don't awaken me./

Tell the doctor/I'm not/feeling well./

Another technique helpful in teaching phrasing is to record a speech sample as the patient is talking about some topic of interest. For example, the patient is discussing going hunting over the weekend. After a few sentences of esophageal speech about hunting, the recorder is stopped and rewound. The speech–language pathologist then writes on a piece of paper or chalkboard the patient's actual language and marks the junctures used in esophageal loading. Whether the break occurred appropriately then can be determined. If it did not, a predetermined pattern of more appropriate phrasing is practiced (Exhibit 7–2).

Usually, patients can improve their speech flow by consciously attending to phrasing. There are no hard rules on this for the esophageal speaker. Rather, pauses should occur at natural breaks in the flow of the speech. It is best, for example, not to pause to load between an article and its noun. By emphasizing the noun and deemphasizing the article, the patient usually can put them together with the same load of esophageal air. Careful attention to appropriate phrasing facilitates better intelligibility in the patient's speech by providing context cues.

Avoidance of Poor Speech Habits

Many aspects of a laryngectomized person's esophageal voice, such as articulation, speech rhythm, and resonance, remain relatively unaffected by the surgery. However, the structural changes resulting from the surgery can have a negative effect on general speech habits and processes. The speech–language pathologist must be aware of any potential bad habits that might become distracting and affect intelligibility. The patient should be helped to eliminate them. The following are common areas of concern.

Facial Distortion

The patient should practice speech tasks in front of a mirror to minimize abnormal facial tics and distortions that often are part of esophageal speak-

Exhibit 7–2 Patterns of Phrasing

Key:
/ = Patient's first pause.
// = Suggested target of pause.
Terry/took the/truck/up the/road to/the camp/site/. We wan/ted a/truck/as/soon as/possible.   *Inadequate*
Terry//took the truck//up the road//to the campsite//. We wanted//the truck//as soon as//possible.   *Improved pause and phrasing*

ing. Eye blinks and lip grimaces during esophageal loading occur often and should be avoided from the beginning of training. This also is true of head jerks as air is taken into the esophagus.

Some patients have had radical neck dissection as part of their laryngeal surgery that can have an effect on head position during speaking. The speech–language pathologist should help the patient become aware of these facial, lip, head, and neck positions and determine whether adjustment during speech training can help eliminate them.

Stoma Management and Stoma Noise. Breathing through the stoma presents many problems to the laryngectomized person. Mucus accumulates at the orifice and must be wiped away constantly. Tissues crust and become dried by the breathing process, often resulting in coughing when pieces fall into the trachea.

Most patients are psychologically concerned about the appearance of the stoma and use neckwear to cover it (Kelly & Welborn, 1980). Patients become excessively "stoma conscious." This is understandable since difficulties are so common.

One primary concern of stoma control involves excessive noise during breathing and speaking. The size of the stoma varies from patient to patient. Some stomas are so small that breathing is impeded to the degree that air rushing into and out of the stoma produces excessive noise. This sound is distracting to the quality of speech. If a patient experiences difficulty with this stoma noise, it will be apparent from the first few utterances. The speech–language pathologist should help the individual become aware of the noise and attempt to reduce it. This can be done by teaching the person to breathe with less effort and not to push so hard with abdominal muscles during speech attempts.

The combination of these factors usually helps solve the problem. Once again, it is important that the speech–language pathologist be aware of this noise from the first moment it occurs so it will not develop into a bad speech habit.

Reduced Loudness of Voice. One of the most perplexing problems a laryngectomized person experiences when using esophageal speech is, as noted earlier, the reduced loudness potential of the voice. It is difficult to communicate in noisy places such as stores, restaurants, nightclubs, sporting events, and cocktail parties. Counseling is necessary to help the patient recognize the loudness limitation. It usually is impossible to compete with the noise of society. To attempt to do so results in reduced articulation control, unintelligibility, stoma noise, injection noise, and general speech ineffectiveness.

Increasing loudness should not be attempted until functional and proficient esophageal speech has been achieved. It is not an early priority in the therapy process. After speech proficiency has been attained, the patient can work to increase loudness by shortening the utterance, loading the esophagus more often, and pushing harder with the abdominal muscles as voice is attempted. However, these adjustments should occur only in unique circumstances. The laryngectomee should be aware that these adjustments for greater loudness diminish quality control.

Another technique that has helped some patients increase loudness is to apply slight digital pressure (one or two fingers) on the tissue of the neck where esophageal vibration can be felt. This can add constriction and tonicity to the vibrating tissue and help increase the loudness of vibration. The speech–language pathologist can experiment with the digital pressure to determine whether the technique is helpful.

A patient also can increase loudness by using an artificial device when going into a social situation with an expected high noise level. A Western Electric, Servox, or similar device can be more effective than an esophageal voice. If a patient has been trained properly to use all possible methods of alaryngeal communication, and has no bias against artificial devices, a difficult communication situation can be improved.

Goal of Functional Esophageal Speech

When has the goal of proficient and functional esophageal speech been reached? The speech–language pathologist and the patient together must evaluate progress to determine when such a goal has been attained. A. E. Aronson (1985) listed several criteria that can be used as a guide:

- Reliable phonation on demand

- Rapid air intake

- Short latency between air intake and phonation

- Four to nine syllables per air charge

- Two to 3 sec of voice duration per air intake
- Eighty-five to 129 words per minute
- Fundamental frequency of 52 to 82 Hz
- Average intensity of 6 to 7 dB below normal
- Good intelligibility

These criteria represent the goal of communication rehabilitation in laryngectomees when esophageal speech is the chosen form of alaryngeal voice.

Case Example of Alaryngeal Phonation

The following case example illustrates both the speech–language pathologist's frustration and satisfaction of working with laryngectomized patients.

L.W., a 49-year-old male, was laryngectomized as a result of cancer of the upper esophagus. His surgery was rather atypical in that both his esophagus and larynx were removed. This required reconstruction of a pseudoesophagus by displacing stomach tissue upward to connect it to his pharynx. He also had extensive radiation to his jaw and neck area.

After an extended stay in the hospital, L.W. was released with little clinical help in restoring communication ability because he lived far from the facility where the surgery was performed. He went for several weeks attempting to communicate by writing on a pad. He was an executive with the Bell Telephone Company and was aware of the electrolarynx but rejected it. On his own, he developed a pharyngeal voice by squeezing air between his tongue and the pharynx and became quite intelligible except on the telephone. He reported that his work required extensive long-distance communication and that operators and clients constantly hung up on him, thinking he was a prank caller.

Six months after his surgery, with pharyngeal speech his only means of communication, I met L.W. Because of his extensive surgery and radiation, the prognosis for learning any other means of communication besides his present method was unclear. I introduced him to several artificial devices, which he rejected. It was decided to attempt "esophageal" speech to determine whether his displaced stomach tissue could be vibrated in the typical sense.

After 3 weeks of this therapy, L.W. could produce short and rather choppy utterances with the locus of vibration in the pseudoesophagus. Although he was not satisfied with the quality of his voice, it seemed to him better than his pharyngeal voice. He was loading his pseudoesophagus primarily by means of consonant and glossopress injection.

On one occasion, L.W. was speaking with a group of student speech–language pathologists about his experiences with throat cancer, using esophageal voice in a rather slow and choppy manner but with complete intelligibility. During his speech, he put his hand up to press gently on the necktie he was wearing as he attempted to produce voice. A dramatic change in voice quality occurred. Rather than choppy and low in pitch, he produced voice with smoother quality and with less effort. The pitch also was higher.

After his speech, an analysis of the bases of change in his voice indicated that L.W. had begun to take air into his esophagus by inhalation and that the digital pressure, evenly disbursed by the tie, applied just enough pressure to the vibrating site (P-E junction) to allow quality phonation. The goal immediately became to improve this newly found technique of alaryngeal phonation. After 2 weeks of therapy, he had developed a superior voice quality with the following characteristics: $F_0 = 120$ Hz (B_2); 15 syllables per inhalation maximum with a mean of 10 syllables; 120 words spoken per minute with 100% intelligibility.

Several times at work after developing his new voice quality, L.W. reported that when talking on the phone, clients who did not know him asked if he had a slight cold. He considered such remarks as great compliments. He now enjoys addressing youth groups and is in great demand as a speaker. He is a totally rehabilitated person and an inspiration to people who meet him (Case, 1981).

Additional Methods of Rehabilitation

Singer, Blom, and Hamaker (1989) reviewed several additional techniques developed to provide alaryngeal communication to laryngectomized individuals. The various procedures have met with mixed success, but have failed to gain generalized acceptance and usage. Most of these procedures attempted to shunt air from the lungs to vibrate tissue for alaryngeal voice, and most are no longer used. This attempt to shunt air from the lungs and the difficulties involved changed when Blom and Singer (1979) reported an endoscopic technique for shunting air from the trachea into the esophagus, allowing pulmonary air to vibrate the P-E junction after laryngectomy. This procedure involves tracheoesophageal puncture (TEP) and the insertion of a prosthesis.

Blom–Singer TEP Procedure

The Blom–Singer procedure involves a surgically produced TEP that links the trachea and esophagus. The TEP can be done as a primary procedure at the time of laryngectomy (Hamaker, Singer, Blom, & Daniels, 1985; Wenig, Mullooly, Levy, & Abramson, 1989) or as a secondary procedure at any time after primary laryngectomy (Myers & Suen, 1989). Whether done as a primary or secondary procedure, a catheter stent is inserted into the TEP and maintained until healing has occurred. The catheter is then removed and replaced by a silicone (Silastic) prosthesis. The prosthesis functions as a one-way valve which allows air to be shunted from the lungs into the esophagus but prevents liquids, saliva, and food from passing from the esophagus into the trachea. Several manufacturers have developed prostheses for TEP insertion, including American V. Mueller (Chicago, IL) and Bivona (Gary, IN). The original Blom–Singer prosthesis is now distributed by Inhealth Technologies (Santa Barbara, CA).

Once in place, the prosthesis is stabilized by a retention flange or strap (see Figure 7–7). The prosthesis is also held in place by means of a retention collar. At the proximal (esophageal) end of the prosthesis is a razor-thin slit that resembles a duck's bill. This slit constitutes the one-way valve aspect of the prosthesis. Variations of the prosthesis are provided by the various manufacturers and include different lengths/resistances (from duck-bill to low pressure).

To shunt air from the trachea into the esophagus for voice, the laryngectomized person must either manually occlude the stoma or be fitted with an air pressure tracheostoma valve (Figure 7–8) that automatically closes during

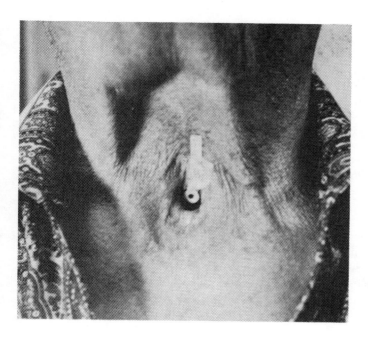

Figure 7–7 TEP Voice Prosthesis.

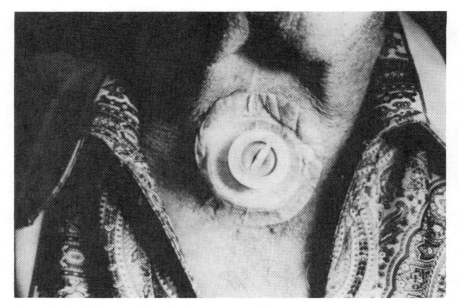

Figure 7–8 TEP Prosthesis with Tracheostoma Valve.

breathing for speech (Hamaker et al. 1985). A kit is available for determining the resistance of the tracheostoma valve so it does not close during normal breathing, but only when speech is intended. The valve chosen must not close easily during normal breathing, even under some conditions of exertion such as walking up stairs, but must be able to withstand the necessary airflow and pressure to shunt air behind it through the prosthesis for voice. A universal housing mechanism accompanies the tracheostoma valve and is held in place within the stoma by tape and a special glue. During coughing, the patient can easily reach up and remove the tracheostoma valve from its housing.

By shunting the air from the lungs into the prosthesis, air is diverted into the esophagus below the P-E junction. This air will vibrate the tissue of the P-E junction to produce esophageal voice. Theoretically, the sound of TEP-produced esophageal voice should not differ in quality from traditional esophageal voice, but does differ in durability since it is driven by 3,000 ml of lung air compared with less than 100 ml of air when the esophagus is the neolung. More will be written later about the actual rather than theoretical differences. The esophageal voice produced is then resonated and articulated into speech in the vocal tract in the same manner as laryngeal or traditional esophageal speech after laryngectomy.

Choosing a Prosthesis After TEP

Juarbe et al. (1989) provided data to indicate that TEP can be used for voice restoration even after extended laryngopharyngectomy. Regardless of whether it is used for extended or typical surgery, several criteria have been established to guide clinicians in determining whether a patient would be a good candidate for TEP alaryngeal phonation. Panje, Van Demark, and McCabe (1981) and Singer et al. (1989) listed the following:

- The stoma should be adequately sized and minimally 1 cm in greatest diameter.

- Patients must be capable of fastidious tracheal hygiene, able to see the stoma, and coordinated enough to insert and maintain the prosthesis.

- If done as a secondary procedure, at least 6 weeks should pass to allow for satisfactory maturation of the tracheostoma and patient ability to maintain hygiene.

- If irradiation is done, at least 6 to 12 weeks should follow before TEP is done to allow the acute effects of radiation therapy to resolve (Trudeau, Schuller, & Hall, 1989).

- Patients should be free of pharyngoesophageal spasm. This can be detected by means of an insufflation test to be described later.

- Patients should be able to meet other TEP speakers in order to understand the pros and cons involved from someone who is involved directly.

- A speech–language pathologist familiar with TEP must be available to facilitate and train the laryngectomized person in usage of the prosthesis.

- Patients must be psychologically stable, free of chronic obstructive lung disease, well motivated to attempt the procedure, and involved in daily communication. A taciturn patient prior to laryngectomy would not be a good candidate for TEP.

Insufflation Test

One factor that will preclude the successful utilization of the TEP procedure for alaryngeal voice is a pharyngoesophageal spasm. Some patients will experience a spasm as pressure is increased in the esophagus. The speech–language pathologist or laryngologist can evaluate a laryngectomized patient for ease of air movement through the P-E junction and identify spasm by means of a transnasal catheter insufflation test.

An ordinary French (14) catheter can be utilized, or an autoinsufflation procedure is available (Blom, Singer, & Hamaker, 1985). When the catheter is inserted sufficiently below the P-E junction, about at the 25 cm mark, the speech–language pathologist blows air into the esophagus through the catheter as the patient opens his or her mouth as if saying an /a/ vowel, or the patient provides the air when autoinsufflation is used. When an autoinsufflation process is used, the speech–language pathologist or patient must manually occlude the valve to shunt the air into the catheter.

Effective voice must be produced for at least 8 sec to pass the insufflation test. Pharyngoesophageal spasm will occur soon after voicing begins and the speech–language pathologist or laryngologist becomes aware of this restricting spastic factor. Lewin, Baugh, and Baker (1987) reported an objective method of measuring air pressures of insufflation by juncturing the tubing from the insufflation air source to the patient and simultaneously to a pressure manometer. Such a procedure helps standardize the pressures involved in insufflation from patient to patient.

When a patient fails the insufflation test but desires to proceed with TEP voice restoration, one of two clinical procedures will likely be necessary to eliminate a spasm (radiologically confirmed; see Singer et al., 1989): pharyngeal constrictor myotomy or pharyngeal plexus neurectomy. For the pharyngeal constrictor myotomy, the surgical intent is to identify and cut (tunnel) the inferior (including cricopharyngeus) and middle pharyngeal constrictor muscles, thereby decreasing their sphincteric contractibility. In the pharyngeal plexus neurectomy, the surgeon identifies the nerves that provided innervation to the constrictor muscles, particularly the middle constrictor, and the nerve supply is sectioned when confirmed by stimulation and observation of muscles involved. Singer et al. (1989) also indicated that such deinnervation can happen as a primary procedure with the laryngectomy. They also recommended that a myotomy of the upper esophagus and cricopharyngeus accompanies the neurectomy. The end result of myotomy and/or neurectomy is to provide a P-E junction that is less likely to spasm under conditions of TEP and prosthetic voice usage.

Steps in TEP Voice Restoration

Once the TEP has been surgically generated and maintained by means of a catheter, it often is the responsibility of the speech–language pathologist to introduce to the patient the actual prosthesis that will be used, and to train the laryngectomized person to use and maintain it. This requires training, skill, confidence, and tender hands. The following steps can serve as guidance, not as a recipe for the procedure.

• The speech–language pathologist must be wearing sterile gloves during the entire procedure of catheter removal and prosthesis insertion and usage. When the catheter is removed, the speech–language pathologist must be prepared to immediately insert the prosthesis. Measurement kits are available from the manufacturers so the proper length of prosthesis can be used.

- When the catheter is removed, the patient should be instructed not to swallow until the prosthesis is in place. With the catheter removed, exposing the open TEP, an attempt can be made to produce voice through the open TEP. Immediately after such an attempt, successful or not, the catheter must be immediately replaced.

- Next, the speech–language pathologist inserts the prosthesis. The catheter is removed, the prosthesis is placed on the inserter stick, the prosthesis strap is held against the inserter, the catheter is removed, and the prosthesis is inserted. As the prosthesis is inserted, a slight amount of pressure will be felt as the retention collar is pushed past the wall of the TEP. Once the prosthesis is securely in place, the difficult part of the procedure is over. The inserter is removed from the prosthesis by holding the strap against the patient's skin while twisting or twirling out the inserter. Before securing the strap with tape, voice can again be attempted. The retention strap can then be secured with tape. This procedure of prosthesis insertion is somewhat uncomfortable for the patient but does not hurt. Coughing may occur since the tissues around the stoma and TEP are sensitive to the touch. After prosthesis insertion and strap retention are completed, the patient should relax for a minute until any coughing is over.

- The patient is now ready to attempt voice usage. It is best for the speech–language pathologist to manually occlude the stoma for air shunting through the prosthesis during these initial voice trials. Instruct the patient to take a deep breath, exhale, and open the mouth as if saying an /a/ sound. During exhalation, the speech–language pathologist should occlude the stoma with as little pressure as necessary to stop all air from escaping out the stoma. If the prosthesis is working well, the patient will produce voice and a clear /a/ sound will be heard during the entire exhalation cycle. A little air escapage around the speech–language pathologist's thumb is not unusual at this point, but should be minimal.

- After a few trials with the speech–language pathologist occluding the stoma, the patient should be allowed to occlude using the thumb of the nondominant hand. The large mirror will help the patient see what is happening. After a few trials of inhaling, occluding during exhaling while producing /a/, then removing the thumb for normal inhalation breathing, the patient should be comfortable with the procedure. Then the patient can be instructed to count, name the days of the week, and say other trite phrases. This can be done with the patient occluding the stoma with his or her thumb.

- Next, the patient is taught to insert the prosthesis without help. The patient must learn to remove the catheter, refrain from swallowing while the TEP is open, then use the inserter stick to insert the prosthesis. The process should be followed for removing a prosthesis and inserting it again as would be done during cleaning. It is important that the patient understand that either a prosthesis or a catheter must be in the TEP all the time, even during the few minutes it might take to clean the prosthesis. Some patients will like to remove the prosthesis for cleaning after a few days, whereas others can go for a few weeks. This is an individual matter and depends on factors such as mucous secretions and general hygiene.

Tracheostomal Valve

With TEP alaryngeal voice, the patient has the option of manually occluding the stoma for voicing or using a tracheostomal valve (see Figure 7–8). The tracheostomal valve allows the patient to shunt lung air into the prosthesis for voicing without hand usage. The Blom–Singer tracheostomal valve (shown in Figure 7–8) involves a latex flapper valve which is open for normal breathing but responds to respiratory pressure and closes for voicing. Instructions are provided with the tracheostomal valve kits, but the following general considerations might be helpful:

- Needed material: brush-on adhesive, tracheostomal valve housing, double-faced adhesive, large mirror, scissors, and valve.

- With the prosthesis in place, the strap not taped, the tracheostomal housing is placed into the area of the stoma in order to test unique skin topography. The housing can be shaped to conform to these unique areas. The area where the housing will be placed is noted and the brush-on adhesive is then applied to that area, including over the prosthesis strap.

- The double-faced adhesive is put onto the housing, which is then placed over the stoma as previously fitted. A blunt instrument can be used to run over the housing to ensure its secure adhesion to the skin of the patient. No leak can occur, including in the area of the prosthesis strap which must be completely under the housing. With the housing secure, once again the patient or speech–language pathologist can manually occlude the stoma to demonstrate voicing.

- The housing is now ready to accommodate the tracheostomal valve, which is easily inserted into the housing in any position. During breathing, the valve flaps will be open to allow the free flow of air. When the patient wants to speak, an abrupt exhalation will immediately close the valve and air will be shunted into the prosthesis to vibrate the P-E junction. The patient can be shown that immediately upon cessation of voicing, the flaps will open for normal breathing. The flaps are available in various thicknesses to accommodate individual patient needs. The flaps must be thick enough to shunt air pressure but not so thin as to close during normal heavy non-speech breathing.

- The tracheostomal valve housing will be secure for 8 to 10 hours. It should be removed at night and reapplied the next day. During daytime naps, the valve should be removed but the housing can remain in place. Should the patient cough, a plastic bar extends over the face of the valve for easy and quick removal. After coughing, the patient should clean mucus from the housing area and around the prosthesis. The prosthesis will not be extruded during coughing and will not interfere with the process in any way.

- The tracheostomal valve need not be worn every day. Should the patient anticipate little talking for the day, he or she might want to forsake the process of fitting the housing for the day, and instead manually occlude the stoma for any voicing. The prosthesis is the only part that must be worn constantly, even at night, or the TEP will spontaneously narrow within minutes and close within hours.

The invention and manufacturing of the various prostheses and tracheostomal valves for TEP speech constitute a remarkable advancement in voice restoration after laryngectomy. Duguay (1989) stated that with the advent of TEP procedures and additional biotechnical developments, esophageal speech is being changed in a revolutionary manner. Lopez, Kraybill, McElroy, and Guena (1987) reported that 88% of surgeons (sample of 1,999) use tracheoesophageal puncture as a voice restoration procedure for an average of 30% of their patients. The younger the surgeon, the more likely it is that he or she will use the procedure. A large body of literature compares the TEP to traditional esophageal speech, artificial devices, and general concerns, and the interested reader is encouraged to investigate this body of knowledge (Gomyo & Doyle, 1989; Pauloski, Fisher, Kempster, & Blom, 1989; Robbins, Christensen, & Kempster, 1986; Sedory, Hamlet, & Connor, 1989; see bibliographies of the above articles for extensive coverage). In any regard, there is little question that the speech–language pathologist who works with laryngectomized individuals must be comfortable with TEP, the prostheses available, the tracheostomal valves, and management concerns.

Challenges in Laryngectomee Rehabilitation

The speech–language pathologist working with laryngectomized persons faces several challenges. The laryngectomized person often has difficulty accepting (a) the loss of communication; (b) the stoma and being a neck-breather; (c) the feeling of being a whole person who still is desirable to others, particularly members of the opposite sex; (d) intimate physical contact with a spouse; and (e) changes in the ability to smell, taste, swim, shower, and bathe. The person also may be unable to continue in a profession, may have problems with alcohol or drug dependence, and may live with the daily threat that all of the cancer was not removed and that it may return at any time. The speech-language pathologist must recognize that all of these factors can have an impact on progress.

A laryngectomized woman once received treatment from a graduate trainee in my clinic. This woman had terminal cancer and was expected to die soon. She knew it, the professionals knew it, her husband knew it, and her children knew it. Yet she continued to strive for improvement in her ability to communicate. She said, "I have to be able to plead my case with St. Peter!"

To ignore the psychological state of this client or others like her would be tantamount to clinical faux pas. The laryngectomized person is not "a speech defect," or "a stoma," or "a missing larynx," or "a P-E segment," or "an esophageal speaker," or "a Blom–Singer prosthesis speaker," or "a terminal client," but is a person, a human being, a father or mother, grandparent, lover. In all cases, the person is more significant than a laryngeal amputee.

In clinical work, these attributes must be considered as significant factors in the rehabilitation process. Careful interaction between psychology and physiology is required (Shanks, 1979). Only when these attributes are allowed to influence clinicians' attitudes about the nature of laryngectomized clients can clinicians be effective in facilitating general and communicative rehabilitation.

Summary

This chapter has provided the speech–language pathologist with background sufficient to understand the changes involved in laryngectomy and how they relate to rehabilitation of the laryngectomized person. General aspects of surgical alteration have been detailed. Considerable attention has been given to various forms of alaryngeal phonation, both extrinsic (electrolarynx, etc.) and intrinsic (esophageal and shunting procedures). Characteristics of esophageal speech have been discussed and specific instructions provided to the speech–language pathologist on how to teach the laryngectomized person to communicate again.

The philosophy of this chapter has been that the speech–language pathologist must provide information regarding all forms of alaryngeal phonation to the patient so the individual can make appropriate decisions as to communication choice. I hope that the speech–language pathologist will feel confident and competent in facilitating alaryngeal communication regardless of what form a particular patient might choose, whether it is an electrolarynx, esophageal speech, shunting procedure, or some combination.

8

Resonance and Miscellaneous Disorders

This chapter covers the resonance disorders of hypernasality, hyponasality, voice quality of deaf and hearing-impaired persons, and miscellaneous vocal disorders, such as laryngeal papillomatosis, webs, cysts, polyps, laryngomalacia, ventricular dysphonia, trauma, Mongolism, and cri du chat—a potpourri of disorders not discussed earlier. The main focus here, however, is on resonance disorders. One of the most significant areas of coverage will be disorders of the velopharyngeal mechanism.

It is appropriate to define some terminology surrounding the velopharyngeal mechanism:

- *Velopharyngeal Inadequacy*: This is a generic term that covers any type of abnormal velopharyngeal functioning, whether organically or structurally based.

- *Velopharyngeal Insufficiency*: Any structurally based malfunctioning that results in imperfect closure of the velopharyngeal mechanism.

- *Velopharyngeal Incompetency*: Imperfect closure of the velopharyngeal apparatus that is caused by a defect in neuromuscular functioning rather than a deficit of tissue.

- *Velopharyngeal Mislearning*: Functionally based abnormal velopharyngeal closure, such as in the case of phonological errors, poor modeling influence, deafness or hearing impairment, or any other nonstructural cause.

These definitions are somewhat consistent with those of of Loney and Bloem (1987), but are in complete accordance with Trost-Cardamone (1989), who recognized that the literature is filled with inconsistent usage of these terms. I will hold to the above definitions except when quoting other researchers, in which case their terms will be maintained as written with added editorial clarification in parentheses.

Disorders of Resonance

As explained in Chapter 1, many of the voice quality dimensions of human phonation result from resonance of the glottal sound in the vocal tract. Three types of vocal resonance abnormalities are hypernasality, hyponasality, and those resulting from deafness or hearing impairment.

Hypernasality

Hypernasality is a general term with several synonyms in the literature: nasality, hyperrhinolalia, hyperrhinophonia, rhinolalia aperta, and assimilated nasality. The condition involves excessive resonance in the nasal cavity during voice production because of coupling of the oral and nasal cavities via the velopharyngeal port.

As mentioned, the speech articulation structure that regulates the extent of nasal cavity participation in the resonance of voice is the velopharyngeal mechanism (also called palatopharyngeal mechanism), comprising the velum (soft palate) and pharyngeal muscles at the same level (superior constrictor). In Chapter 1, the anatomical and physiological bases to velopharyngeal closure were reviewed; Figure 8–1 shows a lateral view of the velopharyngeal port in both open and closed states.

Under normal conditions, velopharyngeal closure is sufficient to completely separate the oral and nasal cavities so that no airflow is allowed to escape nasally during speech production of nonnasal consonants (A. E. Thompson & Hixon, 1979). With 112 normal subjects ranging in age from 3 to 37, Thompson and Hixon reported nasal flow to be zero during all oral consonant and vowel utterances, suggesting airtight velopharyngeal closure. Flow occurred during all nasal consonants /m/, /n/ and /ŋ/ and during vowels adjacent to nasal consonants (assimilation). It is clear, therefore, that the normal

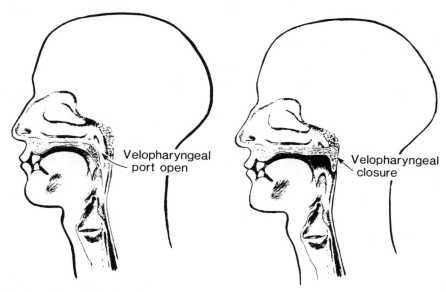

Figure 8–1 Velopharyngeal Port—Two Stages.

velopharyngeal mechanism should be completely closed for nonnasal speech sounds and sufficiently open to allow resonance coupling and airflow for the nasal consonants.

Before describing the various conditions that can affect the velopharyngeal port and produce speech phenomena that in the past were labeled "cleft palate speech" forms, I want to establish my philosophy regarding the role of the speech–language pathologist in such cases. Since this chapter focuses on the resonance disorders surrounding velopharyngeal insufficiency, and not the articulatory and non–voice-related aspects, it is appropriate to define the limits of voice therapy in cases of velopharyngeal insufficiency, incompetency, and inadequacy.

When a child or adult has a hypernasal voice quality, the nasal cavity is participating as a resonator in the production of vowel sounds and voice consonants. Under normal conditions, adequate velopharyngeal closure would prevent such resonance. In the majority of cases, such consistent nasal resonation on vowels and voiced consonants is evidence of velopharyngeal inadequacy. Depending on the extent of inadequacy, articulation processes are likely affected, and nasal air emission and reduced oral pressure would also occur consistently to some degree across all pressure sounds. In such cases, the speech–language pathologist should direct efforts toward objective evaluation of the mechanism and not toward therapy to change speech or voice. When nasal air emission is heard on only isolated pressure sounds, such as the /s/ phoneme, therapy should be directed toward its elimination. No hypernasality (consistent nasal quality on vowels and voiced consonants) will likely be heard. Should a child have excessive nasality on vowels and voice consonants but normal articulation, therapy might be helpful in reducing the nasality but is unlikely to eliminate it. Physical management should be taken in such instances, as explained in this chapter (Peterson-Falzone, 1984).

Several clinical conditions can disrupt functioning of the velopharyngeal port, including orofacial clefting; structural abnormalities other than clefting, such as a deep pharynx, short soft palate, improper muscle attachment as in a submucous cleft, or short hard palate; posttonsillectomy and postadenoidec-tomy deficiency; paresis from central or peripheral nerve damage; maxillary advancement; and miscellaneous factors.

Orofacial Clefting

Several researchers have provided data on the presence of speech and voice abnormalities secondary to orofacial clefting of the velum and other related structures (Bzoch, 1989a; McWilliams, Morris, & Shelton, 1990). Even after primary surgical correction of an orofacial cleft, residual velopharyngeal insuf-ficiency can remain to produce a deleterious effect on speech development.

When the velopharyngeal insufficiency is significant, articulation abnor-malities occur on pressure consonants. If the insufficiency is slight or border-line, articulation of consonants is usually normal unless affected by some other etiology such as dental malocclusion, hearing loss, or poor oral sensation. However, a slight or borderline insufficiency produces a nasal quality to the voice.

Perceptual judgments of hypernasality ranging from slight to severe can be made utilizing the Voice Profile (F. B. Wilson & Rice, 1977) (see Exhibit 3–2). A rating of 1 indicates normal resonance. Resonance ratings of +2, +3, or +4 reflect the range from slight (assimilation) to severe (nasal resonance on the vowels and nasal airflow on the pressure consonants). Children born with orofacial clefts can have normal speech or any one of these categories of hypernasality.

Many excellent references exist to guide the speech–language pathologist in the management of clients born with orofacial clefts, including:

- Etiological endogenous factors of genetics and exogenous environmental factors (Jung, 1989)

- Primary surgical considerations (Ross, 1987a, 1987b, 1987c)

- Dental, orthodontic, and prosthodontic concerns (McWilliams et al., 1990)

- Audiological and otological problems (Kemker & Zarajczyk, 1989)

- Communication disorder associated with orofacial clefting (Bzoch, 1989a; Marsh, 1986; McWilliams et al., 1990; Riski, 1979; Schneider & Shprintzen, 1980; Thorogood & Tickle, 1988)

The nature of the clinical problems resulting from orofacial clefting is beyond the scope of this chapter, with the exception of the associated voice disorder, specifically the nasal resonance aspect. Only this aspect is covered in sufficient detail to provide management techniques for the speech–language pathologist. Clinical management techniques are presented later following the discussion of additional etiological considerations of hypernasality.

Other Structural Abnormalities

Several oral anomalies other than orofacial clefting can have a deleterious effect on velopharyngeal closure and produce hypernasality. Some of these are described by Bradley (1989). Examples of palatopharyngeal (velopharyngeal) insufficiencies in the absence of overt cleft palate include (a) a short but intact hard palate; (b) a short but intact velum; (c) a deep pharynx, making closure difficult; (d) congenital palatal webbing of tissue that tethers the velum downward, impeding the movements of the velum during closure (Warren, Beven, & Winslow, 1978); and (e) abnormal muscle attachment in the velum as in the submucous cleft (Velasco, Ysunza, Hernandez, & Marquez, 1988). Any one of these conditions can alter velopharyngeal closure enough to allow coupling of the oral and nasal cavities to produce hypernasal resonance.

Posttonsillectomy and Postadenoidectomy

Hypernasality has resulted from the surgical removal of the lymphatic tissue that comprises the pharyngeal (adenoid) and palatine tonsils in the nasopharynx and oropharynx, respectively (L. I. Lawson et al., 1972). The procedure is called tonsillectomy (palatine tonsils) or adenoidectomy (pharyngeal tonsils). Although the number of cases resulting in hypernasality after surgery is small compared with the number of children who undergo the procedure—1 in 1,450 surgical cases (Gibb, 1958)—there usually are clear indications before the operation of the possibility of residual hypernasality, making it imperative that surgeons screen for that potentiality in advance (Mason, 1973). Lubit (1967) reported that 71% of the children who had adenoidectomies resulting in hypernasality had clear symptoms of speech defect prior to the operation.

However, Croft, Shprintzen, and Ruben (1981) presented data to indicate that many children in their study showed no significant abnormal speech patterns before adenotonsillectomy and still ended up with postoperative persistent hypernasality and associated speech disorder. They reported that of 120 patients with hypernasality following the surgery, 48 had no evidence of preoperative abnormal speech. The largest number of subjects had classic submucous cleft palate (35, or 29%), whereas 20 (or 17%) had the occult submucous cleft palate (described later). The remaining patients had a variety of neurological disorders, functional abnormalities, and idiopathic etiologies of insufficiency that were unmasked by the surgery.

Removal of adenoid tissue will not produce persistent hypernasality unless a congenital structural abnormality is unmasked by the surgery. In other words, in such cases, the presence of the adenoid tissue adds bulk to the pharynx against which the muscles of velopharyngeal closure move. When the bulk is removed surgically, a congenital insufficiency is unmasked, making normal velopharyngeal closure impossible.

Mason and Warren (1980) reported a similar problem with regard to hypernasality developing in cleft palate children because of adenoid involution. In two cases of cleft palate studied longitudinally, these researchers demonstrated the gradual involution (decrease in amount of tissue), of the adenoid tissue, causing the development of hypernasality. The effect is documented by longitudinal radiography and aeromechanical flow studies. This research also can help the speech–language pathologist understand the anatomical and physiological functions of adenoid tissue and the implications of adenotonsillectomy.

A significant concern to professionals in voice disorder management with regard to the question of nasality and denasality has to do with the concept of nasal resistance. Nasal resistance affects the patency of the nasal cavity for respiration (Hairfield, Warren, & Seaton, 1988; Warren, Hairfield, & Dalston, 1990) and nasal resonation (Dalston & Warren, 1986; Fox, Lynch, & Cronin, 1988). Several factors affect the patency of nasal airway for these respiratory and resonatory phenomena, including nostril closure or restricted anterior nasal opening, collapsed liminal valve, hypertrophied turbinates, deviated nasal septum, nasal polypoid development or other growths such as cysts, misplaced foreign objects such as beans or pencil erasers, and the common occupance of hypertrophied adenoids. Nasal airway resistance can also be affected by abnormalities at the velopharyngeal port itself in the case of pharyngeal flap pharyngoplasty, webbing, or large palatine tonsils. These factors can act singularly or in combination to decrease the patency of the nasal cavity for its intended purposes.

Considerable attention has been given by clinicians and researchers to nasal airway patency or obstruction. General references regarding the usage of aeromechanical pressure and flow measurements (see Chapter 3) are found in McWilliams et al. (1990) and Warren (1989). Allison and Leeper (1990) reported on several variables that might affect such measurement, including tongue posture, respiratory pattern, and repeated measures over time. Since aeromechanical measurement is often used to assess indirectly the size and adequacy of the velopharyngeal port for speech and voice purposes, it is important to understand the contribution of nasal airway resistance to such assessment.

Paresis from Nerve Damage

Several of the dysarthrias discussed in Chapter 4 involve dysfunction of the velopharyngeal mechanism, producing hypernasality and additional articulation disorder. Dysarthrias, for example, can produce palatal paresis, resulting in hypernasality (Johns, 1985).

Maxillary Advancement

Many craniofacial anomalies are being treated with various forms of surgery in which large segments of the facial skeleton are brought into harmony and balance. One common procedure by oral surgeons is the LeFort I maxillary advancement osteotomy. This is performed when there is maxillary micrognathia resulting from childhood injury, cleft palate, specific craniofacial syndromes (e.g., Crouzon's), and other miscellaneous anomalies. The technique is outlined by S. A. Wolfe & Berkowitz (1989). The entire maxillary segment is advanced in relation to the mandible, including the soft tissue of the velum. Because of the anteriorly directed velum relative to the pharynx, velopharyngeal insufficiency can result from this procedure, producing hypernasality.

A review of the literature and my clinical experience indicate that maxillary advancement is unlikely to cause a deterioration of velopharyngeal functioning in non–cleft palate patients or patients who have had excellent palatopharyngeal closure. Patients who have denasality and articulation disorder often demonstrate significant improvement in resonance and articulation following maxillary advancement. However, patients with clefts or borderline velopharyngeal closure are likely to manifest deterioration of velopharyngeal valving after advancement, and their voice quality will increase in nasal resonation. Also, individual patient variation and surgical technique in maxillary advancement make it difficult to predict whether advancement will produce velopharyngeal insufficiency. The report by Kummer, Strife, Grau, Creaghead, and Lee (1989) and the commentary by Witzel (1989) will help the speech–language pathologist to appreciate the polemics of maxillary advancement as they pertain to speech and voice. Several additional references are recommended in the case of maxillary advancement as part of Le Fort procedures in the treatment of the craniofacial dysostoses seen in Crouzon's, Apert's, and other craniofacial anomalies (Bachmayer & Ross, 1986; Kaban, Conover, & Mulliken, 1986; Kreiborg & Aduss, 1986).

Case Study

M.A.H. is a woman born with Apert's syndrome (acrocephalosyndactyly). As a result of this autosomal dominant mutation, M.A.H. was born with craniosynostosis (premature closure of cranial sutures producing significant head growth deformity), midfacial hypoplasia which caused eye protrusions (exopthalmia), dental malocclusion (Class III with severe openbite), and syndactyly (fusion of fingers and toes). Her oral cavity configurations, besides the malocclusion, included an abnormal palatal vault and velopharyngeal abnormalities. Her midfacial hypoplasia produced a small nasopharyngeal space forcing an open-mouth breathing posture, and her voice quality was hyponasal. Her velopharyngeal insufficiency added a component of hypernasality mixed with her denasality. She also had articulation abnormalities, but her speech was quite intelligible.

Because of the severity of her craniofacial and general body differences, M.A.H. was thought to be significantly retarded at birth and was institutionalized as mentally retarded for 14 years. However, she was later discovered to have essentially normal intelligence and learned to live successfully as an adult outside the institution. Her significant craniofacial differences continued to make life difficult for her.

In 1989, M.A.H. was evaluated by the Southwest Craniofacial Team (of which I am a member). It was determined that craniofacial surgery could be done on M.A.H., and a plan was generated that involved two major surgeries, one on her cranium and another on her midfacial area. These were done in 1989.

The surgeries significantly helped M.A.H.'s speech and voice. The Le Fort III osteotomy provided the opportunity to improve nasal airway for respiration and nasal resonance, and to correct her dental malocclusion and openbite. Her voice quality significantly improved as the hyponasality factor was reduced. M.A.H. continues to improve with time. In her case, a highly specialized team of physicians and nonmedical specialists have worked harmoniously to reduce the impact of nature's often cruel effects in terms of her cosmetic appearance, her speech and voice, and her sense of hope and future. (For information on Apert's and similar craniofacial syndromes, see Bzoch, 1989a; Jung, 1989; McWilliams et al., 1990.)

Miscellaneous Factors

Several additional factors can alter the functional relationships of the velum and pharynx to produce hypernasality:

- Cancer of the oral cavity resulting in ablative surgery of a critical part involved in velopharyngeal closure (Tardy, Toriumi, & Broadway, 1989)

- Prolonged wearing of spinal brace for the treatment of scoliosis (Skelly, Donaldson, Scheer, & Guzzardo, 1971)

- Abnormal regional growth abnormalities affecting velopharyngeal closure (Bradley, 1989)

- The "occult" submucous cleft in which the classic triad associated with the traditional submucous cleft is missing (notching of the bony hard palate, midline separation of muscles in the velum, and bifid or split uvula) but that nevertheless involves abnormal muscle attachment of the velum (Bradley, 1989; E. M. Kaplan, 1977)

Phoneme-specific nasal emission without velopharyngeal inadequacy can often be mistaken for nasality and nasal emission patterns that require physical management. It is important that the speech–language pathologist recognize the difference. An excellent reference for helping in that discrimination is Peterson-Falzone and Graham (1990).

The significant usage of cocaine in some populations is beginning to take its toll on the noses and pharyngeal structures of those who use/abuse this drug. Deutsch and Millard (1989) reported cases in which cocaine usage has caused significant deterioration of nasal and pharyngeal structures, including a retracted and asymmetric velum, absent uvula, and ulceration on the superior border of the palate down to the pharyngeal wall involved in velopharyngeal closure.

Treatment of Hypernasality Disorders

Treatment of hypernasality often involves both physical management of the velopharyngeal mechanism (pharyngeal flap surgery, prosthetic obturation, Teflon pharyngoplasty) and various forms of voice therapy. One of the most important clinical tasks facing the speech–language pathologist in management of the hypernasal client is to determine whether the velopharyngeal mechanism is adequate, incompetent, insufficient, or inadequate. Several techniques can help in this diagnostic process. Several surveys have sampled the attitudes of speech–language pathologists with regard to this evaluation process (Pannbacker et al., 1984; Pannbacker, Lass, & Stout, 1990; Schneider & Shprintzen, 1980). Since the earlier survey of Schneider and Shprintzen, speech–language pathologists have begun to turn more toward instrumentation to aid perceptual judgments. As Pannbacker et al. (1990) stated, however, the number of speech–language pathologists who do not use any sort of instrumentation is unknown.

Table 8–1 lists the significant perceptual and instrumentation processes that are currently being used by speech–language pathologists in the evalua-

TABLE 8–1
Velopharyngeal Evaluation Techniques

Technique	References
Listener judgment of voice	(a)
Oral examination of orofacial structures	(b)
Articulation testing	(c)
Radiological assessment	(d)
Videofluoroscopy	(e)
Multiview	(f)
Base and Towne views	(g)
Tomography	(h)
Magnetic resonance imaging	(i)
Endoscopy (oral and nasopharyngoscopy)	
Rigid endoscopy	(j)
Flexible fiber optic endoscopy	(k)
Simultaneous radiological/endoscopic assessment	(l)
Aeromechanical (airflow and pressure)	(m)
Nasometer	(n)
Miscellaneous techniques	(o)

References on Technique

a. McWilliams & Philips, 1990
b. Bateman & Mason, 1984; Bradley, 1989; Pannbacker, 1985
c. Bzoch, 1989a
d. Bzoch, 1989a; Isberg, Julin, Kraepelien, & Henrikson, 1989; McWilliams et al., 1990; W. N. Williams, 1989
e. Skolnick & Cohn, 1989
f. Skolnick & Cohn, 1989
g. Skolnick & Cohn, 1989
h. McWilliams et al., 1990
i. McWilliams et al., 1990
j. Witzel & Posnick, 1989
k. D'Antonio, Marsh, Province, Muntz, & Phillips, 1989; Shprintzen, 1989
l. Stringer & Witzel, 1989
m. Allison & Leeper, 1990; Dalston, Warren, Morr, & Smith, 1988; McWilliams et al., 1990; Morr, Warren, Dalston, & Smith, 1989; Warren, 1989
n. Kay Elemetrics Corporation, 12 Maple Avenue, Pine Brook, NJ 07058. Telephone: (201) 227-2000.
o. Horiguchi & Bell-Berti, 1987; Reich & Redenbaugh, 1985

tion process, as well as useful references. Techniques that have rather limited or merely experimental usage are not listed.

The studies of Pannbacker et al. (1984), Pannbacker et al. (1990), and Schneider and Shprintzen (1980) all indicated that the speech–language pathologist has many techniques available to assess the adequacy or inadequacy of the velopharyngeal mechanism for speech and voice. Clinicians continue to use techniques that require little instrumentation, such as articulation testing and listener judgment, but a growing trend is to utilize objective assessment. It is imperative that speech–language pathologists who are evaluating many children and adults with possible velopharyngeal insufficiency obtain the necessary training to utilize objective measurement to complement their clinical judgments. Those speech–language pathologists who evaluate few such clients must be prepared to refer to centers where objective assessment is available when the velopharyngeal mechanism is suspect in the client's speech or voice. Excellent books are dedicated to an understanding of speech and voice sequelae of velopharyngeal concerns (e.g., Bzoch, 1989a; McWilliams et al., 1990), and the reader is encouraged to investigate these references for comprehensive guidance in the evaluation and treatment of persons who have speech and voice disorder due to velopharyngeal insufficiency.

When the speech–language pathologist determines that the mechanism is functionally incompetent, it is appropriate to engage the client in therapy designed to eliminate its functional misuse. Therapy is appropriate only when there is functional incompetency, since there is little evidence that voluntary effort is capable of overcoming a velopharyngeal insufficiency in continuous speech (Shelton, Chisum, Youngstrom, Arndt, & Elbert, 1969). Efforts to produce velopharyngeal closure with an insufficient mechanism can lead to abnormal compensations in terms of laryngeal adjustment (Shelton, Paesani, McClelland, & Bradfield, 1975), glottal stops and velar and pharyngeal fricatives (McWilliams & Philips, 1990), and abnormal articulation placement (Shelton et al., 1969).

A person with velopharyngeal insufficiency often is capable of demonstrating closure during nonspeech activities, such as blowing, sucking, whistling, and swallowing (Shprintzen, McCall, & Skolnick, 1975), and even during isolated phoneme production, without being able to execute the complete movements of closure during continuous speech. The speech–language pathologist should not be deceived into thinking that a client who can close the mechanism for some isolated behavior also should be able to close it in continuous speech with some amount of training. Such a decision leads to prolonged trial therapy that may last years without achieving functional closure during continuous speech. The analogy is appropriate that most people can take a ''giant step,'' but it is impossible functionally to walk that way. Too often, clinicians ask clients with velopharyngeal insufficiency to take giant steps in attempting velopharyngeal closure.

The question remains as to what action is appropriate for the speech–language pathologist and other professionals (plastic surgeons, radiologists, oral surgeons, prosthodontists) in the management of clients with speech–voice disorder resulting from the velopharyngeal mechanism. The most appropriate step should be to evaluate the mechanism thoroughly, using methodology that is as objective as possible, and recommend physical management of the mechanisms when an insufficiency exists.

Besides speech or voice therapy, speech–language pathologists and team members commonly use four secondary physical management procedures to treat velopharyngeal insufficiency: (a) pharyngeal flap pharyngoplasty, (b) speech appliance (bulb or obturator) including lift, (c) Teflon injection as a form of pharyngoplastic implant, and (d) palatal lift prostheses.

Pharyngeal Flap

Pharyngeal flap pharyngoplasty is the most common form of physical management for velopharyngeal inadequacy (McWilliams et al., 1990), although additional methodologies exist. Teflon pharyngoplasty has been used for many years but has not as yet received Food and Drug Administration approval. Furlow, Block, and Williams (1986) reviewed the many studies of Teflon pharyngoplasty and also one case in which sleep apnea became a surgical consequence. Cartilage has also been implanted to build the necessary mass for adequate closure (Trigos, Ysunza, Gonzalez, & Vazquez, 1988). Jarvis and Trier (1988) also reported the usage of intravelar veloplasty (establishment of normal levator veli palatini muscle course) as part of pharyngeal flap surgery, but indicated that speech results show no significant improvement of this added surgical procedure to the basic flap. New techniques will continue to be attempted, but the current state-of-the-art technique remains the traditional superior- or inferior-based pharyngeal flap pharyngoplasty.

The basic procedure, which has changed little over the years (McWilliams et al., 1990; S. A. Wolfe & Berkowitz, 1989), involves isolating a variable-width section of tissue from the posterior pharyngeal wall, maintaining either an inferior or superior attachment, then connecting the sectioned end to the velum. The flap produces a midline bridge between the velum and the pharynx leaving lateral portals for nasal respiration. These portals remain open for breathing but are closed by residual velopharyngeal closure for speech or swallowing. The size of these lateral portals is a critical factor in the success of the surgery (McWilliams et al., 1990). When successful, inadequate closure efforts prior to surgery have sufficient tissue to achieve the necessary closure. One significant variation on pharyngoplasty called the orticochea flap involves the reverse of the midline flap in which tissue is modified to narrow the lateral pharyngeal walls leaving a small central orifice.

Pharyngeal flap pharyngoplasty has been done as a primary procedure at the time of basic palatoplasty to close the cleft, usually around 1 year of age (Dalston & Stuteville, 1975). More typically, it is done as a secondary procedure following the determination that further surgery after palatoplasty is needed for improved velopharyngeal valving.

The number of cleft palate patients achieving adequate velopharyngeal closure after initial palatal closure varies from less than 50% (Fara et al., 1970) to close to 100%. The typical number is around 33% (Dalston & Stuteville, 1975). Critics of primary pharyngeal flap surgery contend that many patients undergo the operation unnecessarily. However, if the decision on primary pharyngoplasty carefully projects the adequacy of the mechanism following palatoplasty, many unnecessary pharyngoplasties would be avoided.

The technique of the pharyngeal flap involves a transverse flap, an inferiorly based vertical flap, or the superiorly based vertical flap (S. A. Wolfe & Berkowitz, 1989). Improved results can be obtained regardless of flap procedures when the flaps are tailor-made to fit the particularities of each patient. Because flaps tend to become passive rather than dynamic tissue obturators, the surgeon should construct them with sufficient width to allow the lateral pharyngeal wall tissues to move medially against them to achieve closure. When the lateral wall motion is insufficient to close the lateral ports created by the flap, a velopharyngeal insufficiency remains and the patient's speech and voice remain distorted and hypernasal. Sometimes pharyngeal flap surgery is done simultaneously with tonsillectomy (Reath, LaRossa, & Randall, 1987).

Nasality and Flap Pharyngoplasy

The work reported by Fletcher (1978) on speech development of cleft palate subjects in whom nasality was a factor indicated that speech development was enhanced by early surgery. Fletcher found that children who had had primary surgery early had better articulation, resonance (nasality factor), and intelligibility than did those whose surgery was delayed.

Riski (1979) compared the speech sound acquisition and oral–nasal balance of 52 children who had had pharyngeal flaps for velopharyngeal incompetency (insufficiency) with 48 children with cleft palates who had not required secondary management. Riski reported that the children who later would require flap surgery demonstrated virtually no improvement in oral–nasal resonance balance and remained at an unacceptable level until after the operation. Following surgery, ratings of acceptable resonance increased 35% in children with clefts of the lip and palate and 63% in children with only clefts of the palate following the flap.

Riski's results paralleled Fletcher's regarding the early effects of management. Children who had had flaps before they were 6 had achieved acceptable oral–nasal resonance by age 7. However, those who received flaps after age 7 were delayed significantly in acquiring acceptable resonance.

Fox et al. (1988) reported a concern about judging the adequacy of primary surgical results on the basis of nasality alone. They rechecked 20 patients from a large sample of 92 patients who had been judged as having abnormal resonance during a previous study in 1985, and found that over half of the 20 had normal resonance. Fox et al. indicated that, although the need for pharyngeal flap pharyngoplasty can be determined as early as 4 years of age when articulation is considered, this judgment should be delayed until after age 6 when resonance is the critical factor.

Speech Appliances

Pannbacker et al. (1990) reported that few speech–language pathologists utilize the services of dental specialists (prosthodontists) for the treatment of velopharyngeal inadequacy or insufficiency. Surveying 296 speech–language pathologists who were members of the American Cleft Palate Association (return rate of 58.4%), only 4 speech–language pathologists (2.3%) indicated they would treat velopharyngeal insufficiency with prosthesis followed by therapy. None of the speech–language pathologists indicated that they would treat with prosthesis alone, without therapy. Although these data indicate a growing trend toward surgical management followed by therapy (90 speech–language pathologists or 52%) or surgery alone (12 speech–language pathologists or 6.9%), some patients are unable to be treated by surgery or for other reasons are viable candidates for prosthetic management. Riski, Hoke, and Dolan (1989) reported on two cases in which obturators were used on patients who had significant velopharyngeal inadequacy and for whom surgery was contraindicated. Pressure and flow coupled with endoscopic examination of the velopharyngeal port aided in the proper fitting of the obturator. (Figure 8–2 shows a speech obturator.)

Gonzalez and Aronson (1970) presented data on 35 patients with palatopharyngeal insufficiency in the absence of an overt cleft palate who were treated with a palatal lift or lift-obturator prosthesis. Nineteen of these clients had insufficiency resulting from neurologic disease, and the other 16 had anatomic palatopharyngeal deficiency. Cineradiographic analysis of velopharyngeal closure processes and audiotape recordings of contextual speech were obtained on each subject before and after prosthetic placement.

The neurologically involved patients demonstrated improvement in speech intelligibility after placement of the prostheses, but, because of a more generalized dysarthria, their gains were less than those of the palatal deficiency patients. All 35 showed immediate improvement in speech with the prostheses in place. This occurred in the areas of reduced hypernasality and nasal emission on pressure consonant articulation, increased rate of articulation, and over-

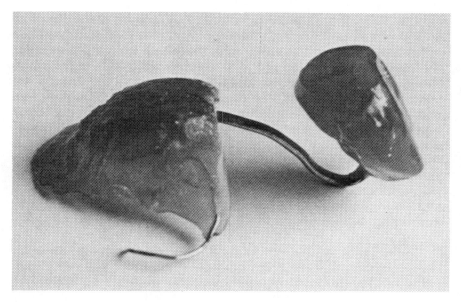

Figure 8–2 Example of a Speech Obturator.

all intelligibility improvement. Since all the patients tolerated the prostheses well, Gonzalez and Aronson (1970) recommended prosthetic management as either a temporary or permanent procedure.

Beery, Rood, and Schramm (1983) studied the lateral and posterior pharyngeal wall activity of 5 adults with cleft palate history who had worn a prosthetic speech appliance for more than 20 years. Rigid fiber optic nasoendoscopy was used to evaluate the muscular activity. The hypothesis was that prosthetic usage stimulates activity in surrounding muscles in cases of velopharyngeal incompetency (insufficiency). The subjects tended to have the greatest activity in the area of the levator veli palatini muscle and what traditionally is described as "Passavant's ridge" (anterior bulging of pharyngeal wall) (Skolnick & Cohn, 1989, p. 25), while no gross activity was observed in the area of the auditory tube. The researchers speculated that the mechanism of closure could occur at several vertical and horizontal levels in these patients as a result of the presence of the prostheses. The data affirmed the concept that prosthetic management of velopharyngeal insufficiency has positive long-term benefits.

Teflon Injection for Pharyngoplasty

Since Teflon became common in plastic surgery in the 1960s, it has been used to build up the posterior pharyngeal wall to aid in velopharyngeal closure when an insufficiency exists. The technique involved in this form of pharyngoplasty is similar to the procedure used in Teflon laryngoplasty described in Chapter 5 for the treatment of laryngeal paralysis. However, the use of Teflon in the pharynx is not approved by the Federal Drug Administration.

Kuehn and Van Demark (1978), in a report on 69 subjects who had undergone Teflon pharyngoplasty, developed a database for comparison that involved preoperative and postoperative speech samples and X-rays. The X-ray data indicated little change in velopharyngeal closure as a function of either treatment or time. Following the Teflon treatment, however, the speech results showed dramatic and significant improvement as a function of time.

Little improvement occurred in speech immediately following the Teflon pharyngoplasty, but by 3 months later there were significant advances. Kuehn and Van Demark stated that patients who have mobile palates, who achieve a velopharyngeal gap of less than 2 mm (lateral X-ray), and who are rated on a velopharyngeal competency scale as exhibiting mild to moderate difficulty make excellent candidates for Teflon pharyngoplasty.

Furlow, Williams, Eisenbach, and Bzoch (1982) presented data on the long-term results of Teflon pharyngoplasty for 35 patients with velopharyngeal insufficiency, 8 of them with failed pharyngeal flaps. These subjects were followed postoperatively for an average of 3 years. Speech evaluations, including nasality judgments and cinefluorography, constituted the database of this longitudinal study.

An overall success rate of 74% was achieved, with the criterion for success being the total elimination of abnormal symptoms. Success rates for various insufficiency etiologies ranged from a high of 100% for submucous cleft patients to a low of 62% for failed pharyngeal flap subjects. These researchers also stressed the importance of determining presurgically that the velum is mobile and that it has appropriate but insufficient movement during contextual speech.

Although Teflon continues to be used in patients to treat velopharyngeal insufficiency, the usage of this material needs careful monitoring. Furlow et al. (1986) reported on a case in which, 6 years after the Teflon was injected, significant obstructive sleep apnea developed. Daytime hypersomnolence and tiredness became a severe problem for him and interfered with his work. Partial revision of the Teflon implant improved his sleep respiration and eliminated his symptoms while maintaining his velopharyngeal adequacy.

Voice Therapy for Hypernasality

Etiologies of several disorders cause communication problems of articulation, resonance, or voice (e.g., the neurogenic dysarthrias of Chapter 5). The etiologies of hypernasality also can involve articulation disorder and hypernasal resonance, but no specific information is provided here on articulation management. References are available on articulation management for cleft palate and other palatal abnormalities (Bzoch, 1989a; Fletcher, 1978; Hahn, 1989; Karnell & Van Demark, 1986; McWilliams et al., 1990; Van Demark & Hardin, 1986). The following discussion focuses on the clinical management of residual hypernasality (resonance) only after any significant articulation disorders associated with the velopharyngeal valving difficulty have been controlled.

Voice therapy for hypernasality can be done with simple feedback devices such as a nasal listening tube. This tube, inserted into the client's nostril, can be used to evaluate and rate the nasality heard on each vowel sound (Figure 8-3). The nostril into which the tip is inserted should be the one through which breathing occurs most easily (should there be a difference between the two). The speech–language pathologist should rate each of the following vowels: /i/, /ɪ/, /e/, /ɛ/, /æ/, /a/, /o/, /ʊ/, /u/, /ʌ/, and /ɚ/. The following ordinal scale can be used to rate each vowel:

0 = Normal, no nasality heard

1 = Slight nasality

2 = Moderate nasality

3 = Severe nasality

When the vowels have been rated, the listening tube can be used to help clients identify their own hypernasality. By inserting the listening tube into their own ear as they produce the vowels, they can differentiate between those that the speech–language pathologist judges to be normal or only slightly nasal and those that are more severe. When clients can discriminate the differences, it is appropriate to begin modification of the moderately and severely judged vowels.

The following steps can be used in teaching the client to produce voice devoid of hypernasality:

- The speech–language pathologist directs the client to say monosyllabic words in consonant–vowel–consonant (CVC) relationships, beginning with vowels rated as normal (0) or only slightly nasal (1). The client listens to these sounds with the tube, then produces vowels rated as moderate (2) or severe (3) in the same CVC relationships so the contrast can be heard between the mildly nasal and the more severely nasal. The client then should be drilled to produce the severely nasal vowels in the CVC relationships until they are like the mild or normal vowels. This should be done by pairing the contrasting CVCs together, for example, /tat/ (1) with /tit/ (3).

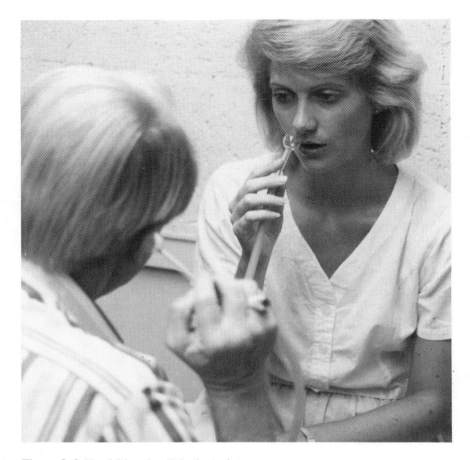

Figure 8–3 Nasal Listening Tube in Action.

- The speech–language pathologist, once the client can produce monosyllabic words or CVC relationships without nasality using the nasal listening tube to discriminate, begins drilling on other words and phrases that do not contain nasal consonants while maintaining the normal or only slightly nasal rating of 0 or 1.

- The speech–language pathologist introduces nasal consonants into the phrases by ending them on a nasal consonant (e.g., ''see the ice cream,'' ''put up the beam''). If the client can maintain voice without moderate or severe nasality even with the presence of a nasal consonant, the clinician should begin to scatter a few nasal consonants in other word positions in the phrases (e.g., ''some of us care,'' ''I am at my school''). The presence of the nasal consonants should not have a significant effect on the vowels in the phrase, which should remain nonnasal.

- When the client is able to say these phrases without excessive nasality on the vowels while listening on the tube, the speech–language pathologist removes the tube to determine whether the client can tell when the voice is nasal or nonnasal without the tube. If the client can, and also can eliminate the excessive nasality, the clinician introduces consonants, then longer phrases, then context reading, and finally conversation. At each increase in task difficulty, the speech–language pathologist should determine that proper discrimination and production of voice without nasality are occurring by spot-checking with the nasal listening tube rather than using it constantly.

- The speech–language pathologist should find negative practice helpful at any of these steps. The client can be asked to speak the sound, word, phrase, or sentence with excessive and deliberate nasality. When the client learns to handle the resonance voluntarily in either a negative or positive manner, the carryover into everyday voice production is more likely to occur because the individual is in control of the process—instead of the reverse.

The above therapy steps are significantly enhanced by the use of instrumentation designed to detect nasal resonance, such as the Kay Elemetrics Nasometer (Figure 8–4) or the PERCI aeromechanical system explained in Chapter 3 and shown here in Figure 8–5.

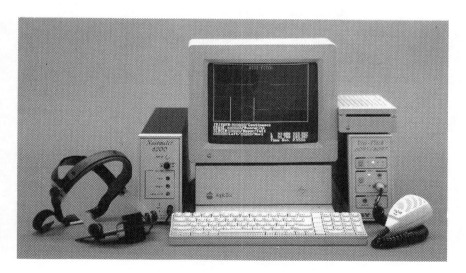

Figure 8–4 Kay Elemetrics Nasometer.

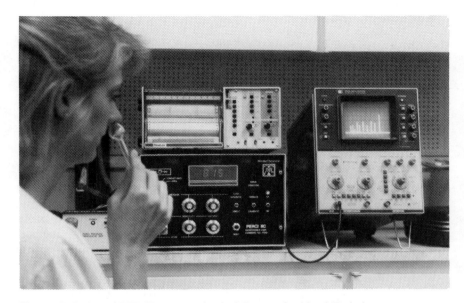

Figure 8–5 Use of PERCI Aeromechanical System for Nasal Emission.

A similar approach for the modification of hypernasality in young children is presented by Andrews, Tardy, and Pasternak (1984). In this program, the See-Scape™ (available from PRO-ED, Inc., 8700 Shoal Creek Boulevard, Austin, Texas 78758) is used as a feedback source indicating nasal resonance (flow). The program is divided into the following phases:

Phase 1: Discrimination between oral and nasal sounds in CVs and VCs

Phase 2: Spontaneous production of sentences produced with appropriate oral resonance (words made up only of vowels and oral consonants)

Phase 3: Production of oral and nasal sounds in structured phrases

Phase 4: Production of oral and nasal sounds in self-generated sentences

The program is designed to shape the child into appropriate production of self-generated sentences containing oral and nasal sounds with 90% accuracy. Although this program is designed to modify hypernasality in the young child, with minor modifications it is suitable for any aged child.

An alternative method of eliminating hypernasality (Shprintzen et al., 1975) involves pairing whistling and blowing with phonation to achieve improved velopharyngeal valving. The rationale for this procedure is based on the finding that normal speakers demonstrate the same velopharyngeal closure pattern during blowing, whistling, and speech as revealed by multiview videofluoroscopic observation.

When objective tests such as fluoroscopic or endoscopic examination reveal that closure mechanisms for blowing and whistling are normal but that speech closure is aberrant, this technique can facilitate improved closure for speech by pairing it with blowing or whistling. Utilizing successive approximation under principles of operant conditioning, Shprintzen et al. were able to shape normal speech closure in 4 subjects with velopharyngeal incompetence for speech.

It seems clear that hypernasality as a voice disorder can be modified clinically using available techniques and instruments. Two positive effects of such reduction are speaker intelligibility and improved social acceptability. Whether the etiology of the hypernasality is one of cleft palate, mental retardation, palate abnormalities, or hearing loss and deafness (discussed later), the speech-language pathologist must consider hypernasality as a vocal parameter to be modified, particularly after any needed physical management of the velopharyngeal mechanisms of closure has been accomplished (Andrews, 1986).

Hyponasality

Hyponasality, also called denasality, is the opposite of hypernasality. It is a vocal quality that occurs when the nasal cavity has some condition that prevents it from participating normally as a resonance chamber. The English consonants /m/, /n/, and /ŋ/ require oral and nasal coupling for normal production. The velopharyngeal port is open to allow this to occur. Under coupling conditions, the chambers of the nasal cavity resonate these nasal consonants by allowing sound to enter. If some condition in the nasal cavity reduces resonance potential, the /m/ phoneme will be perceived more as a /b/, the /n/ phoneme as a /d/, and the /ŋ/ phoneme as a /g/.

Several conditions in the nasal cavity—diseases of the nasopharynx—produce hyponasality (DeWeese & Saunders, 1982). The following conditions can have a significant effect on the resonance potential of the nasal cavity to produce hyponasality:

- *Tonsils and Adenoids*: The lymphatic tissue in the form of pharyngeal tonsils (adenoid) and palatine tonsil tissue can produce hyponasality and cause difficulty breathing through the nose (Rastatter & Hyman, 1984). When the pharyngeal and palatine tonsilar masses (called Waldeyer's ring when added to the lingual tonsil) become infected, a condition known as pharyngitis or tonsillitis is present, requiring medical and often surgical attention (tonsillectomy and/or adenoidectomy).

- *Diseases of the Turbinates*: Any disease caused by infection or allergy can cause the nasal turbinates (conchae) to become swollen or hypertrophied, thereby decreasing the space available in the nasal cavity for vocal resonance and nasal breathing.

- *Allergic Rhinitis*: Many persons have severe allergies to environmental substances (smoke, grasses, pollen, dust, dairy products, etc.) and experience tissue reaction in the form of swelling and inflammation when exposed to them. Some individuals have acute experiences with intermittent effects; others have chronic difficulty, with almost constant nasal congestion. They can have persistent hyponasality as a voice quality and also become mouth breathers (Rastatter & Hyman, 1984).

- *Nasal Polyps*: Several types of nasal polyps can develop in the cavity and obstruct space for resonance and breathing. Nasal polyps are seen most often in patients with allergic rhinitis. They may be large or numerous enough to completely occlude the nasal cavity. The typical nasal polyp is soft, pale gray, nontender, and mobile and is attached by a pedunculated base.

- *Papillomas*: Papillomas are small wartlike growths that may develop in the squamous epithelium of the nasal cavity. Their cause is unknown, although a viral etiology is suspected. (More information is provided later.)

- *Foreign Bodies*: Children enjoy putting objects in the cavities of the body and the nasal orifice is no exception. These objects include buttons, beans, pebbles, and eraser tips. The object often is put into the nasal cavity inadvertently, then forgotten until some tissue reaction causes pain, swelling, or inflammation.

- *Neoplasm or Malignant Growth*: Although rare, malignant growths can develop in the nasal cavity, producing bloody discharge, pain or tenderness, difficulty in nasal breathing, and hyponasality.

- *Acute Rhinitis*: Acute rhinitis (the common cold) is a high-incidence condition that has afflicted most people. The plethora of over-the-counter medicines designed to eliminate or reduce the symptoms of acute rhinitis is evidence of its commonality. The symptoms of this condition include nasal discharge, nasal inflammation and edema, difficulty with nasal breathing, and hyponasality.

- *Deviated Nasal Septum*: The nasal septum formed by the perpendicular plate of the ethmoid bone and the vomer divides the nasal cavity into right and left chambers. Through birth injury, trauma, or aging, the septum can deviate to one side, causing nasal obstruction on the convex side of the deviation and occluding the passageway unilaterally, possibly producing a hyponasal voice quality. However, Rastatter and Hyman (1984) found these patients able to produce normal resonance. Therefore, the presence of a deviated nasal septum does not automatically cause hyponasal resonance.

- *Patulous Eustachian Tubes*: The eustachian tubes leading from the posterior nasopharynx to the middle ear space normally are closed, opening only during the act of swallowing or yawning. Abnormal patency (openness) of the eustachian tubes can cause significant discomfort and anxiety since any change in acoustic or static pressure will be transmitted immediately to the ears. Some persons with patulous eustachian tubes have learned to eliminate some of the acoustic effect by maintaining constant velopharyngeal closure so that much of the acoustic energy is kept from the tubes. The effect is functional hyponasality since the velopharyngeal port remains closed for the nasal consonants. Batza and Parker (1971) reported 1 case in which patulous eustachian tubes were responsible for the development of hyponasality. (They also reviewed several other cases.)

Hypernasality Versus Hyponasality

A speech–language pathologist may listen to a person's voice and detect a nasal factor but have difficulty determining whether it is hypernasality, hyponasality, or a combination of both. This is not an easy decision in some cases because of the possible combination of factors. For example, a person can have velopharyngeal insufficiency or incompetency that allows nasal resonance but, because of nasal congestion from an allergy, cold, or some other factor, also manifests decreased resonance on the nasal consonants. In another case, a child visiting the speech–language pathologist for an evaluation of velopharyngeal functioning might be upset and cry before the examination, causing nasal edema and congestion.

The best method for a clinician to discriminate between hypernasality and hyponasality from a perceptual point of view is to have the client read words, phrases, or sentences that are either loaded with or lacking nasal consonants (Exhibit 8–1). By listening carefully to how these phrases sound, the speech–language pathologist can judge whether the voice quality heard is hypernasality or hyponasality. The person with a hypernasal voice quality will sound excessively nasal while reading nonnasal phrases and nearly normal on phrases loaded with nasal consonants. The hyponasal individual will manifest nearly normal voice quality on the nonnasal phrases and evidence the problem mainly on the nasally loaded phrases. In these phrases, the person with hyponasality will distort the nasal consonants, so the /m/ will sound like a /b/, the /n/ like a /d/, and the /ŋ/ like a /g/.

The person with mixed hypernasality and hyponasality manifests these same differences, but the discrimination process usually is more difficult. Hypernasality is heard on the nonnasal phrases, but not noticeably so. Hyponasality is as apparent in a mixed state as it is in its pure form; that is, the nasal consonants do not sound nasal.

Exhibit 8–1 Nonnasal and Nasal Phrases

Nonnasal Phrases	*Nasally Loaded Phrases*
See what I do to it	My mom can be mean
If you see what I did	Mama made lemon jam
Carry it to the truck	Many men came home then
The cars are parked at the arcade	May I plan my menu?
Look at the truck over there	Ten times ten is one hundred
Be here at 6 o'clock	My time can never be turned back
Will you go to the store?	Ten men came when I sang

Hyponasality and Nasal Breathing

It is important to determine how easily a person with resonance disorder can breathe through the nose. If sufficient nasal congestion is present to restrict airflow through the nose for respiration, it is likely that nasal resonance for the nasal consonants also will be dampened. Hairfield, Warren, Hinton, and Seaton (1987) reviewed significant aspects of nasal breathing in inspiratory and expiratory maneuvers. They also reviewed the literature on nasal respiration in normal and cleft palate populations.

The speech–language pathologist can have the person run in place for a minute or so until slightly out of breath, then sit down and attempt to achieve normal breathing cycles using only the nose. If the client has difficulty doing that and must open the mouth to catch up on breathing, it is reasonable to expect a nasal congestion factor sufficient to produce a hyponasal voice quality.

It is a good idea to determine whether breathing is better through one nostril than the other. Congestion on only one side still is sufficient to generate hyponasal resonance.

Cul-de-Sac Resonance

The closed tube cul-de-sac resonance phenomenon can help the speech–language pathologist detect hypernasality. Cul-de-sac resonance occurs in humans when the nostrils are pinched together as a vowel sound is produced and prolonged if there is oral and nasal coupling through the velopharyngeal port. Under these conditions, the client emitting an /i/ as the nostrils are pinched experiences a sudden change in the nature of the sound.

An extension of this is the nasal flutter test (Bzoch, 1989a). It is performed by the client's alternately pinching and releasing the nostrils while prolonging the vowels /i/ or /u/. The rapidly alternated pattern makes the changes produced by cul-de-sac resonance more noticeable. If no such change is heard, there probably is no excessive or hypernasal resonance in the speech signal.

One of the most helpful clinical devices available for detecting hypernasal or hyponasal resonance is the nasal listening tube (Figure 8–3). It is a simple device constructed of rubber tubing with glass or plastic tips on each end that can be placed in either a nostril or an external auditory meatus. When one tip is placed in the client's nostril and the other tip in the speech–language pathologist's ear, amplified sound is heard when present in the nasal cavity. Hyponasality is detected by having the client alternate saying a /b/ and an /m/ sound in a CVC phonemic relationship. For example, /bib/ and /mim/ do not sound significantly different through the listening tube when hyponasality is present—both essentially sound close to /bib/. Both CVCs would be dampened in intensity. With hypernasality, however, both /bib/ and /mim/ sound similar but closer to /mim/. Rather than the dampening of sound heard in hyponasality, the hypernasality productions through the listening tube seem quite loud. It also is possible to discern when air is escaping into the nasal cavity on the pressure consonants.

The nasal listening tube can be a helpful device in making some clinical perception judgments. The speech–language pathologist must remember that, using the listening tube, no objective information is obtained regarding the sufficiency or insufficiency of the velopharyngeal structures. However, the tube may help the speech–language pathologist in perceptual judgments of speech and resonance patterns that would be part of the administration of any test of articulation. It also may be of assistance in clinical judgments as to the presence or absence of hypernasality, hyponasality, or combinations. It may be useful in providing feedback in therapy to a client on articulation and voice productions that involve nasal airflow and resonance.

However, the tube should not be used by the speech–language pathologist to determine whether therapy or physical management is the procedure of choice. This decision should be based on information provided by more objective procedures, such as videofluoroscopy, aeromechanical data, and endoscopic examination coupled with clinical evaluations of oral examination, articulation, and voice testing.

Hyponasality and the Speech–Language Pathologist

When an evaluation of resonance determines that a client has a hyponasal voice disorder, the only appropriate management action the speech–language pathologist should take is to facilitate a referral for medical examination. The physician then can determine the specific cause of the hyponasality (adenoids, allergy, polyps, deviated septum, etc.). Once medical or surgical treatment has been provided, the hyponasality will be eliminated and no further speech–language therapy will be needed. The rare exception to this is the functional hyponasality caused by patulous eustachian tubes. Stated simply, hyponasality is a medical problem, and the speech–language pathologist should not try to modify it.

Velopharyngeal Examination

When examining the velopharyngeal port of clients suspected of having abnormal velopharyngeal valving, the speech–language pathologist should be aware that head position can affect the efficiency of closure. McWilliams, Musgrave, and Crozier (1968) demonstrated that many cleft palate clients were able to achieve velopharyngeal closure when the head was in a normal upright position looking straight forward but were unable to achieve closure with the head extended as though looking upward. Extending the head upward appears to add a factor of difficulty to velopharyngeal closure. In examining children's oral structures, speech–language pathologists are seated in such a position that they are looking down into the client's mouth. If the child's head is extended upward significantly, the examination of movements of the velopharyngeal structures could produce spurious results. The client should be positioned so the examiner can obtain a direct frontal view in a horizontal plane. Inspection of velopharyngeal structures should be done under normal speech production conditions. For example, the clinician should not have the client extend the tongue significantly to assess velopharyngeal functioning. Such excessive protrusion alters normal anatomical and physiological relationships and restricts full motion of the structures.

The mouth also should not be opened excessively during this examination. The speech–language pathologist should ask the client to open the mouth slightly as an /a/ vowel is prolonged. By shining a light directly into the oral cavity during this vowel prolongation effort, the clinician should be able to view the palatal movements; if not, the client should be instructed to continue prolonging the vowel as the mouth gradually is opened more until the structures can be viewed easily. A tongue depressor can be used during this vowel prolongation, but the speech–language pathologist must be aware that its presence is bothersome to many people, can produce a gagging effect, and can alter the normal closure pattern.

Although normal velopharyngeal closure processes vary from person to person, they are essentially sphincteric in nature. The velum does not merely move up against the posterior pharyngeal wall; rather, it usually lifts upward and backward, the lateral walls of the pharynx move medially, and the posterior wall of the pharynx moves slightly forward to completely close the port between the oral and nasal cavities (see Chapter 1 on movement patterns).

It is difficult to analyze these sphincteric movements from direct oral inspection, particularly since closure occurs above the level of the uvula near or above the palatal plane (the line intersecting the anterior nasal spine and the posterior nasal spine). However, direct oral inspection can reveal some general patterns of movement, and extreme velopharyngeal insufficiency often can be identified. Subtle patterns of closure, including its adequacy in border- line cases, in all likelihood cannot be determined by oral inspection.

Considerable information can be gained by visual inspection of the color of velopharyngeal structures. A bluish or slightly purple soft palate midline indicates a possible submucous cleft. When this is noted, the hard palate struc- tures must be inspected carefully to determine whether there is a notch in the posterior aspect of the hard palate covered by mucosa. This can be noted during velar movements. If it is suspected, the speech–language pathologist should cover a finger with an inspection rubber and feel along the margin of the hard palate and velum. If a well-defined hard palate margin, including the presence of the posterior nasal spine, is felt, a submucous cleft of the hard palate can be ruled out.

However, this does not preclude the possibility of an occult submucous cleft of the soft tissues. Although a bifid uvula has been highly correlated with submucous clefting (Bzoch, 1989a), these abnormalities can be present when the structures appear normal in superficial inspection. Only surgical inspection reveals the abnormal muscle attachment associated with the occult submucous cleft. However, speech, voice, and facial abnormalities are asso- ciated with occult submucous cleft (Kaplan, 1977).

The speech–language pathologist should inspect the velopharyngeal mechanisms as carefully as possible to determine whether any obvious abnor- malities exist in length, color, pharyngeal depth, and movement patterns. These observations should be correlated with judgments about voice quality and artic- ulation accuracy. A decision then can be made as to whether further diagnostic procedures need to be instituted or whether therapy to modify aberrant speech and voice characteristics can be started.

A complete oral examination format has been provided by Mason (1980). By following this format while keeping in mind the suggestions of this chapter, the speech–language pathologist can make many judgments about the status of the velopharyngeal structures that support voice and articulation. Should such judgment indicate that further diagnostic evaluation is necessary, a referral would be appropriate for videofluoroscopic, aeromechanical, or endoscopic examination to obtain more objective information regarding the adequacy of the velopharyngeal mechanisms.

Voices of the Hearing Impaired and Deaf

Deafness or severe hearing loss has a direct impact on the voice, an effect that is paralleled by the degree of hearing loss and how early in speech development it occurs. The voice is affected in breath support; in control of pitch, stress, loudness, and general quality; and in particular subtle prosodic elements of speech.

Horii (1982b) compared the fundamental frequency (F_0) of 12 hard-of-hearing young women with normal control subjects during reading and conversational speech. On the average, the hard-of-hearing persons had a higher mean F_0 (oral reading, 256.7; spontaneous speech, 264.1) than the normals (oral reading, 213.2; spontaneous speech, 203.5) and showed little difference in F_0. The normals tended to increase their F_0 during oral reading. Smaller standard deviations also were observed for the hard-of-hearing regardless of speaking conditions. Similar findings were reported by Leder, Spitzer, and Kirchner (1987) for profoundly deaf adult men.

An extensive study of acoustic and perceptual qualities in voice samples of young hearing-impaired children was reported by Monsen (1979). Twenty-four hearing-impaired and 6 normal hearing children (near age 5) were subjected to both a gross (spectrographic) and fine (computer-aided) acoustic analysis of five voice parameters: (a) mean fundamental frequency, (b) duration of word production, (c) mean period-to-period changes in intensity and in fundamental frequency, (d) spectral energy ratio above and below 1000 Hz, and (e) intonation contour patterns of speech. A major finding was that the intonation contours were the most significant characteristics separating the better from the poorer deaf speakers. Those perceptually judged to be poorer speakers tended to have intonation contours that were either flat or excessively changing. However, the average fundamental frequency was found to be 297 Hz, which was within normal limits for normal hearing subjects at the age studied.

Thus, it seems probable that the higher pitch noted by Horii (1982b) develops later in life in deaf and hard-of-hearing persons. In other words, the lowering of pitch associated with puberty does not occur as naturally in deaf or hearing-impaired children.

Monsen (1979) speculated that many of the voice quality patterns heard in this study that were acoustically or perceptually abnormal were related to aberrant respiration patterns. Forner and Hixon (1977) said that hearing-impaired subjects had normal tidal respiration patterns but abnormal respiration function when speaking. Monsen noted Forner and Hixon's study and felt that young hearing-impaired children often simply relied on whatever air supply was present in the lungs the moment they decided to speak and did not inhale naturally in preparation for speech.

The typical voice quality of deaf or severely hearing-impaired persons probably is a combination of poor respiratory control, inadequate laryngeal valving, and abnormal posturing of the tongue in the hypopharynx that produces a marked cul-de-sac resonance effect (Boone & McFarlane, 1988). These effects are coupled with the marked hypernasality also characteristic of deaf speakers.

Subtelny, Li, Whitehead, and Subtelny (1989) studied the physiological basis for abnormal resonance in hearing-impaired speakers by means of cephalometric and cineradiographic analysis. They analyzed many vocal tract configurations including postures of the lips, tongue, mandible, velum, hyoid bone, epiglottis, and laryngeal sinus. These authors found that hearing-impaired speakers, compared with normal speakers, manifested greater variation in basic tongue posture during vowel production, a significant retrusion of the tongue for front vowels, and consistent retrusion of the dorsum or root of the tongue during contextual speech. These postures affected the resonance of the speakers' voices and provided support for Boone and McFarlane's (1988) notions about the physiological bases for hearing-impaired speech.

Stevens, Nickerson, Boothroyd, and Rollins (1976) described a technique of detection of hypernasality in deaf speakers using a small (1.8 g) accelerometer attached to the surface of the nose. The vibrations associated with nasal resonance provide data on the presence of velopharyngeal incompetency and associated hypernasality. These researchers also utilized the accelerometer and its signal to provide feedback in the management of hypernasality in these deaf subjects. D. K. Wilson (1987) suggested that hyponasality may contribute to the typical voice quality of hearing-impaired children.

Voice Therapy in Hearing Loss

Several therapy techniques are recommended for modifying the voice quality of deaf and hearing-impaired persons under conditions of proper amplification.

Pitch. Visual feedback of the F_0 produced by a hearing-impaired speaker makes it rather easy to evaluate the pitch used and modify it when it is found to be aberrant. The Kay Visi-Pitch or similar instrumentation can provide easy modification of significantly high pitch patterns in these subjects.

Since the visual display also provides feedback on pitch inflection patterns, the speech–language pathologist can use this instrument to demonstrate normal prosodic elements of speech. The split-screen potential of the Visi-Pitch allows the clinician to provide a model for hearing-impaired clients to use in attempting to produce a more normal inflection pattern.

Loudness. The intensity mode of the Visi-Pitch or a volume unit meter also can provide feedback to the hearing-impaired client on the appropriateness of voice loudness. There are significant loudness factors in normal vocal prosody: These can be taught more effectively with the visual feedback provided by this instrument.

D. K. Wilson (1987) offered many techniques for modifying pitch and loudness in hearing-impaired children that can be used with the feedback potential of the Visi-Pitch or similar instrumentation. These techniques are more appropriate for children, but they can be modified for older clients.

Resonance.   To modify nasality in hearing-impaired subjects, it is important to remember that such a characteristic is poorly perceived by persons with hearing impairment and that special amplification is needed. As Ling (1975) pointed out, amplification in the 300 Hz range is necessary to discriminate the acoustics of nasality. A high-quality group amplifier will be more successful for this problem than most individual systems, which often do not amplify the low frequencies well. When an auditory training system is used to help the client discriminate nasality productions, the speech–language pathologist must remember that the person's own hearing aid eventually must be sufficient for these discriminations. The group trainer merely provides initial support for the training process.

Boone and McFarlane (1988) stated that much of the unusual voice quality heard in deaf speakers is cul-de-sac resonance resulting from a backward tongue placement. Voice quality can be improved by teaching the hearing-impaired client to carry the tongue in a more forward position during speech. Drill on CV combinations that involve forward placement of the tongue, such as /ta/ and /da/, can help the client learn this forward placement. Boone added that such approaches as (a) chewing, (b) open mouth, (c) relaxation training, (d) yawn–sigh, and (e) negative practice can be helpful in teaching voice quality that is more normally resonated in the oral cavity. When the voice quality of the hearing-impaired client is hypernasal as a result of velopharyngeal dysfunction, rather than the cul-de-sac resonance described by Boone, the speech–language pathologist can teach the client to monitor the nasality by resting a finger lightly on the side of the nose to feel the vibrations of nasal resonance. These vibrations can be determined more objectively with an accelerometer (Stevens et al., 1976).

Miscellaneous Disorders of Voice

Many miscellaneous conditions produce dysphonia. Some of these are treated only medically, and the speech–language pathologist generally is not involved in their management. However, it is imperative that the speech–language pathologist be aware of these conditions to be effective in voice management.

Papillomas

The most common benign laryngeal tumor in children is the squamous cell juvenile papilloma or papillomas (multiple forms) (Ogura & Thawley, 1980).

Papillomas take the form of fingers of connective tissue growths covered with squamous epithelium lying on a basement of intact membrane. These have a warty appearance in both single and multiple forms. Their etiology is considered viral in nature, resulting from one or more of the human papilloma viruses commonly found throughout the body. Although DeWeese and Saunders (1982) seemed to indicate that juvenile papillomas occur only in young boys, Cohen, Geller, Seltzer, and Thompson (1980) reported data on 90 children with this disease, including 43 females.

Papillomas have a well-identifiable appearance under laryngoscopic inspection: white to pinkish red, glistening nodules with either sessile (broad-based) or pedunculated (stem) attachment. They are highly vasculated and bleed easily upon removal (Ogura & Thawley, 1980). Notwithstanding this appearance, Cohen et al. (1980) commented that less than one-third of the 90 patients they reviewed had been diagnosed correctly before direct laryngoscopy; the erroneous diagnoses were vocal nodules, obstructive tonsils and adenoids, or laryngomalacia. Two of these patients actually underwent tonsillectomies and adenoidectomies for airway obstruction, when in fact the problem was caused by laryngeal papillomas.

The symptomatology of laryngeal papillomatosis depends on the site of lesion. The most common symptom is hoarseness. Cohen et al. (1980) reported that 90% of the patients studied presented hoarseness that usually was moderate but progressive in severity. Some children had aphonia. Airway obstruction, a critical and life-threatening concern, was documented in 44% of the children they studied. For example, one child had a normal larynx but had severe stridor that had been diagnosed as emphysema. Bronchoscopy disclosed that her trachea was almost totally obstructed by large papillomatous masses. Some patients with airway obstruction require tracheotomy. In adults, hoarseness usually is the only significant symptom.

Treatment of Papillomas

Since papillomas have a tendency to reappear after treatment, the most effective method of dealing with them has been meticulous surgical removal. Even so, some children have had numerous surgeries for removal. One child reported by Cohen et al. (1980) had undergone 110 operations and another child 109 before succumbing to bronchogenic carcinoma that developed long after the arrest of papillomatosis.

Treatment consists of either cup forceps surgery, CO_2 laser surgery (Wetmore, 1987), or interferon (Benjamin et al., 1988). Additional procedures used against papillomas include ultrasound and cryosurgery, as well as steroid, antibiotic, and radiologic treatments. Dedo and Jackler (1982) stated that the CO_2 laser clearly was superior to cup forceps surgery in 109 patients with recurrent laryngeal papillomas. These patients were treated at 2-month intervals until they entered remission; thereafter, they were seen at longer intervals. Remission was achieved in 41% of them, many of whom had not achieved that state after multiple cup forceps procedures. These researchers reported an average of five CO_2 procedures per patient leading to remission; forceps treatments averaged 10 per patient. As part of the CO_2 treatment, the involved area was painted with podophyllum, a topical agent that causes destruction of tissue at the site of application. With this combination of CO_2 laser removal and podophyllum painting, Dedo and Jackler felt that more complications (tracheotomy, voice quality effect, morbidity, and recurrence) could be avoided.

Interferon Therapy

A more recently developed treatment that shows promise is interferon therapy. Interferons are polypeptides produced by virtually all higher organism cells in response to viral and nonviral stimuli. Microquantities of interferon are required for the development of the antiviral state. The actual antiviral process is incompletely understood but is known to be extremely complex. Interferons are classified into Type 1 (alpha and beta) and Type 2 (gamma), depending on the cell of origin or type of inducer.

Lim and Chang (1986) presented the case of a 34-year-old male who was treated for severe laryngeal obstruction including progressive dyspnea, stridor, and loss of voice for 3 years. The tissues in his larynx were biopsied and found to be papilloma with atypical manifestations. Because of the extensiveness of his involvement, this man was laryngectomized. Histologic sectioning disclosed a diffused papillomatosis and the presence of a well-differentiated squamous cell carcinoma. Abitbol, Mathe, and Battista (1988) also reported data suggesting a relationship between adults with different types of human papillomavirus and malignant lesions. These authors suggested that even though gynecologic research has been more aggressive in determining the relationship between genital or venereal warts and uterine cervical carcinoma, laryngologists are only beginning to study the possible relationship of human papillomavirus and laryngeal carcinoma. These studies add to the importance of encouraging potential speech–language clients, particularly hoarse adults, to obtain a medical diagnosis and referral for therapy.

A physician evaluating a patient with laryngeal papilloma will prescribe a treatment (i.e., surgery or a medical application such as interferon) that in all probability will not involve a speech–language pathologist. However, the speech–language pathologist must understand laryngeal papillomatosis clearly since, through screening or other referral processes, a patient might be evaluated as having hoarseness or other dysphonia prior to medical examination. It would be easy, for example, for a school speech–language pathologist screening a child with persistent hoarseness to notice that the client is a yelling, screaming, vocally aggressive person and assume the hoarseness is caused by vocal abuse. Without medical referral safeguards, such a child might receive inappropriate therapy.

Even when the speech–language pathologist performs indirect laryngoscopy, as many commonly do, it would be inappropriate to enroll any child with persistent hoarseness without medical consultation. The disease of laryngeal papillomatosis is one of the main reasons why this safeguard is so valuable. Vocal nodules are not responsible for juvenile death, but laryngeal papillomas can be (Cohen et al., 1980). The many misdiagnoses reported in this chapter, even when the larynx was inspected medically, must alert the speech–language pathologist to be wary of diagnosing any child's or adult's voice solely by vocal symptoms and without medical consultation.

For another reason, the speech–language pathologist must be aware of laryngeal papillomatosis. When surgery is done on these patients, the speech–language pathologist can help reestablish vocalizations after the postsurgery recovery period. The techniques described in Chapter 4, on vocal abuse and surgical treatment of vocal nodules and ulcers of the larynx, can be helpful in this treatment.

Laryngeal Polyps

Although vocal nodules (Chapter 4) are classified as laryngeal polyps, many additional polyps develop in the laryngeal area that are unique and distinct, with different histological characteristics and etiology. Polyps of this kind often are unilateral and can be found anywhere within the larynx. They usually are attached to a sessile (broad) base but can be pedunculated (stem or small stalk). They may be blood filled and appear reddish, as in a hematoma. The term angioma often is used to describe blood-filled polyps. Excellent photographs of various laryngeal pathologies, including polpys, is found in Colton and Casper (1990) and Shaw and Lancer (1987).

Several precipitating and aggravating factors that have been related to the development of laryngeal polyps: allergies, thyroid imbalance, emotional imbalance, change of life, upper respiratory infections, sinus disease, cigarette smoking, alcohol consumption, and vocal abuse (Lucente, 1987; Shaw & Lancer, 1987).

The management of laryngeal polyps requires elimination of precipitating and aggravating factors and, usually, surgical removal. The speech–language pathologist may be called in on cases involving vocal abuse or misuse.

Ventricular Dysphonia

Ventricular dysphonia is the most common name of a disorder known under several names, including dysphonia plicae ventricularis, dysphonia ventricularis, or false vocal fold phonation. It is a voice disorder that results when the false or ventricular folds are involved in the generation of sound. The vocal symptoms heard in ventricular dysphonia include hoarseness, reduced intensity, aperiodicity, diplophonia, and hyperfunctional tension.

In the case of a nonpathological larynx, the ventricular folds could not be responsible for phonation independent of the true folds; rather, both vibrating structures would be involved in ventricular dysphonia. However, in the case of laryngeal paralysis or dysphonia resulting from dysarthria, the ventricular folds may be responsible for a significant amount of the laryngeal tone. After cordectomy or hemilaryngectomy for cancer, the ventricular folds may contribute greatly to the sound generated in the larynx. Ventricular dysphonia probably is responsible for the vocal quality heard in many persons with Down's syndrome (A. E. Aronson, 1985).

Most diagnoses of ventricular dysphonia result from indirect laryngoscopy. Typically, the physician will see the overhanging ventricular folds meeting at midline during phonation and identify ventricular dysphonia. Technically, however, ventricular dysphonia should be diagnosed by means of frontal radiography (tomograms) to establish the contribution of the ventricular as well as true vocal folds.

There are several therapies for improving the voice quality in cases of ventricular dysphonia, as discussed in the following sections.

Pitch Establishment.   When the pitch of the voice is varied, a pitch often can be found that involves improved quality and vocal effort. This also is a means of eliminating any diplophonia.

Relaxation Training.   When ventricular phonation involves hyperfunctional effort, rather than paralysis or surgical ablation, training the client to phonate with less physical effort can reduce the involvement of the ventricular folds. After a more relaxed state has been achieved, the client should produce vocal efforts as they are being recorded, perhaps on a loop-tape. When an improved vocal quality is heard, the recorded sample can become the target model for continued therapy.

Digital Pressure.   When the ventricular folds are used following surgical removal of tissue, a slight amount of pressure applied to the laryngeal area in various places during phonation can result in improved vocal quality. As this is done, the phonation effort should be recorded to document the effort and help establish a target voice quality. Once the client hears the improved voice under digital pressure, and internalizes the feeling involved in producing it, the quality can be maintained by internal adjustment as the digital pressure is eliminated.

Laryngeal Webs

Several degrees of webbing across the glottal space can be responsible for laryngeal stenosis. These can range from a small web across the anterior commissure to complete agenesis of the glottis. Embryologically, the glottis is formed by tissue resorption that establishes the glottal lumen. Failure of this resorption results in a congenital web of some degree. When webbing is extensive in neonates, their lives are severely compromised and, unless emergency treatment (tracheotomy) is performed, there is a great chance the result will become another infant-death statistic.

The symptoms that should alert the attending physician that a neonate might have laryngeal stenosis from webbing or other malformation include cyanosis, stridor, restlessness, or other signs of respiratory distress. Direct laryngoscopy would be necessary to confirm suspicions of laryngeal stenosis. A bronchoscope then could be passed into the laryngeal area to allow palpation of the web to determine its extent and thickness. Severe stenosis or extensive webbing requires either cricothyrotomy or tracheostomy to provide an airway (Lucente, 1987). Webs can also occur as a result of laryngeal trauma (Colton & Casper, 1990).

Surgical correction of a web requires the placement of a keel between the vocal folds to keep the web from reforming during the reepithelialization stage of healing. Without the keel, the constant contact of the healing vocal folds regenerates the web. Although it would appear that a web could be corrected easily, the dynamic nature of vocal fold movement makes it difficult for easy management, and the client with a congenital laryngeal web may have to undergo several procedures of management, including dilations and surgical excision, the latter performed recently by means of the CO_2 laser.

Congenital Chondromalacia

Another congenital condition that can produce immediate symptoms of stridor, dyspnea, and cyanosis is congenital chondromalacia, which involves flaccidity of the cartilaginous structures of the larynx. Because of this flaccidity, the epiglottis and aryepiglottal folds are easily pulled down over the opening to the glottis, causing respiratory difficulty. It is thought to be caused by a calcium deficiency and usually is treated successfully by diet control. It does not usually present such a problem that tracheostomy or intubation is required (Cody, Kern, & Pearson, 1981).

Cri du Chat Syndrome

Cri du chat (cry of the cat) syndrome was named because infants born with this condition have a high-pitched cry that sounds more like a kitten than a baby crying. It involves chromosome abnormality (partial deletion of a group B chromosome).

Several additional characteristics associated with the cri du chat infant include mental retardation, a rounded facies, a beaklike profile, microcephaly, hypotonia, hypertelorism, anti-Mongoloid palpebral fissures, epicanthal folds, strabismus, midline oral clefts, and generally poor development (A. E. Aronson, 1985).

Other Laryngeal Conditions

Several other conditions that can occur in the laryngeal area are worth mentioning, although the speech–language pathologist usually is not involved in the rehabilitation. A laryngeal cyst is a growth occurring in multifocal or singular form. It usually is found on the false vocal folds and in the larynx and develops secondary to abnormalities in the ductal system of the mucous glands. Cysts generally are removed surgically. Some cases have needed the services of a speech–language pathologist in vocal rehabilitation (Bais, Uppal, & Logani, 1989; Colton & Casper, 1990; Shaw & Lancer, 1987). Another abnormality is the laryngocele, an air sac connected to the laryngeal ventricle as well as to other locations. Laryngoceles often are seen following laryngectomy in the area of the pharyngoesophageal junction (P-E junction). Laryngoceles differ from cysts in that they are filled with air, whereas cysts are filled with mucus.

Laryngeal Trauma. Some persons have become dysphonic as a result of an automobile accident, a blow to the larynx in a fight, or a penetrating wound such as from a bullet or knife. Each such form of laryngeal trauma is different, and the speech–language pathologist must evaluate every case on the basis of residual status of the larynx following all medical and reconstructive treatment. The principles of evaluation and treatment for many of the disorders covered in this book apply to the person with dysphonia following laryngeal trauma (Sataloff et al., 1988; Schaefer & Close, 1989).

Dysphonia Presenting as Asthma. Christopher et al. (1983) presented information on a functional voice disorder that mimics attacks of bronchial asthma. They reported on 5 patients who presented symptoms of dramatic episodes of wheezing who had been diagnosed as having uncontrolled asthma. Paroxysms (sudden recurrence or intensification) of wheezing and dyspnea persisted despite aggressive medical management, including bronchodilators and long-term steroid therapy.

Loudon, Lee, and Holcomb (1988) studied 10 healthy subjects and compared them with 14 patients with varying degrees of asthma. Their protocol involved conversation, monologue, and counting at two loudness levels while measuring respiration patterns with a Respitrace. These authors found that asthma patients used a greater percentage of their reduced vital capacities, had slower inspiratory flow rates, faster expiratory flow rates, and spent a greater amount of the total respiratory cycle time on inspiration. When necessary, asthma patients favored respiratory needs over communication needs and would cease speaking in order to maintain necessary ventilation.

Multidisciplinary analyses, including physiologic, psychiatric, laryngologic, and speech pathologic evaluations, provided the correct diagnosis of a functional spasm of the vocal folds that the authors interpreted as a conversion disorder. The patients responded uniformly and dramatically to voice and psychiatric therapies that taught them how to relax and reduce the laryngeal spasm and to understand the nature of the disorder. Because this vocal phenomenon has been only recently understood, more patients can be expected to be found with it.

AIDS and the Speech–Language Pathologist

The speech–language pathologist is often involved in the evaluation and treatment of patients with AIDS (acquired immunodeficiency syndrome). It is therefore imperative that the speech–language pathologist be concerned about infection and the possible spreading of any virus including the human immunodeficiency virus of AIDS. Hadderingh, Tange, Danner, and Schattenkerk (1987) reported 43 of 63 (68%) cases of AIDS had otolaryngological manifestations, including neck masses, a greater incidence of shortness of breath, and chronic cough. Care should be taken by speech–language pathologists to use gloves in the examination of all patients in which the exchange of body fluids is possible, such as orolaryngeal and endoscopic examinations. An excellent reference for clinicians practicing in hospitals and clinics in which there is a greater probability of such examinations occurring is provided by R. M. Miller and Groher (1990).

Summary

The main focus of this chapter has been a description of resonance disorders of the voice, including degrees of hypernasality, mixed nasality, and hearing impairment. The nature of these disorders, etiology, evaluation, medical and rehabilitation therapies, and general consideration of management have been discussed. Several miscellaneous laryngeal disorders, including papillomas, polyps, ventricular dysphonia, laryngeal webs, chondromalacia, cri du chat, cysts, and laryngocele, also have been described.

References

Abitbol, J., de Brux, J., Millot, G., Masson, M.-F., Mimoun, O. L., Pau, H., & Abitbol, B. (1989). Does a hormonal vocal cord cycle exist in women? Study of vocal premenstrual syndrome in voice performers by videostroboscopy-glottography and cytology on 38 women. *Journal of Voice, 3,* 157–162.

Abitbol, J., Mathe, G., & Battista, C. (1988). Preliminary report on detection of papillomaviruses types 6, 11, 16, and 18 in laryngeal benign and malignant lesions. *Journal of Voice, 2,* 334–337.

Allison, D. L., & Leeper, H. A., Jr. (1990). A comparison of noninvasive procedures to assess nasal airway resistance. *Cleft Palate Journal, 27*(1), 40–45.

American Joint Committee for Cancer Staging and End-Results Reporting: Manual for stages of cancer (2nd ed.). (1983). Philadelphia: J. B. Lippincott.

American Psychiatric Association. (1987). *The diagnostic and statistical manual of mental disorders* (3rd ed. rev.). Washington, DC: Author.

Andrews, M. L. (1986). *Voice therapy for children.* New York: Longman.

Andrews, M., Tardy, S., & Pasternak, L. (1984). The modification of hypernasality in young children: a programming approach. *Language Speech and Hearing Services in Schools, 15,* 37–43.

Arnold, G. E. (1980). Disorders in laryngeal function. In M. M. Paparella & D. A. Shumrick (Eds.), *Otalaryngology* (Vol. 3). Philadelphia: W. B. Saunders.

Aronson, A. E. (1971). Early motor unit disease masquerading as psychogenic breathy dysphonia: A clinical case presentation. *Journal of Speech and Hearing Disorders, 36*(1), 115–124.

Aronson, A. E. (1973). *Audio seminars in speech pathology: Psychogenic voice disorders: An interdisciplinary approach to detection diagnosis, and therapy.* Philadelphia: Saunders.

Aronson, A. E. (1985). *Clinical voice disorders: An interdisciplinary approach* (2nd ed.). New York: Thieme-Stratton.

Aronson, A. E., & DeSanto, L. W. (1983). Adductor spastic dysphonia: Three years after recurrent laryngeal nerve resection. *Laryngoscope, 93,* 1–8.

Aronson, A. E., & Hartman, D. E. (1981). Adductor spastic dysphonia as a sign of essential (voice) tremor. *Journal of Speech and Hearing Disorders, 46*(1), 52–58.

Aronson, L. R., & Cooper, M. L. (1979). Amygdaloid hypersexuality in male rats reexamined. *Physiology and Behavior, 22,* 257–265.

Bachmayer, D., & Ross, R. B. (1986). Stability of Le Fort III advancement surgery in children with Crouzon's, Apert's, and Pfeiffer's syndromes. *Cleft Palate Journal, 23*(Suppl. 1), 69–74.

Baer, T., Titze, I. R., & Yoshioka, H. (1983). Multiple simultaneous measures of vocal fold activity. In D. B. Bless & J. H. Abbs (Eds.), *Vocal fold physiology: Contemporary research and clinical issues.* San Diego: College-Hill.

Bailey, B. J., & Biller, H. F. (1985). *Surgery of the larynx.* Philadelphia: Saunders.

Bais, A. S., Uppal, K., & Logani, K. B. (1989). Congenital cysts of the larynx. *Journal of Laryngology and Otology, 103,* 966–967.

Baken, R. J. (1987). *Clinical measurement of speech and voice.* Austin, TX: PRO-ED.

Barnhart, E. R. (Ed.). (1990). *Physician's desk reference* (44th ed.). Oradell, NJ: Medical Economics.

Bassich, C. J., & Ludlow, C. L. (1986). The use of perceptual methods by new clinicians for assessing voice quality. *Journal of Speech and Hearing Disorders, 51,* 125–133.

Bateman, H. E., & Mason, R. M. (1984). *Applied anatomy and physiology of the speech and hearing mechanism.* Springfield, IL: Charles C. Thomas.

Batza, E. M., & Parker, W. (1971). Hyponasality associated with patulous eustachian tubes: Report of a case. *Journal of Speech and Hearing Disorders, 36,* 410–413.

Beery, Q. C., Rood, S. R., & Schramm, V. L. (1983). Pharyngeal wall motion in prosthetically managed cleft palate adults. *Cleft Palate Journal, 20*(1), 7–14.

Bell-Berti, F. (1976). Electromyographic study of velopharyngeal function in speech. *Journal of Speech and Hearing Research, 19,* 225–240.

Benjamin, B., & Croxson, G. (1987). Vocal nodules in children. *Annals of Otology, Rhinology, and Laryngology, 99,* 530–533.

Benjamin, B. N., Gatenby, P. A., Kitchen, R., Harrison, H., Cameron, K., & D'Phil, A. B. (1988). Alpha-interferon (wellferon) as an adjunct to standard surgical therapy in the management of recurrent respiratory papillomatosis. *Annals of Otology, Rhinology, and Laryngology, 97,* 376–380.

Berke, G. S., Hanson, D. G., Trapp, T. K., Moore, D. M., Gerratt, B. R., & Natividad, M. (1989). Office-based system for voice analysis. *Archives of Otolaryngology: Head and Neck Surgery, 115,* 74–77.

Berry, W. R., Darley, F. R., Aronson, A. E., & Goldstein, N. P. (1974). Dysarthria in Wilson's disease. *Journal of Speech and Hearing Research, 17,* 169–183.

Bevan, K., Griffiths, M. V., & Morgan, M. H. (1989). Cricothyroid muscle paralysis: Its recognition and diagnosis. *Journal of Laryngology and Otology, 103,* 191–195.

Biller, H. F., & Lawson, W. (1981). Bilateral vertical partial laryngectomy for bilateral vocal cord carcinoma. *Annals of Otolaryngology, 90,* 489–491.

Bless, D. M., & Abbs, J. H. (Eds.). (1983). *Vocal fold physiology.* San Diego: College-Hill.

Blitzer, A. B., Brin, M. F., Fahn, S., & Lovelace, R. E. (1988). Localized injections of botulinum toxin for the treatment of focal laryngeal dystonia (spastic dysphonia). *Laryngoscope, 98,* 193–197.

Blitzer, A., Brin, M. F., Green, P. E., & Fahn, S. (1989). Botulinum toxin injection for the treatment of oromandibular dystonia. *Annals of Otology, Rhinology, and Laryngology, 98,* 93–97.

Blom, E. D., & Singer, M. L. (1979). Surgical-prosthetic approaches for postlaryngectomy voice restoration. In R. L. Keith & F. L. Darley (Eds.), *Laryngectomee rehabilitation.* Austin, TX: PRO-ED.

Blom, E. D., Singer, M. I., & Hamaker, R. C. (1982). Tracheostoma valve for post-laryngectomy voice rehabilitation. *Annals of Otology, Rhinology, and Laryngology, 91,* 576–578.

Blom, E. D., Singer, M. I., & Hamaker, R. C. (1985). An improved esophageal insufflation test. *Archives of Otolaryngology, 111,* 211–213.

Bocca, E., Pignataro, O., & Oldini, C. (1983). Supraglottic laryngectomy: 30 years of experience. *Annals of Otology, Rhinology, and Laryngology, 92,* 14–18.

Boone, D. R. (1966). Treatment of functional aphonia in a child and an adult. *Journal of Speech and Hearing Disorders, 31,* 69–74.

Boone, D. R. (1977). *The voice and voice therapy* (2nd ed.). Englewood Cliffs, NJ: Prentice-Hall.

Boone, D. R. (1980). *The Boone voice program for children.* Austin, TX: PRO-ED.

Boone, D. R. (1982). *The Boone voice program for adults.* Austin, TX: PRO-ED.

Boone, D. R. (1988). Respiratory training in voice therapy. *Journal of Voice, 2,* 20–25.

Boone, D. R., & McFarlane, S. (1988). *The voice and voice therapy* (4th ed.). Englewood Cliffs, NJ: Prentice-Hall.

Bradley, D. P. (1989). Congenital and acquired velopharyngeal inadequacy. In K. R. Bzoch (Ed.). *Communicative disorders related to cleft lip and palate.* Austin, TX: PRO-ED.

Bralley, R. C., Bull, G. L., Gore, C. H., & Edgerton, M. T. (1978). Evaluation of vocal pitch in male transsexuals. *Journal of Communication Disorders, 11,* 443–449.

Brantigan, C. O., Brantigan, T. A., & Joseph, N. (1982). Effect of beta blockade and beta stimulation on stage fright. *American Journal of Medicine, 72,* 88–94.

Brin, M. F., Blitzer, A., Fahn, S., Gould, W., & Lovelace, R. E. (1989). Adductor laryngeal dystonia (spastic dysphonia): Treatment with local injections of botulinum toxin (Botox). *Movement Disorders, 4,* 287–296.

Brodnitz, F. S. (1961). Contact ulcer of the larynx. *Archives of Otolaryngology, 74,* 70–75.

Brodnitz, F. S. (1975). The age of the castrato voice. *Journal of Speech and Hearing Disorders, 40,* 290–291.

Brodnitz, F. S. (1981). Psychological considerations in vocal rehabilitation. *Journal of Speech and Hearing Disorders, 46,* 21–26.

Brown, W. S., Morris, R. J., & Michel, J. F. (1989). Vocal jitter in young adult and aged female voices. *Journal of Voice, 3,* 113–119.

Bzoch, K. R. (Ed.). (1989a). *Communicative disorders related to cleft lip and palate* (3rd Ed.) Austin, TX: PRO-ED.

Bzoch, K. R. (1989b). Measurement and assessment of categorical aspects of cleft palate language, voice and speech disorders. In K. R. Bzoch (Ed.). *Communicative disorders related to cleft lip and palate* (3rd Ed.) Austin, TX: PRO-ED.

Campbell, S. L., Reich, A. R., Klockars, A. J., & McHenry, M. A. (1988). Factors associated with dysphonia in high school cheerleaders. *Journal of Speech and Hearing Disorders, 53,* 175–185.

Cannon, C. R., & McLean, W. C. (1982). Laryngectomy for chronic aspiration. *American Journal of Otolaryngology, 3,* 145–149.

Carpenter, R. J., McDonald, T. J., & Howard, F. M. (1979). The otolaryngologic presentation of myasthenia gravis. *Laryngoscope, 89,* 922–928.

Case, J. L. (1981, November). *Excellent pharyngeal to superior pseudoesophageal phonation after laryngoesophagectomy: A case study.* Paper presented at the convention of the American Speech–Language–Hearing Association, Los Angeles.

Case, J. L. (1982a). Applications in behavior therapy. In D. E. Mowrer, *Methods of modifying speech behaviors* (2nd ed.). Columbus, OH: Merrill.

Case, J. L. (1982b). Case example of vocal nodules with serious complications. In D. E. Mowrer & J. L. Case, *Clinical management of speech disorders.* Austin, TX: PRO-ED.

Case, J. L. (1987, November). *Puberphonia: Before and after therapy. Acoustic analysis of pitch.* Paper presented at the Annual Convention of the American Speech–Language–Hearing Association, New Orleans.

Case, J. L., Beaver, V. L., & Nenaber, P. J. (1978, November). *A longitudinal study of a high-risk population for vocal abuse—University cheerleaders.* Paper presented at the convention of the American Speech–Language–Hearing Association, San Francisco.

Case, J. L., & Cleary, K. (1976, November). *Psychogenic falsetto associated with surgically induced vocal fold paralysis.* Paper presented at the convention of the American Speech–Language–Hearing Association, Houston.

Case, J. L., & Holen, D. (1976). *A survey of attitudes of Arizona laryngologists regarding alaryngeal rehabilitation.* Paper presented at the convention of the Arizona Speech–Language–Hearing Association, Tucson.

Case, J. L., LaPointe, L. L., & Duane, D. D. (1990, March). *Speech and voice characteristics in spasmodic torticollis.* Paper presented at the International Congress of Movement Disorders, Washington, DC.

Case, J. L., Thome, J., & Kohler, S. (1979, November). *A longitudinal study of vocal abuse among cheerleaders.* Paper presented at the Convention of the American Speech–Language–Hearing Association, Atlanta.

Casper, J. K., Brewer, D. W., & Colton, R. H. (1987). Variations in normal human laryngeal anatomy and physiology as viewed fiberscopically. *Journal of Voice, 1,* 180–185.

Casper, J. K., Brewer, D. W., & Colton, R. H. (1988). Pitfalls and problems in flexible fiberoptic videolaryngoscopy. *Journal of Voice, 1,* 347–352.

Christensen, J. M., & Weinberg, B. (1976). Vowel duration characteristics of esophageal speech. *Journal of Speech and Hearing Research, 19,* 678–689.

Christensen, J. M., Weinberg, B., & Alfonso, P. J. (1978). Productive voice onset time characteristics esophageal speech. *Journal of Speech and Hearing Research, 21,* 56–62.

Christopher, K. L., Wood, R. P., Eckert, R. C., Blager, F. B., Raney, R. A., & Souhrada, D. F. (1983). Vocal cord dysfunction presenting as asthma. *The New England Journal of Medicine, 308,* 1566–1570.

Cody, D. T. R., Kern, E. B., & Pearson, B. W. (1981). *Diseases of the ears, nose, and throat: A guide to diagnosis and management.* Chicago: Year Book Medical Publishers.

Cohen, S. R., Geller, K. A., Birns, J. W., & Thompson, J. W. (1982). Laryngeal paralysis in children: A long-term retrospective study. *Annals of Otology, Rhinology, and Laryngology, 91,* 417–424.

Cohen, S. R., Geller, K. A., Seltzer, S., & Thompson, J. W. (1980). Papilloma of the larynx and tracheobronchial tree in children: A retrospective study. *Annals of Otolaryngology, 89,* 497–502.

Coleman, R. F. (1987). Performance demands and the performer's vocal capabilities. *Journal of Voice, 1,* 209–216.

Colton, R. H., & Casper, J. K. (1990). *Understanding voice problems. A physiological perspective for diagnosis and treatment.* Baltimore: Williams and Wilkins.

Cooper, D. S., & Titze, I. R. (1985). Generation and dissipation of heat in vocal fold tissue. *Journal of Speech and Hearing Research, 28,* 207–215.

Cornut, G., & Bouchayer, M. (1989). Phonosurgery for singers. *Journal of Voice, 3,* 269–276.

Crissman, J. D. (1982). Laryngeal keratosis preceding laryngeal carcinoma. *Archives of Otolaryngology, 108,* 445–448.

Croft, C. B., Shprintzen, R. J., & Ruben, R. J. (1981). Hypernasal speech following adenotonsillectomy. *Otolaryngology Head and Neck Surgery, 89,* 179–188.

Crysdale, W. S., Feldman, R. I., & Naito, K. (1988). Tracheotomies: A 10-year experience in 319 children. *Annals of Otology, Rhinology, and Laryngology, 97,* 439–443.

Dalston, R. M., & Keefe, M. J. (1988). Digital, labial, and velopharyngeal reaction times in normal speakers. *Cleft Palate Journal, 25,* 203–209.

Dalston, R. M., & Stuteville, O. H. (1975). A clinical investigation of the efficacy of primary nasopalatal pharyngoplasty. *Cleft Palate Journal, 12,* 177–191.

Dalston, R. M., & Warren, D. W. (1986). Comparison of Tonar II, pressure flow, and listener judgments of hypernasality in assessment of velopharyngeal function. *Cleft Palate Journal, 23,* 108–115.

Dalston, R. M., Warren, D. W., Morr, K. E., & Smith, L. R. (1988). Intraoral pressure and its relationship to velopharyngeal inadequacy. *Cleft Palate Journal, 25,* 210–219.

Damsté, P. H. (1958). *Oesophageal speech.* Groningen, The Netherlands.

Daniloff, R., Schuckers, G., & Feth, L. (1980). *The physiology of speech and hearing: An introduction.* Englewood Cliffs, NJ: Prentice-Hall.

D'Antonio, L. L., Marsh, J. L., Province, M. A., Muntz, H. R., & Phillips, C. J. (1989). Reliability of flexible fiberoptic nasopharyngoscopy for evaluation of velopharyngeal function in a clinical population. *Cleft Palate Journal, 26,* 217–225.

Darley, F. L. (1940). *A normative study of oral reading rate.* Unpublished master's thesis, State University of Iowa, Iowa City.

Darley, F. L., Aronson, A. E., & Brown, J. R. (1969a). Clusters of deviant speech dimensions in the dysarthrias. *Journal of Speech and Hearing Research, 12,* 462–496.

Darley, F. L., Aronson, A. E., & Brown, J. R. (1969b). Differential diagnostic patterns of dysarthria. *Journal of Speech and Hearing Research, 12,* 246–269.

Darley, F. L., Aronson, A. E., & Brown, J. R. (1975). *Audio seminars in speech pathology: Motor speech disorders.* Philadelphia: Saunders.

Darley, F. L., Aronson, A. E., & Brown, J. R. (1975b). *Motor-speech disorders.* Philadelphia: Saunders.

Darley, F. L., Brown, J. R., & Goldstein, N. P. (1972). Dysarthria in multiple sclerosis. *Journal of Speech and Hearing Research, 15,* 229–245.

Deal, R. E., McClain, B., & Sudderth, J. F. (1976). Identification, evaluation, therapy, and follow-up for children with vocal nodules in a public school setting. *Journal of Speech and Hearing Disorders, 41,* 390–397.

Dedo, D. D., & Dedo, H. H. (1980). Vocal cord paralysis. In M. M. Paparelle & D. A. Shumrick (Eds.), *Otolaryngology: Vol. 3. Head and neck.* Philadelphia: Saunders.

Dedo, H. H. (1976). Recurrent laryngeal nerve section for spastic dysphonia. *Annals of Otology, Rhinology, and Laryngology, 85,* 1–9.

Dedo, H. H. (1988). Avoidance and treatment of complications of Teflon injection of the vocal cord. *Journal of Voice, 2,* 90–92.

Dedo, H. H., & Izdebski, K. (1983a). Intermediate results of 306 recurrent laryngeal nerve sections for spastic dysphonia. *Laryngoscope, 93,* 9–15.

Dedo, H. H., & Izdebski, K. (1983b). Problems with surgical (RLN section) treatment in spastic dysphonia. *Laryngoscope, 93,* 268–271.

Dedo, H. H., & Jackler, R. K. (1982). Laryngeal papilloma: Results of treatment with the CO_2 laser and podophyllum. *Annals of Otology, Rhinology, and Laryngology, 91,* 425–430.

DeSanto, L. W., Holt, J. J., Beahrs, O. H., & O'Fallon, M. W. (1982). Neck dissection: Is it worthwhile? *Laryngoscope, 92,* 502–509.

DeSanto, L. W., Pearson, B. W., & Olsen, K. D. (1989). Utility of near-total laryngectomy for supraglottic, pharyngeal, base-of-tongue, and other cancers. *Annals of Otology, Rhinology, and Laryngology, 99,* 2–6.

Deutsch, H. L., & Millard, D. R. (1989). A new cocaine abuse complex: Involvement in the nose, septum, palate, and pharynx. *Archives of Otolaryngology: Head & Neck Surgery, 115,* 235–237.

DeWeese, D. D., & Saunders, W. H. (1982). *Textbook of otolaryngology* (6th ed.). St. Louis: Mosby.

Dey, F. L., & Kirchner, J. A. (1961). The upper esophageal sphincter after laryngectomy. *Laryngoscope, 71,* 99–115.

Dickens, W. J., Cassisi, N. J., Million, R. R., & Boa, F. J. (1983). Treatment of early vocal cord carcinoma: A comparison of apples and apples. *Laryngoscope, 93,* 216–219.

Dickson, D. R., & Dickson, W. M. (1972). Velopharyngeal anatomy. *Journal of Speech and Hearing Research, 15,* 372–381.

Dickson, D. R., & Dickson, W. M. (1982). *Anatomical and physiological bases of speech.* Austin, TX: PRO-ED.

Dickson, S., Barron, S., & McGlone, R. E. (1978). Aerodynamic studies of cleft palate speech. *Journal of Speech and Hearing Disorders, 43,* 160–167.

Diedrich, W. M., & Youngstrom, K. A. (1966). *Alaryngeal speech.* Springfield, IL: Charles C. Thomas.

Directory of residency training programs. (1989). Chicago: American Medical Association.

Doherty, T. E., & Shipp, T. (1988). Tape recorder effects on jitter and shimmer extraction. *Journal of Speech and Hearing Research, 31,* 485–490.

Donald, P. J. (1982). Voice change surgery in the transsexual. *Otolaryngology Head and Neck Surgery, 4,* 433–437.

Drudge, M. K. M., & Philips, B. J. (1976). Shaping behavior in voice therapy. *Journal of Speech and Hearing Disorders, 41,* 398–411.

Duane, D. D. (1988). Spasmodic torticollis: Clinical and biologic features and their implications for focal dystonia. In S. Fahn, C. D. Marsden, & D. B. Calne (Eds.). *Advances in neurology: Vol. 50. Dystonia 2.* New York: Raven Press.

Duguay, M. (1979). Special problems of the alaryngeal speaker. In R. L. Keith & F. L. Darley, *Laryngectomee rehabilitation.* Austin, TX: PRO-ED.

Duguay, M. J. (1989). Esophageal voice: An historical review. *Journal of Voice, 3,* 264–268.

Eckel, F. C., & Boone, D. R. (1981). The s/z ratio as an indicator of laryngeal pathology. *Journal of Speech and Hearing Disorders, 46,* 147–149.

Emanuel, F. W., & Whitehead, R. L. (1979). Harmonic levels and vowel roughness. *Journal of Speech and Hearing Research, 22,* 829–840.

Emerick, L. L., & Hatten, J. T. (1974). *Diagnosis and evaluation in speech pathology.* Englewood Cliffs, NJ: Prentice-Hall.

Fahn, S., Marsden, C. D., & Calne, D. B. (Eds.). (1988). *Advances in neurology: Vol. 50. Dystonia 2.* New York: Raven Press.

Fairbanks, G. (1960). *Voice and articulation drillbook* (2nd ed.). New York: Harper and Brothers.

Fara, M., Dedlackova, E., Klaskova, O., Hrivnakova, J., Chemelova, A., & Supacek, I. (1970). Primary pharyngofixation in cleft palate repair: A survey of 46 years' experience with an evaluation of 2,073 cases. *Plastic and Reconstructive Surgery, 45,* 449–458.

Feder, R. J. (1983). Varix of the vocal cord in the professional voice user. *Otolaryngology Head and Neck Surgery, 91,* 435–436.

Fendler, M., & Shearer, W. M. (1988). Reliability of the S/Z ratio in normal children's voices. *Language Speech and Hearing Services in Schools, 19,* 2.

Finitzo, T., & Freeman, F. (1989). Spasmodic dysphonia, whether and where: Results of seven years of research. *Journal of Speech and Hearing Research, 32,* 541–555.

Fletcher, S. G. (1978). *Diagnosing speech disorders from cleft palate.* New York: Grune and Stratton.

Flores, T. C., Wood, B. G., Levine, H. L., Koegel, L., & Tucker, H. M. (1982). Factors in successful deglutition following supraglottic laryngeal surgery. *Annals of Otology, Rhinology, and Laryngology, 91,* 579–583.

Ford, C. N. & Bless, D. M. (1987). Collagen injection in the scarred vocal fold. *Journal of Voice, 1,* 116–118.

Forner, L. L., & Hixon, T. J. (1977). Respiratory kinematics in profoundly hearing impaired speakers. *Journal of Speech and Hearing Research, 20,* 373–408.

Fox, D. R., Lynch, J. I., & Cronin, T. D. (1988). Change in nasal resonance over time: A clinical study. *Cleft Palate Journal, 25,* 245–247.

Froeschels, E., Kastein, S., & Weiss, D. A. (1955). A method of therapy for paralytic conditions of the mechanisms of phonation, respiration, and glutination. *Journal of Speech and Hearing Disorders, 20,* 365–370.

Furlow, L. T., Jr., Block, A. J., & Williams, W. N. (1986). Obstructive sleep apnea following treatment of velopharyngeal incompetence by Teflon injection. *Cleft Palate Journal, 23,* 153–158.

Furlow, L. T., Williams, W. N., Eisenbach, C. R., & Bzoch, K. R. (1982). A long term study on treating velopharyngeal insufficiency by Teflon injection. *Cleft Palate Journal, 19,* 47–56.

Gacek, R. R. (1987). Botulinum toxin for relief of spasmodic dysphonia (To the Editor). *Archives of Otolaryngology—Head and Neck Surgery, 113,* 1240.

Gallivan, G. J., Dawson, J. A., & Robbins, L. D. (1989). Videolaryngoscopy after endotracheal intubation: Implications for voice. *Journal of Voice, 3,* 76–80.

Garfinkle, T. J., & Kimmelman, C. P. (1982). Neurological disorders: Amyotrophic lateral sclerosis, myasthenia gravis, multiple sclerosis, and poliomyelitis. *American Journal of Otolaryngology, 3,* 204–212.

Gates, G. A., & Hearne, E. M. (1982). Predicting esophagal speech. *Annals of Otology, Rhinology, and Laryngology, 91,* 454–457.

Gates, G. A., & Montalbo, P. J. (1987). The effects of low-dose beta-blockade on performance anxiety in singers. *Journal of Voice, 1,* 105–108.

Gay, T., & Hirose, H. (1972). Electromyography of the intrinsic laryngeal muscles during phonation. *Annals of Otology, Rhinology, and Laryngology, 81,* 401–409.

Gelfer, M. P. (1988). Perceptual attributes of voice: Development and use of rating scales. *Journal of Voice, 2,* 320–326.

Gibb, A. G. (1958). Hypernasality (*rhinolalia aperta*) following tonsil and adenoid removal. *Journal of Laryngology and Otology, 72,* 433–451.

Gilbert, H. R., & Weismer, G. G. (1974). The effects of smoking on the speaking fundamental frequency of adult women. *Journal of Psycholinguistic Research, 3,* 225–231.

Gilman, A. G., Goodman, L. S., & Gilman, A. (Eds.). (1980). *Goodman and Gilman's The Pharmacological Basis of Therapeutics* (6th ed.). New York: Macmillan.

Gomyo, Y., & Doyle, P. G. (1989). Perception of stop consonants produced by esophageal and tracheoesophageal speakers. *Journal of Otolaryngology, 18,* 184–188.

Gonzalez, J. B., & Aronson, A. E. (1970). Palatal lift prosthesis for treatment for anatomic and neurologic palatopharyngeal insufficiency. *Cleft Palate Journal, 7,* 91–104.

Goudie, A. J., & Emmett-Oglesby, M. W. (1989). *Psychoactive drugs: Tolerance and sensitization.* Clifton, NJ: Humana Press.

Gould, W. J. (1987). The clinical voice laboratory: Clinical application of voice research. *Journal of Voice, 1,* 305–309.

Gould, W. J., & Lawrence, V. L. (1984). Surgical care of voice disorders. New York: Springer-Verlag.

Gramming, P., Sundberg, J., Ternstrom, S., Leanderson, R., & Perkins, W. H. (1988). *Journal of Voice, 2,* 118–126.

Green, G., & Huylts, M. (1982). Preferences for three types of alaryngeal speech. *Journal of Speech and Hearing Disorders, 47,* 141–145.

Greene, M. C. L. (1980). *The voice and its disorders* (4th ed.). Philadelphia: Lippincott.

Griffiths, C., & Bough, I. D., Jr. (1989). Neurological diseases and their effect on voice. *Journal of Voice, 3,* 148–156.

Haber, K. (1987). *Common abbreviations in clinical medicine.* New York: Raven Press.

Hadderingh, R. J., Tange, R. A., Danner, S. A., & Schattenkerk, J. K. M. E. (1987). Otorhinolaryngological findings in AIDS patients: A study of 63 cases. *Archives of Otorhinolaryngology, 244,* 11–14.

Hahn, E. (1989). Directed home language stimulation program for infants with cleft lip and palate. In K. R. Bzoch (Ed.). *Communicative disorders related to cleft lip and palate* (3rd ed.). Austin, TX: PRO-ED.

Hairfield, W. M., Warren, D. W., Hinton, V. A., & Seaton, D. L. (1987). Inspiratory and expiratory effects of nasal breathing. *Cleft Palate Journal, 24,* 183–189.

Hairfield, W. M., Warren, D. W., & Seaton, D. L. (1988). Prevalence of mouth-breathing in cleft lip and palate. *Cleft Palate Journal, 25,* 135–138.

Hamaker, R. C., Singer, M. I., Blom, E. D., & Daniels, H. A. (1985). Primary voice restoration at laryngectomy. *Archives of Otolaryngology, 111,* 182–186.

Hammarberg, B., Fritzell, B., & Schiratzki, H. (1984). Teflon injection in 16 patients with paralytic dysphonia: Perceptual and acoustic evaluations. *Journal of Speech and Hearing Disorders, 49,* 72–82.

Hartman, D. E., & Aronson, A. E. (1983). Psychogenic aphonia masking mutational falsetto. *Archives of Otolaryngology, 109,* 415–416.

Hartman, D. E., Daily, W. W., & Morin, K. N. (1989). A case of superior laryngeal nerve paresis and psychogenic dysphonia. *Journal of Speech and Hearing Disorders, 54,* 526–529.

Harvey, N., & Howell, P. (1980). Isotonic vocalis contraction as a means of producing rapid decreases in F_0. *Journal of Speech and Hearing Research, 23,* 576–592.

Hess, D. A. (1976). A new experimental approach to assessment of velopharyngeal adequacy: Nasal manometric bleed testing. *Journal of Speech and Hearing Disorders, 41,* 427–443.

Hicks, J. N., Walker, E. E., & Moor, E. E. (1982). Diagnosis and conservative surgical management of chondrosarcoma of the larynx. *Annals of Otology, Rhinology, and Laryngology, 91,* 389–391.

Higgins, M. B., & Saxman, J. H. (1989). Variations in vocal frequency perturbation across the menstrual cycle. *Journal of Voice, 3,* 233–243.

Hillman, R. E., Holmberg, E. B., Perkell, J. S., Walsh, M., & Vaughan, C. (1989). Objective assessment of vocal hyperfunction: An experimental framework and initial results. *Journal of Speech and Hearing Research, 32,* 373–392.

Hirano, M. (1980). *The regulatory mechanism of voice in singing.* New York: Voice Foundation.

Hirano, M. (1981). *Clinical examination of voice.* New York: Springer-Verlag.

Hirano, M. (1990). Surgical and medical management of voice disorders. In R. H. Colton & J. K. Casper, *Understanding voice problems.* Baltimore: Williams & Wilkins.

Hirano, M., Feder, R., & Bless, D. M. (1983). *Clinical evaluation of patients with voice disorder: Stroboscopic evaluation.* Paper presented at the Convention of the American Speech–Language–Hearing Association, Cincinatti, OH.

Hirano, M., Kakita, Y., Kawasaki, H., Gould, W. J., & Lambiase, A. (1981). Data from high-speech motion picture studies. In K. N. Stevens & M. Hirano (Eds.), *Vocal fold physiology.* Tokyo: University of Tokyo Press.

Hirano, M., & Kurita, S. (1986). Histological structure of the vocal fold and its normal and pathological variations. In J. A. Kirchner (Ed.), *Vocal fold histopathology: A symposium.* San Diego: College-Hill.

Hirano, M., Kurita, S., & Matsuoka, H. (1987). Vocal function following hemilaryngectomy. *Annals of Otology, Rhinology, and Laryngology, 96,* 586–589.

Hirano, M., Kurita, S., & Nakashima, T. (1981). The structure of the vocal chords. In K. N. Stevens & M. Hirano (Eds.), *Vocal fold physiology.* Tokyo: University of Tokyo Press.

Hirano, M., Kurita, S., & Sakaguchi, S. (1989). Aging of the vibratory tissue of human vocal folds. *Acta Otolaryngology, 107,* 428–433.

Hirose, H., Kiritani, S., & Sawashima, M. (1982). Patterns of dysarthria movements in patients with amyotrophic lateral sclerosis and pseudobulbar palsy. *Folia Phoniatrica, 34,* 106–112.

Hixon, T. J., Bless, D. M., & Netsell, R. (1976). A new technique for measuring velopharyngeal orifice area during sustained vowel production: An application of aerodynamic forced oscillation principles. *Journal of Speech and Hearing Research, 19,* 601–607.

Hixon, T. J., Goldman, M. D., & Mead, J. (1973). Kinematics of the chest wall during speech production: Volume displacement of the rib cage, abdomen, and lungs. *Journal of Speech and Hearing Research, 16*(1), 78–115.

Hixon, T. J., Hawley, J. L., & Wilson, K. J. (1982). An around-the-house device for the clinical determination of respiratory driving pressure: A note on making simple even simpler. *Journal of Speech and Hearing Disorders, 47,* 413–415.

Hixon, T. J., Watson, P. J., Harris, F. P., & Pearl, N. B. (1988). Relative volume changes of the rib cage and abdomen during prephonatory chest wall posturing. *Journal of Voice, 2,* 13–19.

Hodge, M. M., & Rochet, A. P. (1989). Characteristics of speech breathing in young women. *Journal of Speech and Hearing Research, 32,* 466–480.

Holbrook, A., Rolnick, M. I., & Bailey, C. W. (1974). Treatment of vocal abuse disorders using a vocal intensity controller. *Journal of Speech and Hearing Disorders, 39,* 298–303.

Hollien, H. (1987). Old voices: What do we really know about them? *Journal of Voice, 1,* 2–17.

Hollien, H., Dew, D., & Phillips, P. (1971). Phonational frequency ranges of adults. *Journal of Speech and Hearing Research, 14,* 755–760.

Hollien, H., & Muller, E. (1973). Perceptual responses in infant crying: Identification of cry types. *Journal of Child Language, 1,* 89–95.

Hoops, H. R., & Noll, J. D. (1969). Relationship of selected acoustic variables to judgments of esophageal speech. *Journal of Communication Disorders, 2,* 1–13.

Hoover, L. A., Wortham, D. G., Lufkin, R. B., & Hanafee, W. N. (1987). Magnetic resonance imaging of the larynx and tongue base: Clinical applications. *Otolaryngology—Head and Neck Surgery, 97,* 245–256.

Horiguchi, S., & Bell-Berti, F. (1987). The velotrace: A device for monitoring velar position. *Cleft Palate Journal, 24,* 104–111.

Horii, Y. (1982a). Jitter and shimmer differences among sustained vowel phonations. *Journal of Speech and Hearing Research, 25,* 12–14.

Horii, Y. (1982b). Some voice fundamental frequency characteristics of oral reading and spontaneous speech by hard-of-hearing young women. *Journal of Speech and Hearing Research, 25,* 608–610.

Horii, Y. (1989). Frequency modulation characteristics of sustained /a/ sung in vocal vibrato. *Journal of Speech and Hearing Research, 32,* 829–836.

Horn, K. L., & Dedo, H. H. (1980). Surgical correction of the convex vocal cord after Teflon injection. *Laryngoscope, 90,* 281–286.

Horsley, I. A. (1982). Hypnosis and self-hypnosis in the treatment of psychogenic dysphonia: A case report. *The American Journal of Clinical Hypnosis, 24,* 277–283.

Hubbard, D. J., & Kushner, D. (1980). Comparison of speech intelligibility between esophageal and normal speakers via three modes of presentation. *Journal of Speech and Hearing Research, 23,* 909–916.

Hudson, A. I., & Holbrook, A. (1981). A study of the reading fundamental vocal frequency of young black adults. *Journal of Speech and Hearing Research, 24,* 197–201.

Hufnagle, J., & Hufnagle, K. K. (1988). S/Z ratio in dysphonic children with and without vocal cord nodules. *Language Speech and Hearing Services in Schools, 19,* 418–422.

Hutchinson, B. B., Hanson, M. L., & Mecham, M. J. (1979). *Diagnostic handbook of speech pathology.* Baltimore: Williams and Wilkins.

Isberg, A., Julin, P., Kraepelien, T., & Henrikson, C. O. (1989). Absorbed doses and energy imparted from radiographic examination of velopharyngeal function during speech. *Cleft Palate Journal, 26,* 105–109.

Isshiki, N., Taira, T., & Tanabe, M. (1983). Surgical alteration of the vocal pitch. *The Journal of Otolaryngology, 12,* 335–340.

Isshiki, N., Yanagihara, N., & Morimoto, M. (1966). Approach to the objective diagnosis of hoarseness. *Folia Phoniatrica, 18,* 393–400.

Izdebski, K., Ross, J. C., & Klein, J. C. (1990). Transoral rigid laryngovideostroboscopy (phonoscopy). In *Seminars in Speech and Language 11*(1), S. C. McFarlane (Ed.). New York: Thieme Medical.

Jacobson, E. (1978). *You must relax* (5th ed.). New York: McGraw-Hill.

Jarvis, B. L., & Trier, W. C. (1988). The effect of intravelar veloplasty on velopharyngeal competence following pharyngeal flap surgery. *Cleft Palate Journal, 25,* 389–394.

Johns, D. F. (Ed.). (1985). *Clinical management of neurogenic communicative disorders* (2nd ed.). Austin, TX: PRO-ED.

Johnson, T. S. (1976). *Vocal abuse reduction program.* Logan, UT: Utah State University, Department of Communication Disorders.

Johnson, T. S. (1983). Treatment of vocal abuse in children. In W. H. Perkins (Ed.), *Voice disorders: Current therapy of communication disorders.* New York: Thieme-Stratton.

Juarbe, C., Shemen, L., Wang, R., Anand, V., Eberle, R., Sirovatka, A., Malanaphy, K., & Klatsky, I. (1989). Tracheoesophageal puncture for voice restoration after extended laryngopharyngectomy. *Archives of Otolaryngology: Head and Neck Surgery, 115,* 356–359.

Jung, J. H. (1989). *Genetic syndromes in communication disorders.* Austin, TX: PRO-ED.

Kaban, L. B., Conover, M., & Mulliken, J. B. (1986). Midface position after Le Fort III advancement: A long-term follow-up study. *Cleft Palate Journal, 23*(Suppl. 1), 75–77.

Kahane, J. C. (1982). Growth of the human prepubertal and pubertal larynx. *Journal of Speech and Hearing Research, 25,* 446–455.

Kahane, J. C. (1987). Connective tissue changes in the larynx and their effects of voice. *Journal of Voice, 1,* 27–30.

Kahane, J. C., & Mayo, R. (1989). The need for aggressive pursuit of healthy childhood voices. *Language Speech & Hearing Services in Schools, 20*(1), 102–107.

Kalat, J. W. (1981). *Biological psychology.* Belmont, CA: Wadsworth.

Kalb, M. B., & Carpenter, M. A. (1981). Individual speaker influence on relative intelligibility of esophageal speech and artificial larynx speech. *Journal of Speech and Hearing Disorders, 46,* 77–80.

Kaplan, E. M. (1977). The occlut submucous cleft palate. *Cleft Palate Journal, 14,* 356–368.

Kaplan, S. L. (1982). Mutational falsetto. *Journal of the American Academy of Child Psychiatry, 21,* 82–85.

Karnell, M. P. (1989). Synchronized videostroboscopy and electroglottography. *Journal of Voice, 3,* 68–75.

Karnell, M. P., & Van Demark, D. L. (1986). Longitudinal speech performance in patients with cleft palate: Comparisons based on secondary management. *Cleft Palate Journal, 23,* 278–288.

Kay, N. J. (1982). Voice nodules in children—Aetiology and management. *Journal of Laryngology and Otology, 96,* 731–736.

Kelly, D. H., & Welborn, P. (1980). *The cover-up: Neckwear for the laryngectomee and other neck breathers.* Houston: College-Hill.

Kemker, F. J., & Zarajczyk, D. R. (1989). Audiological management in patients with cleft palate. In K. R. Bzoch, *Communicative disorders related to cleft lip and palate* (3rd ed.). Austin, TX: PRO-ED.

Kempster, G. B., Larson, C. R., & Kistler, M. K. (1988). Effects of electrical stimulation of cricothyroid and thyroarytenoid muscles on voice fundamental frequency. *Journal of Voice, 2,* 221–229.

Kendall, P. C., & Norton-Ford, J. D. (1982). *Clinical psychology: Scientific and professional dimensions.* New York: Wiley.

Kent, R. D., Netsell, R., & Abbs, J. H. (1979). Acoustic characteristics of dysarthria associated with cerebellar disease. *Journal of Speech and Hearing Research, 22,* 627–648.

Key, M. R. (1975). *Male/female language.* Metuchen, NJ: Scarecrow Press.

Kirchner, J. A. (1986). *Vocal fold histopathology: A symposium.* San Diego: College-Hill.

Kleinsasser, O. (1986). Microlaryngoscopic and histologic appearances of polyps, nodules, cysts, Reinke's edema, and granulomas of the vocal cords. In J. A. Kirchner (Ed.), *Vocal fold histopathology: A symposium.* San Diego: College-Hill.

Koufman, J. A. (1988). Letter to the Editor. *Journal of Voice, 2,* 269.

Koufman, J. A. (1989). Surgical correction of dysphonia due to bowing of the vocal cords. *Annals of Otology, Rhinology, and Laryngology, 98,* 41–45.

Koufman, J. A., & Blalock, P. D. (1982). Classification and approach to patients with functional voice disorders. *Annals of Otology, Rhinology, and Laryngology, 91,* 372–377.

Kozak, F. K., Freeman, R. D., Connolly, J. E., & Riding, K. H. (1989). Tourette syndrome and otolaryngology. *Journal of Otolaryngology, 18*(6), 279–282.

Kreiborg, S., & Aduss, H. (1986). Pre- and post-surgical facial growth in patients with Crouzon's and Apert's syndromes. *Cleft Palate Journal, 23*(Suppl. 1), 78–90.

Kuehn, D. P., & Van Demark, D. R. (1978). Assessment of velopharyngeal competency following Teflon pharyngoplasty. *Cleft Palate Journal, 15*(2), 145–149.

Kummer, A. W., Strife, J. L., Grau, W. H., Creaghead, N. A., & Lee, L. (1989). The effects of Le Fort I osteotomy with maxillary movement on articulation, resonance, and velopharyngeal function. *Cleft Palate Journal, 26,* 193–199.

Laing, A. (1989). *Speaking as a woman.* King of Prussia, PA: Creative Design Services.

Lancer, J. M., Syder, O., Jones, A. S., & LeBoutillier, A. (1988). Vocal cord nodules: A review. *Clinical Otolaryngology, 13*(1), 43–51.

Large, J. (1980). *Contributions of voice research in singing.* Houston: College-Hill.

Larson, C. R. (1988). Brain mechanisms involved in the control of vocalization. *Journal of Voice, 4,* 301–311.

Larson, C. R., Kempster, G. B., & Kistler, M. K. (1987). Changes in voice fundamental frequency following discharge of single motor units in cricothyroid and thyroarytenoid muscles. *Journal of Speech and Hearing Research, 30,* 552–558.

Lauder, E. (1985). *Self-help for the laryngectomee.* (Available from Edmund Lauder, 11115 Whisper Hollow, San Antonio, TX 78230.)

Lawson, L. I., Chierici, G., Castro, A., Harvold, E. P., Miller, E. R., & Owsley, J. Q. (1972). Effects of adenoidectomy on the speech of children with potential velopharyngeal dysfunction. *Journal of Speech and Hearing Disorders, 37,* 390–402.

Lawson, W., Biller, H. F., & Suen, J. Y. (1989). Cancer of the larynx. In E. N. Myers & J. Y. Suen, *Cancer of the head and neck* (2nd ed.). New York: Churchill Livingstone.

Leanderson, R., & Sundberg, J. (1988). Breathing for singing. *Journal of Voice, 2*(1), 2–12.

Leder, S. B., Spitzer, J. B., & Kirchner, J. C. (1987). Speaking fundamental frequency of postlingually profoundly deaf adult men. *Annals of Otology, Rhinology, and Laryngology, 96,* 322–324.

Lewin, J. S., Baugh, R. F., & Baker, S. R. (1987). An objective method for prediction of tracheoesophageal speech production. *Journal of Speech and Hearing Disorders, 52,* 212–217.

Lieberman, P. (1963). Some measures of the fundamental periodicity of normal and pathological larynges. *Journal of the Acoustical Society of America, 35,* 344–353.

Lieberman, P. (1977). *Speech physiology and acoustic phonetics.* New York: Macmillan.

Lieberman, P., Harris, K., Woolff, P., & Russell, L. (1971). Newborn infant cry and nonhuman primate vocalization. *Journal of Speech and Hearing Research, 14,* 718–727.

Lim, R. Y., & Chang, H. H. (1986, September). *Malignant degeneration of a laryngeal papilloma.* Paper presented at the Annual Meeting of the American Academy of Otolaryngology—Head and Neck Surgery, San Antonio, TX.

Lindstrom, J. M., Seybold, M. W., Lennon, V. A., Whittingham, S., & Duane, D. D. (1976). Antibody to acetylcholine receptor in myasthenia gravis: Prevalence, clinical correlates and diagnostic value. *Neurology* (Minneapolis), *26,* 1054–1059.

Ling, D. (1975). Amplification for speech. In D. R. Calvert & S. R. Silverman (Eds.), *Speech and deafness.* Washington, DC: Alexander Graham Bell Association for the Deaf.

Linville, S. E., Skarin, B. D., & Fornatto, E. (1989). The interrelationship of measures related to vocal function, speech rate, and laryngeal appearance in elderly women. *Journal of Speech and Hearing Science, 32,* 323–330.

Lippman, R. P. (1981). Detecting nazalization using a low-cost miniature accelerometer. *Journal of Speech and Hearing Research, 24,* 314–317.

Lisak, R. P. (1980). Multiple sclerosis: Evidence for immunopathogenesis. *Neurology,* *30,* 99–105.

Logemann, J. A., Fisher, H. B., Boshes, B., & Blonsky, R. (1978). Frequency and cooccurance of vocal tract dysfunctions in the speech of a large sample of Parkinson patients. *Journal of Speech and Hearing Disorders, 43*(1), 59–75.

Loney, R. W., & Bloem, T. J. (1987). Velopharyngeal dysfunction: recommendations for use of nomenclature. *Cleft Palate Journal, 24,* 334–335.

Lopez, M. J., Kraybill, W., McElroy, T. H., & Guena, O. (1987). Voice rehabilitation practice among head and neck surgeons. *Annals of Otology, Rhinology, and Laryngology, 96,* 261–263.

Loudon, R. G., Lee, L., & Holcomb, B. J. (1988). Volumes and breathing patterns during speech in healthy and asthmatic subjects. *Journal of Speech and Hearing Research, 31,* 219–227.

Lubit, E. C. (1967). Before an adenoidectomy stop! look! and listen! *New York State Journal of Medicine, 67,* 681–684.

Lucente, F. E. (Ed.). (1987). *Essentials of otolaryngology* (2nd ed.). New York: Raven Press.

Ludlow, C. L., & Conner, N. P. (1987). Dynamic aspects of phonatory control in spasmodic dysphonia. *Journal of Speech and Hearing Research, 30,* 197–206.

Lumpkin, S. M. M., Bishop, S. G., & Katz, P. O. (1989). Chronic dysphonia secondary to gastroesophageal reflux (GERD): Diagnosis using simultaneous dual-probe prolonged pH monitoring. *Journal of Voice, 4,* 351–355.

Maccomb, W. S., & Fletcher, G. H. (1967). *Cancer of the head and neck.* Baltimore: Williams and Wilkins.

Maniglia, A. J., Dodds, B., Sorensen, K., Kumar, N., & Katirji, M. B. (1989). Newer techniques of laryngeal reinnervation. *Annals of Otology, Rhinology, and Laryngology, 98,* 8–14.

Marsh, J. L. (1986). Long-term results of craniofacial surgery: A supplement to the Cleft Palate Journal. *Cleft Palate Journal, 23,* 1–128.

Martin, F. G. (1988). Tutorial: Drugs and vocal function. *Journal of Voice, 2,* 338–344.

Mason, R. (1973). Preventing speech disorders following adenoidectomy of preoperative examination. *Clinical Pediatrics, 12,* 405–414.

Mason, R. M. (1980). Principles and procedures of orofacial examination. *International Journal of Orofacial Myology, 6*(2), 3–16.

Mason, R. M., & Warren, D. W. (1980). Adenoid involution and developing hypernasality in cleft palate. *Journal of Speech and Hearing Disorders, 45,* 469–480.

Mason, R. M., & Zemlin, W. (1969). The phenomenon of vocal vibrato. *National Association of Teachers of Singing Bulletin, 22,* 12–17.

Mattson, P. J. (1980). *Vocal abuse from cheerleading: A case study.* Unpublished master's project, Arizona State University, Tempe.

McFarlane, S. C., & Watterson, T. L. (1990). Vocal nodules: Endoscopic study of their variations and treatment. In *Seminars in Speech and Language, 11*(1), S. C. McFarlane (Ed.). New York: Thieme Medical.

McKerns, D., & Bzoch, K. R. (1970). Variations in velopharyngeal valving: The factor of sex. *Cleft Palate Journal, 7,* 652–662.

McWilliams, B. J., Morris, H. L., & Shelton, R. L. (1990). *Cleft palate speech* (2nd ed.). Philadelphia: B. C. Decker.

McWilliams, B. J., Musgrave, R. H., & Crozier, P. A. (1968). The influence of head position upon velopharyngeal closure. *Cleft Palate Journal, 5,* 117–124.

McWilliams, B. J., & Philips, B. J. (1990). *Velopharyngeal incompetence: An audio seminar.* Philadelphia: B. C. Decker.

Mihashi, S., Okado, M., Kurita, S., Nagata, K., Oda, M., Hirano, M., & Nakashima, T. (1981). In K. N. Stevens & M. Hirano (Eds.), *Vocal fold physiology.* Tokyo: University of Tokyo Press.

Miller, R. H., Woodson, G. E., & Jankovic, J. (1987). Botulinum toxin injection for vocal fold for spastic dysphonia. *Archives of Otolaryngology–Head and Neck Surgery, 113,* 603–605.

Miller, R. M., & Groher, M. E. (1990). *Medical speech pathology.* Rockville, MD: Aspen.

Monsen, R. B. (1979). Acoustic qualities of phonation in young hearing-impaired children. *Journal of Speech and Hearing Research, 22,* 270–288.

Montgomery, W. W. (1979). Laryngeal paralysis Teflon injection. *Annals of Otolaryngology, 88,* 647–657.

Moore, P., & von Leden, H. (1958). *The function of the normal larynx* [Film]. Los Angeles: Wexler Film Productions.

Moore, P., & von Leden, H. (1962). Ultra-high speed photography in laryngeal physiology. *Journal of Speech and Hearing Disorders, 27,* 165–171.

Moran, M. J., & Pentz, A. L. (1987). Otolaryngologists' opinions of voice therapy for vocal nodules in children. *Language Speech and Hearing Services in Schools, 18,* 172–178.

Morr, K. E., Warren, D. W., Dalston, R. M., & Smith, L. R. (1989). Screening of velopharyngeal inadequacy by differential pressure measurements. *Cleft Palate Journal, 26,* 42–45.

Moses, P. J. (1954). *The voice of neurosis.* New York: Grune and Statton.

Mowrer, D. E. (1982). *Methods of modifying speech behaviors* (2nd ed.). Columbus, OH: Merrill.

Mowrer, D. E., & Case, J. L. (1982). *Clinical management of speech disorders.* Austin, TX: PRO-ED.

Murdoch, B. E., Chenery, H. J., Bowler, S., & Ingram, J. C. L. (1989). Respiratory function in Parkinson's subjects exhibiting a perceptible speech deficit: A kinematic and spirometric analysis. *Journal of Speech and Hearing Disorders, 54,* 610–626.

Murphy, A. T. (1964). *Functional voice disorders.* Englewood Cliffs, NJ: Prentice-Hall.

Murry, T., & Doherty, E. T. (1980). Selected acoustic characteristics of pathologic and normal speakers. *Journal of Speech and Hearing Research, 23,* 361–369.

Myers, E. N., & Suen, J. Y. (Eds.). (1989). *Cancer of the head and neck* (2nd ed.). New York: Churchill Livingstone.

Mysak, E. D. (1983). Cerebral palsy. In G. H. Shames & E. H. Wiig (Eds.), *Human communication disorders: An introduction.* Columbus, OH: Merrill.

Narcy, P., Contencin, P., & Viala, P. (1990). Surgical treatment for laryngeal paralysis in infants and children. *Annals of Otology, Rhinology, and Laryngology, 99,* 124–128.

Neel, H. B., & Unni, K. K. (1982). Cartilaginous tumors of the larynx: A series of 33 patients. *Otolaryngology Head and Neck Surgery, 90,* 201–202.

Netsell, R., & Hixon, T. J. (1978). A noninvasive method for clinically estimating subglottal air pressure. *Journal of Speech and Hearing Disorders, 43,* 326–330.

Netter, F. H. (1983). *The CIBA collection of medical illustrations: Vol. I. The nervous system, Part I, anatomy and physiology.* West Caldwell, NJ: CIBA Pharmaceutical.

Newman, R. K., & Byers, R. M. (1982). Squamous carcinoma of the larynx in patients under the age of 35 years. *Otolaryngology Head and Neck Surgery, 90,* 431–433.

Offer, D. (1980). Normal adolescent development. In H. I. Kaplan, A. M. Freedman, & B. J. Saddock (Eds.), *Comprehensive textbook of psychiatry* (3rd ed.) (Vol. 3). Baltimore: Williams and Wilkins.

Ogura, J. H., & Thawley, E. E. (1980). Cysts and tumors of the larynx. In M. M. Paparella & D. A. Shumrick (Eds.), *Otolaryngology: Vol. 3. Head and neck* (2nd ed.) Philadelphia: Saunders.

Ohlsson, A.-C., Brink, O., & Lofqvist, A. (1989). A voice accumulator-validation and application. *Journal of Speech and Hearing Research, 32,* 451–457.

Pabon, J. P. H., & Plomp, R. (1988). Automatic phonetogram recording supplemented with acoustical voice-quality parameters. *Journal of Speech and Hearing Research, 31,* 710–722.

Panje, W. R., Van Demark, D., & McCabe, B. F. (1981). Voice button prosthesis rehabilitation of the laryngectomee. *Annals of Otolaryngology, 90,* 503–505.

Pannbacker, M. (1985). Common misconceptions about oral pharyngeal structure and function. *Language, Speech, and Hearing Services in Schools, 16*(1), 29–33.

Pannbacker, M., Lass, N., Middleton, G., Crutchfield, E., Trapp, D., & Scherbick, K. (1984). Current clinical practices in the assessment of velopharyngeal closure. *Cleft Palate Journal, 21,* 33–37.

Pannbacker, M., Lass, N. J., & Stout, B. M. (1990). Speech-language pathologists' opinions on the management of velopharyngeal insufficiency. *Cleft Palate Journal, 27,* 68–71.

Paparella, M. M., & Shumrick, D. A. (Eds.). (1980). *Otolaryngology: Vol. 3. Head and neck* (2nd ed.). Philadelphia: Saunders.

Pauloski, B. R., Fisher, H. B., Kempster, G. B., & Blom, E. D. (1989). Statistical differentiation of tracheoesophageal speech produced under four prosthetic/occlusion speaking conditions. *Journal of Speech and Hearing Research, 32,* 591–599.

Pearson, B. W., Woods, J., & Hartman, D. (1980). Extended hemilaryngectomy for T3 glottic carcinoma with preservation of speech and swallowing. *Laryngoscope, 90,* 1950–1961.

Perkins, W. H. (1983). Quantification of vocal behavior: A foundation for clinical management of voice. In D. M. Bless & J. H. Abbs (Eds.), *Vocal fold physiology: Contemporary research and clinical issues.* San Diego: College-Hill.

Pershall, K. E., & Boone, D. R. (1987). Supraglottal contribution to voice quality. *Journal of Voice, 1,* 186–190.

Peterson-Falzone, S. J. (1984). Hypernasality: Comments on article by Andres, Tardy, and Pasternak. *Language, Speech, and Hearing Services in Schools, 15,* 222–223.

Peterson-Falzone, S. J., & Graham, M. S. (1990). Phoneme-specific nasal emission in children with and without physical anomalies of the velopharyngeal mechanism. *Journal of Speech and Hearing Disorders, 55,* 132–139.

Portnoy, R. A., & Aronson, A. E. (1982). Diadochokinetic syllable rate and regularity in normal and in spastic and ataxic dysarthric subjects. *Journal of Speech and Hearing Disorders, 47,* 324–328.

Prator, R. J., & Swift, R. W. (1984). *Manual of voice therapy.* Austin, TX: PRO-ED.

Prosek, R. A., Montgomery, A. A., Walden, B. E., & Schwartz, D. M. (1978). EMG biofeedback in the treatment of hyperfunctional voice disorders. *Journal of Speech and Hearing Disorders, 47,* 324–328.

Ptacek, P. H., & Sander, E. K. (1963). Maximum duration of phonation. *Journal of Speech and Hearing Disorders, 28,* 171–182.

Ramig, L. A., Scherer, R. C., Klasner, E. R., Titze, I. R., & Horii, Y. (1990). Acoustic analysis of voice in amyotrophic lateral sclerosis: A longitudinal case study. *Journal of Speech and Hearing Disorders, 55,* 2–14.

Ramig, L. A., Scherer, R. C., Titze, I. R., & Ringel, S. P. (1988). Acoustic analysis of voices of patients with neurologic disease: Rationale and preliminary data. *Annals of Otology, Rhinology, and Laryngology, 97,* 164–171.

Ramig, L. A., & Shipp, T. (1987). Comparative measures of vocal tremor and vocal vibrato. *Journal of Voice, 1,* 162–167.

Rastatter, M. P., & Hyman, M. (1982). Maximum phoneme duration of /s/ and /z/ by children with vocal nodules. *Language, Speech and Hearing Services in Schools, 13,* 197–199.

Rastatter, M. P., & Hyman, M. (1984). Effects of selected rhinologic disorders on the perception of nasal resonance in children. *Language, Speech and Hearing Services in Schools, 15,* 44–50.

Reath, D. B., LaRossa, D., & Randall, P. (1987). Simultaneous posterior pharyngeal flap and tonsillectomy. *Cleft Palate Journal, 24,* 250–253.

Redenbaugh, M. A., & Reich, A. R. (1989). Surface EMG and related measures in normal and vocally hyperfunctional speakers. *Journal of Speech and Hearing Disorders, 54,* 68–73.

Reich, A. R., & Lerman, J. W. (1978). Teflon laryngoplasty: An acoustical and perceptual study. *Journal of Speech and Hearing Disorders, 43,* 496–505.

Reich, A. R., Mason, J. A., Frederickson, R. R., & Schlauch, R. S. (1989). Factors influencing fundamental frequency range estimates in children. *Journal of Speech and Hearing Disorders, 54,* 429–438.

Reich, A., & McHenry, M. (1987). Respiratory volumes in cheerleaders with a history of dysphonic episodes. *Folia Phoniatrica, 39,* 71–77.

Reich, A., McHenry, M., & Keaton, A. (1986). A survey of dysphonic episodes in high school cheerleaders. *Language, Speech, and Hearing Services in Schools, 17,* 63–71.

Reich, A. R., & Redenbaugh, M. R. (1985). Relation between nasal/voice accelerometric values and interval estimates of hypernasality. *Cleft Palate Journal, 22,* 237–245.

Rekart, D. M., & Begnal, C. F. (1989). Acoustic characteristics of reticent speech. *Journal of Voice, 3,* 324–336.

Riski, J. E. (1979). Articulation skills and oral–nasal resonance in children with pharyngeal flaps. *Cleft Palate Journal, 16,* 421–428.

Riski, J. E., Hoke, J. A., & Dolan, E. A. (1989). The role of pressure flow and endoscopic assessment in successful palatal obturator revision. *Cleft Palate Journal, 26,* 56–62.

Robbins, J., Christensen, J., & Kempster, G. (1986). Characteristics of speech production after tracheoesophageal puncture: Voice onset time and vowel duration. *Journal of Speech and Hearing Research, 29,* 499–504.

Rollin, W. J. (1987). *The psychology of communication disorders in individuals and their families.* Englewood Cliffs, NJ: Prentice-Hall.

Rosenbek, J. C., & LaPointe, L. L. (1985). The dysarthrias: description, diagnosis and treatment. In D. F. Johns (Ed.), *Clinical management of neurogenic communication disorders*. Austin, TX: PRO-ED.

Ross, R. B. (1987a). Treatment variables affecting facial growth in complete unilateral cleft lip and palate. Part 3: Alveolus repair and bone grafting. *Cleft Palate Journal, 24*, 33–44.

Ross, R. B. (1987b). Treatment variables affecting facial growth in unilateral lip and palate. Part 4: Repair of the cleft lip. *Cleft Palate Journal, 24*, 45–53.

Ross, R. B. (1987c). Treatment variables affecting growth in cleft lip and palate. Part 6: Techniques of palate repair. *Cleft Palate Journal, 24*, 64–70.

Rubin, H. J. (1975). Misadventures with injectionable polytef (Teflon). *Archives of Otolaryngology, 101*, 114–116.

Rubin, W. (1987). Allergic, dietary, chemical, stress, and hormonal influences in voice abnormalities. *Journal of Voice, 1*, 378–385.

Salmon, S. J. (1979). Factors that may interfere with esophageal speech. In R. L. Keith & F. L. Darley, *Laryngectomee rehabilitation*. Austin, TX: PRO-ED.

Salmon, S. J., & Goldstein, L. P. (1978). *The artificial larynx handbook*. New York: Grune and Stratton.

Sander, E. K. (1989). Arguments against the aggressive pursuit of voice therapy for children. *Language Speech and Hearing Services in Schools, 20*, 94–101.

Sataloff, R. T. (1981). Professional singers: The science and art of clinical care. *American Journal of Otolaryngology, 2*, 251–256.

Sataloff, R. T. (1983). Physical examination of the professional singer. *The Journal of Otolaryngology, 12*, 277–281.

Sataloff, R. T. (Ed.). (1987). *Journal of Voice, 1*, 123–171.

Sataloff, R. T. (1988). Editorial: Respiration and singing. *Journal of Voice, 2*, 1–50.

Sataloff, R. T. (in press). *Professional voices: The science and art of clinical care*. New York: Raven Press.

Sataloff, R. T., Feldman, M., Darby, K. S., Carroll, L. M., Spiegel, J. R., & Schiebel, B. R. (1988). Arytenoid dislocation. *Journal of Voice, 1*, 368–377.

Sataloff, R. T., Spiegel, J. R., Carroll, L. M., Schiebel, B. R., Darby, K. S., & Rulnick, R. (1987). Strobovideolaryngoscopy in professional voice users: Results and clinical value. *Journal of Voice, 1*, 359–364.

Schaefer, S. D., & Close, L. G. (1989). Acute management of laryngeal trauma. *Annals of Otology, Rhinology, and Laryngology, 98*, 98–104.

Scherer, R. C., Gould, W. J., Titze, I. R., Meyers, A. D., & Sataloff, R. T. (1988). Preliminary evaluation of selected acoustic and glottographic measures for clinical phonatory function analysis. *Journal of Voice, 2*, 245–249.

Schmidt, P., Klingholz, F., & Martin, F. (1988). Influence of pitch, voice sound pressure, and vowel quality on the maximum phonation time. *Journal of Voice, 2*, 245–249.

Schneider, E., & Shprintzen, R. J. (1980). A survey of speech pathologists: Current trends in the diagnosis and management of velopharyngeal insufficiency. *Cleft Palate Journal, 17*, 249–253.

Scott, S., & Caird, F. I. (1982). Speech therapy for Parkinson's disease. *Journal of Neurology, Neurosurgery, and Psychiatry, 46*, 140–144.

Sedory, S. E., Hamlet, S. L., & Connor, N. P. (1989). Comparisons of perceptual and acoustic characteristics of tracheoesophageal and excellent esophageal speech. *Journal of Speech and Hearing Disorders, 54,* 209–214.

Seibert, R. W., Seibert, J. J., Norton, J. B., & Williams, J. B. (1981). Recurrent laryngeal nerve damage following formalin infiltration of ductus arteriosus. *Laryngoscope, 91,* 392–393.

Shanks, J. C. (1979). Essentials for alaryngeal speech: Psychology and physiology. In R. L. Keith & F. L. Darley, *Laryngectomee rehabilitation.* Austin, TX: PRO-ED.

Shapiro, A. K., Shapiro, E. S., Brauun, R. D., & Sweet, R. D. (1978). *Gilles de la Tourette syndrome.* New York: Raven Press.

Shaw, J. D., & Lancer, J. M. (1987). *A colour atlas of fiberoptic endoscopy of the upper respiratory tract.* Ipswich, England: Wolfe Medical.

Shelton, R. L., Chisum, L., Youngstrom, K. A., Arndt, W. B., & Elbert, M. (1969). Effect of articulation therapy on palatopharyngeal closure, movement of the pharyngeal wall, and tongue posture. *Cleft Palate Journal, 6,* 440–448.

Shelton, R. L., Paesani, A., McClelland, K. D., & Bradfield, S. S. (1975). Panendoscopic feedback in the study of voluntary velopharyngeal movements. *Journal of Speech and Hearing Disorders, 40,* 232–244.

Shin, T., Hirano, M. Maeyama, T., Nozoe, I., & Ohkubo, H. (1981). The function of the extrinsic laryngeal muscles. In K. N. Stevens & M. Hirano (Eds.), *Vocal fold physiology.* Tokyo: University of Tokyo Press.

Shipp, T. (1967). Frequency, duration, and perceptual measures in relation to judgments of alaryngeal speech acceptability. *Journal of Speech and Hearing Research, 10,* 417–427.

Shipp, T. (1987). Vertical laryngeal position: research findings and applications for singers. *Journal of Voice, 1,* 217–219.

Shipp, T., Izdebski, K., Reed, C., & Morrissey, P. (1985). Intrinsic laryngeal muscle activity in a spastic dysphonic patient. *Journal of Speech and Hearing Disorders, 50,* 54–59.

Shprintzen, R. J. (1989). Nasopharyngoscopy. In. K. R. Bzoch (Ed.), *Communicative disorders related to cleft lip and palate* (3rd ed.). Austin, TX: PRO-ED.

Shprintzen, R. J., McCall, G. N., & Skolnick, M. L. (1975). A new technique for the treatment of velopharyngeal incompetence. *Journal of Speech and Hearing Disorders, 40,* 69–83.

Singer, M. I., Blom, E. D., & Hamaker, R. C. (1989). Voice rehabilitation following laryngectomy. In E. N. Myers & J. Y. Suen (Eds.). *Cancer of the head and neck* (2nd ed.). New York: Churchill Livingstone.

Silverman, F. H. (1989). *Communication for the speechless* (2nd ed.). Englewood Cliffs, NJ: Prentice-Hall.

Skelly, M., Donaldson, R. C., Scheer, G. E., & Guzzardo, M. R. (1971). Dysphonias associated with spinal bracing in scoliosis. *Journal of Speech and Hearing Disorders, 36,* 368–376.

Skolnick, M. L., & Cohn, E. R. (1989). *Videofluoroscopic studies of speech in patients with cleft palate.* New York: Springer-Verlag.

Skolnick, M. L., McCall, G. N., & Barnes, M. (1973). The sphincteric mechanisms of velopharyngeal closure. *Cleft Palate Journal, 10,* 286–305.

Smith, B. E., Weinberg, B., Feth, L. L., & Horii, Y. (1978). Vocal roughness and jitter characteristics of vowels produced by esophageal speakers. *Journal of Speech and Hearing Research, 21,* 240–249.

Smitheran, J., & Hixon, T. J. (1981). A clinical method for estimating laryngeal airway resistance during vowel production. *Journal of Speech and Hearing Disorders, 46,* 138–146.

Snidecor, J. C., & Isshiki, N. (1965). Vocal and air use characteristics of a superior male esophageal speaker. *Folia Phoniatrica, 17,* 217–232.

Solomon, N. P., McCall, G. N., Trosset, M. W., & Gray, W. C. (1989). Laryngeal configuration and constriction during two types of whispering. *Journal of Speech and Hearing Research, 32,* 161–174.

Spiegel, J. H., Sataloff, R. T., & Gould, W. J. (1987). The treatment of vocal fold paralysis with injectable collagen: Clinical concerns. *Journal of Voice, 1,* 119–121.

Spiegel, H., & Spiegel, D. (1980). Hypnosis. In H. I. Kaplan, A. M. Freedman, & B. J. Sadock (Eds.). *Comprehensive textbook of psychiatry* (3rd ed., Vol. 2). Baltimore: Williams & Wilkins.

Stevens, K. N., & Hirano, M. (Eds.). (1981). *Vocal fold physiology.* Tokyo: University of Tokyo Press.

Stevens, K. N., Nickerson, R. S., Boothroyd, A., & Rollins, A. M. (1976). Assessment of nasalization in the speech of deaf children. *Journal of Speech and Hearing Research, 19,* 393–416.

Stoller, R. J. (1980). Gender identity disorders. In H. I. Kaplan, A. M. Freedman, & B. J. Saddock (Eds.), *Comprehensive textbook of psychiatry* (3rd ed.) (Vol. 3). Baltimore: Williams and Wilkins.

Stone, R. E., Jr. (1983). Issues in clinical assessment of laryngeal function: Contraindications for subscribing to maximum phonation time and optimal frequency. In D. M. Bless & J. H. Abbs (Eds.), *Vocal fold physiology: Contemporary research and clinical issues.* San Diego: College-Hill.

Stringer, D. A., & Witzel, M. A. (1989). Comparison of multi-view videofluoroscopy and nasopharyngoscopy in the assessment of velopharyngeal insufficiency. *Cleft Palate Journal, 26,* 88–91.

Subtelny, J., Li, W., Whitehead, R., & Subtelny, J. D. (1989). Cephalometric and cineradiographic study of deviant resonance in hearing-impaired speakers. *Journal of Speech and Hearing Disorders, 54,* 249–263.

Tait, N. A., Michel, J. F., & Carpenter, M. A. (1980). Maximum duration of sustained /s/ and /z/ in children. *Journal of Speech and Hearing Disorders, 45,* 239–246.

Tardy, M. E., Jr., Toriumi, D., & Broadway, D. (1989). Facial plastic and reconstructive surgery in an aging population: A critical review. In J. C. Goldstein, H. K. Kashima, & C. F. Koopmann, Jr. (Eds.), *Geriatric otolaryngology.* Toronto: B. C. Decker.

Teter, D. L. (1977). Vocal nodules: Their cause and treatment. *Music Education Journal, 1,* 38–41.

Thompson, A. E., & Hixon, T. J. (1979). Nasal airflow during normal speech production. *Cleft Palate Journal, 16,* 412–420.

Thompson, J. W., Rosenthal, P., & Camilon, F. S., Jr. (1990). Vocal cord paralysis and superior laryngeal nerve dysfunction in Reye's syndrome. *Archives of Otolaryngology: Head and Neck Surgery, 116,* 46–48.

Thorogood, P., & Tickle, C. (Eds.). (1988). *Craniofacial development*. Cambridge, England: Company of Biologists.

Titze, I. R. (1980). Comments on the myoelastic-aerodynamic theory of phonation. *Journal of Speech and Hearing Research, 23*, 495–510.

Titze, I. R. (1988). A framework for the study of vocal registers. *Journal of Voice, 2*, 183–194.

Titze, I. R., Baer, T., Cooper, D., & Scherer, R. (1983). Automated extraction of glottographic waveform parameters and regression to acoustic and physiological variables. In D. M. Bless & J. H. Abbs (Eds.), *Vocal fold physiology: Contemporary research and clinical issues*. San Diego: College-Hill.

Titze, I. R., Luschei, E. S., & Hirano, M. (1989). Role of the thyroarytenoid muscle in regulation of fundamental frequency. *Journal of Voice, 3*, 213–224.

Toohill, R. J. (1975). The psychosomatic aspects of children with vocal nodules. *Archives of Otolaryngology, 101*, 591–595.

Torgerson, J. K., & Martin, D. E. (1976). Acquisition of esophageal speech subsequent to learning pharyngeal speech: An unusual case study. *Journal of Speech and Hearing Disorders, 41*, 233–237.

Trigos, I., Ysunza, A., Gonzalez, A., & Vazquez, M. C. (1988). Surgical treatment of borderline velopharyngeal insufficiency using homologous cartilage implantation with videonasopharyngoscopic monitoring. *Cleft Palate Journal, 25*, 167–170.

Trost-Cardamone, J. E. (1989). Coming to terms with VPI: A response to Loney and Bloem. *Cleft Palate Journal, 26*, 68–70.

Trudeau, M. D., Schuller, D. E., & Hall, D. A. (1989). The effects of radiation on tracheoesophageal puncture. *Archives of Otolaryngology: Head and Neck Surgery, 115*, 1116–1117.

Tucker, H. M. (1980). Vocal cord paralysis—1979. Etiology and management. *Laryngoscope, 90*, 585–590.

Tucker, H. M. (1987). *The larynx*. New York: Thieme Medical.

Tucker, H. M., Rusnov, M., & Cohen, L. (1982). Speech development in aphonia children. *Laryngoscope, 92*, 566–568.

Van Demark, D. L., & Hardin, M. A. (1986). Effectiveness of intensive articulation therapy for children with cleft palate. *Cleft Palate Journal, 23*, 215–224.

Van Riper, C., & Irwin, J. V. (1958). *Voice and articulation*. Englewood Cliffs, NJ: Prentice-Hall.

Velasco, M. G., Ysunza, A., Hernandez, X., Marquez, C. (1988). Diagnosis and treatment of submucous cleft palate: A review of 108 cases. *Cleft Palate Journal, 25*, 171–173.

von Leden, H. (1988). Legal pitfalls in laryngology. *Journal of Voice, 2*, 330–333.

von Leden, H., Abitbol, J., Bouchayer, M., Hirano, M., & Tucker, H. (1989). Phonosurgery. *Journal of Voice, 3*, 175–182.

Warren, D. W. (1989). Aerodynamic assessment of velopharyngeal performance. In K. R. Bzoch (Ed.), *Communicative disorders related to cleft lip and palate*. Austin, TX: PRO-ED.

Warren, D. W., Hairfield, W. M., & Dalston, E. T. (1990). The relationship between nasal airway size and nasal–oral breathing in cleft lip and palate. *Cleft Palate Journal, 27*, 46–52.

Wasz-Hockert, O., Lind, J., Vuorenkoski, V., Partenen, T., & Valanne, E. (1968). *The infant cry*. London: William Heinemann Medical Books.

Watterson, T., Hansen-Magorian, H. J., & McFarlane, S. C. (1990). A demographic description of laryngeal contact ulcer patients. *Journal of Voice, 4*, 71–75.

Watterson, T., McFarlane, S. C., & Menicucci, A. L. (1990). Vibratory characteristics of Teflon-injected and noninjected paralyzed vocal folds. *Journal of Speech and Hearing Disorders, 55*, 61–66.

Weinberg, B. (1980). *Reading in speech following total laryngectomy*. Baltimore: University Park Press.

Weinberg, B., & Bennett, S. (1971). A study of talker sex recognition of esophageal voices. *Journal of Speech and Hearing Research, 14*, 391–395.

Weinberg, B., & Riekena, A. (1973). Speech produced with the Tokyo artificial larynx. *Journal of Speech and Hearing Disorders, 38*, 383–389.

Weiner, H. L., & Levitt, L. P. (1978). *Neurology for the house officer* (2nd ed.). Baltimore: Williams and Wilkins.

Welch, G. F., Sergeant, D. C., & MacCurtain, F. (1988). Some physical characteristics of the male falsetto voice. *Journal of Voice, 2*, 151–163.

Welch, G. F., & Sergeant, D. C., & MacCurtain, F. (1989). Xeroradiographic-electrolaryngographic analysis of male vocal registers. *Journal of Voice, 2*, 244–256.

Wenig, B. L., Mullooly, V., Levy, J., & Abramson, A. L. (1989). Voice restoration following laryngectomy: The role of primary versus secondary tracheoesophageal puncture. *Annals of Otology, Rhinology, and Laryngology, 98*, 70–73.

Wenig, B. L., Stegnjajic, A., & Abramson, A. L. (1989). Glottic reconstruction following conservation laryngeal surgery. *Laryngoscope, 99*, 983–985.

West, R., Kennedy, L., & Carr, A. (1947). *Rehabilitation of speech* (rev. ed.). New York: Harper and Brothers.

Wetmore, S. J. (1987). The course of laryngeal papillomatosis modified by CO_2 laser surgery. *Otolaryngology: Head and Neck Surgery, 90*, 538–541.

Wilcox, K., & Horii, Y. (1980). Age and changes in vocal jitter. *Journal of Gerontology, 35*, 194–198.

Williams, C. E., & Stevens, K. N. (1972). Emotions and speech: Some acoustical correlations. *Journal of the Acoustical Society of America, 52*, 1238–1250.

Williams, W. N. (1989). Radiographic assessment of velopharyngeal function for speech. In K. R. Bzoch (Ed.), *Communicative disorders related to cleft lip and palate* (3rd ed.). Austin, TX: PRO-ED.

Wilson, D. K. (1979). *Voice problems of children* (2nd ed.). Baltimore: Williams and Wilkins.

Wilson, D. K. (1987). *Voice problems of children* (3rd ed.). Baltimore: Williams and Wilkins.

Wilson, F. B., & Rice, M. (1977). *Voice disorders: A programmed approach to voice therapy*. Hingham, MA: Teaching Resources Corp.

Witzel, M. A. (1989). Commentary. *Cleft Palate Journal, 26*, 199–200.

Witzel, M. A., & Posnick, J. C. (1989). Patterns and location of velopharyngeal valving problems: Atypical findings on video nasopharyngoscopy. *Cleft Palate Journal, 26*, 63–67.

Wolfe, S. A., & Berkowitz, S. (1989). *Plastic surgery of the facial skeleton*. San Diego: College-Hill.

Wolfe, V. I., Ratusnik, D. L., Smith, F. H., & Northrop, G. (1990). Intonation and fundamental frequency in male-to-female transsexuals. *Journal of Speech and Hearing Disorders, 55,* 43–50.

Wolfe, V. I., & Steinfatt, T. M. (1987). Prediction of vocal severity within and across voice types. *Journal of Speech and Hearing Research, 30,* 230–240.

Wolski, W. (1967). Hypernasality as the presenting symptom of myasthenia gravis. *Journal of Speech and Hearing Disorders, 32,* 36–38.

Woo, P., Colton, R. H., & Shangold, L. (1987). Phonatory airflow analysis in patients with laryngeal disease. *Annals of Otology, Rhinology, and Laryngology, 96,* 549–555.

Wyke, B. (1983). Neuromuscular control systems in voice production. In D. M. Bless & J. H. Abbs, *Vocal fold physiology: Contemporary research and clinical issues.* San Diego: College-Hill.

Yahr, M. D., & Bergmann, K. J. (Eds.). (1987). *Parkinson's disease.* New York: Raven Press.

Yanagihara, N. (1967). Significance of harmonic changes and noise components of hoarseness. *Journal of Speech and Hearing Research, 10,* 531–541.

Yanagisawa, E., Godley, F., & Muta, H. (1987). Selection of video cameras for stroboscopic videolaryngoscopy. *Annals of Otology, Rhinology, and Laryngology, 96,* 578–585.

Yanagisawa, E., Isaacson, G., Kmucha, S. T., & Hirokawa, R. (1989). Video nasopharyngoscopy: A comparison of fiberscopic, telescopic, and microscopic documentation. *Annals of Otology, Rhinology, and Laryngology, 98,* 15–20.

Yang, S., & Mu, L. (1989). A study on the mechanism of functional dysphonia. *Journal of Voice, 3,* 337–341.

Yorkston, K. M., Beukelman, D. R., & Bell, K. R. (1988). *Clinical management of dysarthric speakers.* Austin, TX: PRO-ED.

Yumoto, E. (1988). Quantitative assessment of the degree of hoarseness. *Journal of Voice, 1,* 310–313.

Zagzebski, J. A. (1975). Ultrasonic measurement of lateral pharyngeal wall motion at two levels in the vocal tract. *Journal of Speech and Hearing Research, 18,* 308–318.

Zemlin, W. R. (1988). *Speech and hearing science: Anatomy and physiology* (3rd ed.). Englewood Cliffs, NJ: Prentice-Hall.

Zitsch, R. P., & Reilly, J. S. (1987). Vocal cord paralysis associated with cystic fibrosis. *Annals of Otology, Rhinology, and Laryngology, 96,* 680–683.

Zwitman, D. H., & Calcaterra, T. C. (1973). The "silent cough" method for vocal hyperfunction. *Journal of Speech and Hearing Disorders, 38,* 119–125.

Zwitman, D. H., & Calcaterra, R. C. (1975). A case against Teflon injection to lower pitch. *Journal of Speech and Hearing Disorders, 40,* 499–501.

Zwitman, D. H., & Disinger, R. S. (1975). Experimental modification of the Western Electric #5 electrolarynx to a mouth-type instrument. *Journal of Speech and Hearing Disorders, 40,* 35–39.

Author Index

Abbs, J. H., 2, 63
Abitbol, B., 51, 107, 300
Abitbol, J., 51, 107, 300
Abramson, A. L., 230, 260
Aduss, H., 275
Alfonso, P. J., 246
Allison, D. L., 274, 278
Aminoff, C., 175
Andrews, M. L., 135, 288, 289
Arndt, W. B., 279
Arnold, G. E., 96, 141
Aronson, A. E., 13, 18, 63, 72, 76, 98,
    114, 120, 131, 135, 141, 163, 164, 165,
    167, 169, 170, 172, 173, 175, 176, 177,
    189, 197, 199, 207, 213, 217, 218, 252,
    258, 282, 283, 302, 304

Bachmayer, D., 275
Baer, T., 78
Bailey, B. J., 54, 135
Bailey, C. W., 54, 135
Bais, A. S., 304
Baken, R. J., 2, 22, 28, 70, 80, 81
Baker, S. R., 162, 264

Barnhart, E. R., 50
Barnes, M., 9
Barron, S., 80
Bassich, C. J., 85, 90
Bateman, H. E., 278
Battista, C., 300
Batza, E. M., 291
Baugh, R. F., 264
Beahrs, O. H., 231
Beaver, V. L., 111
Beery, Q. C., 283
Begnal, C. F., 189
Bell, K. R., 183
Bell-Berti, F., 278
Benjamin, B., 94, 299
Bennett, S., 242
Bergmann, K. J., 165
Berk, G. S., 52
Berkowitz, S., 275, 280, 281
Berry, W. R., 170
Beukelman, D. R., 183
Bevan, K., 156, 273
Biller, H. F., 54, 226, 230

Birns, J. W., 157
Bishop, S. G., 141
Blalock, P. D., 207
Bless, D. B., 2, 63, 162
Bless, D. M., 47, 80, 162
Blitzer, A., 164, 178
Block, A. J., 280
Bloem, T. J., 270
Blom, E. D., 260, 263, 267
Blonsky, R., 165
Boa, F. J., 230
Bocca, E., 230
Boone, D. R., 29, 31, 61, 70, 72, 74, 76, 83, 84, 97, 98, 108, 135, 141, 179, 181, 184, 193, 197, 199, 216, 252, 296, 297, 298
Boothroyd, A., 297
Boshes, B., 165
Bouchayer, M., 51, 132
Bough, I. D., Jr., 163, 166
Bowler, S., 166
Bradfield, S. S., 279
Bradley, D. P., 273, 277, 278
Bralley, R. C., 221, 222
Brantigan, C. O., 222
Brantigan, T. A., 222
Braun, R. D., 171
Brewer, D. W., 22, 45
Brin, M. F., 164, 178
Brink, O., 108
Broadway, D., 276
Brodnitz, F. S., 138, 218, 219, 223
Brown, W. S., 25, 163, 164, 168
Bull, G. L., 221
Byers, R. M., 229
Bzoch, K. R., 10, 272, 273, 276, 278, 279, 284, 285, 292, 295

Caird, F. I., 166
Calcaterra, R. C., 104, 160
Calcaterra, T. C., 104, 160
Calne, D. B., 164
Camilon, F. S., Jr., 156
Campbell, S. L., 112
Cannon, C. R., 158
Carpenter, M. A., 84, 97, 169, 235, 247
Carpenter, R. J., 84, 97, 235, 247

Carr, A., 97
Case, J. L., 72, 96, 111, 112, 125, 156, 165, 211, 226, 231, 236, 250, 260
Casper, J. K., 22, 45, 61, 63, 69, 70, 76, 95, 106, 120, 126, 222, 252, 301, 303, 304
Cassisi, N. J., 230
Chang, H. H., 300
Chenery, H. J., 166
Chisum, L., 279
Christensen, J., 246, 267
Christensen, J. M., 246, 267
Christopher, K. L., 304
Cleary, K., 156
Close, L. G., 304
Cody, D. T. R., 54, 141, 303
Cohen, L., 157, 158, 299, 301
Cohen, S. R., 157, 158, 299, 301
Cohn, E. R., 278, 283
Coleman, R. F., 101
Colton, R. H., 22, 45, 61, 63, 69, 70, 76, 79, 95, 106, 120, 126, 222, 252, 301, 303, 304
Contencin, P., 158
Conner, N. P., 175, 267
Connolly, J. E., 171
Conover, M., 275
Cooper, D. S., 21, 78, 191
Cooper, M. L., 21, 78, 97, 191
Cornut, G., 132
Creaghead, N. A., 275
Crissman, J. D., 228
Croft, C. B., 273
Cronin, T. D., 274
Croxson, G., 94
Crozier, P. A., 294
Crysdale, W. S., 158

Daily, W. W., 156
Dalston, E. T., 10, 274, 278, 281
Dalston, R. M., 10, 274, 278, 281
Damste, P. H., 239
Daniels, H. A., 260
Daniloff, R., 26, 31
Danner, S. A., 305
D'Antonio, L. L., 278
Darley, F. R., 163, 164, 168, 169, 170, 171, 172, 245

Dawson, J. A., 141
Deal, R. E., 126
Dedo, D. D., 157, 159, 160, 162, 177, 299, 300
Dedo, H. H., 157, 159, 160, 161, 162, 175, 176, 299, 300
DeSanto, L. W., 173, 175, 176, 177, 230, 231
Deutsch, H. L., 277
Dew, D., 35
DeWeese, D. D., 230, 289, 299
Dey, F. L., 241
Dickens, W. J., 230
Dickson, D. R., 8, 9, 14, 15, 18, 80
Dickson, S., 9, 80
Dickson, W. M., 8, 14, 15, 18, 80
Diedrich, W. M., 239, 241, 242, 250, 251
Disinger, R. S., 234
Dodds, B., 159
Doherty, E. T., 26, 27, 75
Doherty, T. E., 75
Dolan, E. A., 282
Donald, P. J., 219
Donaldson, R. C., 277
Doyle, P. G., 267
Drudge, M. K. M., 126
Duane, D. D., 164, 165, 169
Duguay, M. J., 225, 236, 267

Eckel, F. C., 84, 97
Edgeron, M. T., 221
Eisenbach, C. R., 284
Elbert, M., 279
Emanuel, F. W., 75
Emerick, L. L., 61
Emmett-Oglesby, M. W., 51

Fahn, S., 164, 178
Fairbanks, G., 70, 83
Fara, M., 281
Feder, R. J., 47, 102
Feldman, M., 158
Feldman, R. I., 158
Fendler, M., 84
Feth, L. L., 26, 245
Finitzo, T., 174
Fisher, H. B., 165, 267

Fletcher, G. H., 140, 281, 285
Fletcher, S. G., 140, 281, 285
Flores, T. W., 230
Ford, C. N., 162
Fornatto, E., 35
Forner, L. L., 296
Fox, D. R., 274, 282
Freeman, F., 171, 174
Freeman, R. D., 171, 174
Fritzell, B., 161
Froeschels, E., 179
Furlow, L. T., Jr., 280, 284

Gacek, R. R., 178
Gallivan, G. J., 141
Garfinkle, T. J., 167, 168, 169
Gates, G. A., 222, 250
Gay, T., 36
Gelfer, M. P., 86, 90
Geller, K. A., 157, 299
Gibb, A. G., 273
Gilbert, H. R., 106
Gilman, A. G., 107, 115, 169, 191
Godley, F., 45
Goldman, M. D., 83
Goldstein, L. P., 168, 170, 234, 235, 250
Goldstein, N. P., 168, 170, 234, 235, 250
Gomyo, Y., 267
Gonzalez, A., 280, 282, 283
Gonzalez, J. B., 280, 282, 283
Goodman, L. S., 107, 191
Gore, C. H., 221
Goudie, A. J., 51
Gould, W. J., 22, 77, 78, 162, 178, 220
Graham, M. S., 277
Grau, W. H., 275
Gray, W. C., 73
Green, G., 164, 247
Green, P. E., 164, 247
Greene, M. C. L., 135
Griffiths, C., 156, 163, 166
Griffiths, M. V., 156, 163, 166
Groher, M. E., 51, 251, 305
Guena, O., 267
Guzzardo, M. R., 277

Haber, K., 51
Hadderingh, R. J., 305
Hahn, E., 285
Hairfield, W. M., 274, 292
Hall, D. A., 263
Hamaker, R. C., 260, 262, 263
Hamlet, S. L., 267
Hammarberg, B., 161
Hanafee, W. N., 49
Hansen-Magorian, H. J., 138
Hanson, D. G., 61
Hanson, M. L., 61
Hardin, M. A., 285
Harris, F. P., 32, 83, 100
Harris, K., 32, 83, 100
Hartman, D. E., 156, 157, 172, 218, 230
Harvey, N., 17
Harvold, E. P., 273
Hatten, J. T., 61
Hawley, J. L., 81
Hearne, E. M., 250
Henrikson, C. O., 278
Hernandez, X., 273
Hess, D. A., 80
Hicks, J. N., 229, 230
Higgins, M. B., 107
Hillman, R. E., 73
Hinton, V. A., 292
Hirano, M., 2, 15, 17, 18, 19, 20, 22, 35, 36, 47, 51, 79, 81, 96, 102, 131, 132, 135, 230
Hirokawa, R., 45
Hirose, H., 36, 167
Hixon, T. J., 27, 78, 79, 80, 81, 83, 83, 100, 270, 296
Hodge, M. M., 83
Hoke, J. A., 282
Holbrook, A., 34, 135
Holcomb, B. J., 304
Holen, D., 250
Hollien, H., 32, 33, 34, 35
Holmberg, E. B., 73
Holt, J. J., 231
Hoops, H. R., 246
Hoover, L. A., 49
Horiguchi, S., 278

Horii, Y., 25, 26, 27, 32, 167, 245, 296
Horn, K. L., 160, 162
Horsley, I. A., 205
Howard, F. M., 169
Howell, P., 17
Hubbard, D. J., 246
Hudson, A. I., 34
Hufnagle, J., 85
Hufnagle, K. K., 85
Hutchinson, B. B., 61
Huylts, M., 247
Hyman, M., 97, 289, 290

Ingram, J. C. L., 166
Irwin, J. V., 97
Isaacson, G., 45
Isberg, A., 278
Isshiki, N., 97, 220, 243, 245
Izdebski, K., 48, 175, 176, 177

Jackler, R. K., 299, 300
Jacobson, E., 181, 205
Jankovic, J., 178
Jarvis, B. L., 280
Johns, D. F., 275
Johnson, T. S., 113, 126, 135
Jones, A. S., 94
Joseph, N., 222
Juarbe, C., 263
Julin, P., 278
Jung, J. H., 272, 276

Kaban, L. B., 275
Kahane, J. C., 13, 32, 35, 57, 207
Kalat, J. W., 191, 209, 219
Kalb, M. B., 235, 247
Kaplan, E. M., 208, 277, 295
Kaplan, S. L., 208, 217, 277, 295
Karnell, M. P., 78, 285
Kastein, S., 179
Katirji, M. B., 159
Katz, P. O., 141
Kawasaki, H., 22
Kay, N. J., 94, 98, 135
Keaton, A., 113
Keefe, M. J., 10
Kelly, D. H., 257

Kemker, F. J., 273
Kempster, G. B., 17, 24, 267
Kendall, P. C., 206
Kennedy, L., 97
Kern, E. B., 54, 141, 303
Key, M. R., 221
Kimmelman, C. P., 167, 168, 169
Kirchner, J. A., 106, 150, 159,
    241, 296
Kirchner, J. C., 106, 150, 159,
    241, 296
Kiritani, S., 167
Kistler, M. K., 17, 24
Klasner, E. R., 167
Klein, J. C., 48
Kleinasser, O., 95
Klingholz, F., 85
Klockars, A. J., 112
Kmucha, S. T., 45
Koegel, L., 230
Kohler, S., 112
Koufman, J. A., 158, 161, 207
Kozak, F. K., 171
Kraepelien, T., 278
Kraybill, W., 267
Kreiborg, S., 275
Kuehn, D. P., 284
Kumar, N., 159
Kummer, A. W., 275
Kurita, S., 18, 19, 35, 96, 131, 230
Kushner, D., 246

Laing, A., 219, 221
Lambiase, A., 22
Lancer, J. M., 45, 94, 301, 304
LaPointe, L. L., 165, 183
Large, J., 102
LaRossa, D., 281
Larson, C. R., 17, 18, 24, 150
Lass, N., 277
Lass, N. J., 277
Lauder, E., 255
Lawrence, V. L., 220
Lawson, L. I., 229, 230, 273
Lawson, W., 226, 229, 230
Leanderson, R., 27, 100
LeBoutillier, A., 94
Leder, S. B., 51, 296

Lee, L., 275, 304
Leeper, H. A., Jr., 274, 278
Lennon, V. A., 169
Lerman, J. W., 161
Levine, H. L., 230
Levitt, L. P., 168
Levy, J., 260
Lewin, J. S., 264
Li, W., 297
Lieberman, P., 28, 32, 75, 77
Lim, R. Y., 300
Lindstrom, J. M., 169
Lind, J., 32
Ling, D., 298
Linville, S. E., 35
Lippman, R. P., 80
Lisak, R. P., 168
Lofqvist, A., 108
Logani, K. B., 304
Logemann, J. A., 165
Loney, R. W., 270
Lopez, M. J., 267
Loudon, R. G., 304
Lovelace, R. E., 178
Lubit, E. C., 273
Lucente, F. E., 301, 303
Ludlow, C. L., 85, 90, 175
Lufkin, R. B., 49
Lumpkin, S. M. M., 141
Luschei, E. S., 17
Lynch, J. I., 274

McCabe, B. F., 263
McCall, G. N., 9, 73, 279
McClain, B., 126
McClelland, K. D., 279
MacComb, W. S., 140
MacCurtin, F., 49, 211
McDonald, T. J., 169
McElroy, T. H., 267
McFarlane, S. C., 31, 48, 61, 70, 73,
    74, 76, 83, 94, 98, 100, 135, 138,
    141, 161, 179, 184, 197, 199, 216,
    252, 296, 297, 298
McGlone, R. E., 80
McHenry, M. A., 112, 113
McKerns, D., 10
McLean, W. C., 158

McWilliams, B. J., 272, 273, 274, 276, 278, 279, 280, 285, 294
Maeyama, T., 15
Maniglia, A. J., 159
Marquez, C., 273
Marsden, C. D., 164
Marsh, J. L., 273, 278
Martin, D. E., 51, 85, 238
Martin, F. G., 51, 85, 238
Mason, J. A., 15, 70, 273, 274, 278, 295
Mason, R. M., 15, 70, 273, 274, 278, 295
Mathe, G., 300
Matsuoka, H., 230
Mattson, P. J., 98
Mayo, R., 57
Mead, J., 83
Mecham, M. J., 61
Menicucci, A. L., 161
Meyers, A. D., 78
Michel, J. F., 25, 84, 97
Mihashi, S., 20
Millard, D. R., 277
Miller, E. R., 251
Miller, R. H., 178, 251
Miller, R. M., 51, 251, 305
Million, R. R., 230
Monsen, R. B., 296
Montalbo, P. J., 222
Montgomery, A. A., 106, 160, 161, 180
Montgomery, W. W., 106, 160, 161, 180
Moor, E. E., 229, 278
Moore, D. M., 22, 93
Moore, P., 93
Moran, M. J., 57
Morgan, M. H., 156
Morimoto, M., 97
Morin, K. N., 156
Morris, H. L., 25, 272
Morris, R. J., 25, 272
Morrissey, P., 175
Moses, P. J., 189
Mowrer, D. E., 72, 123, 125, 231
Mu, L., 188
Muller, E., 32

Mulliken, J. B., 275
Mullooly, V., 260
Muntz, H. R., 278
Murdoch, B. E., 166
Murphy, A. T., 174
Murry, T., 75
Musgrave, R. H., 294
Muta, H., 45
Myers, E. N., 106, 226, 229, 230, 261
Mysak, E. D., 172

Naito, K., 158
Nakashima, T., 18, 19
Narcy, P., 158
Neel, H. B., 228
Nenaber, P. J., 111
Netsell, R., 80, 81
Netter, F. H., 6, 7, 149, 191, 192
Newman, R. K., 229
Nickerson, R. S., 297
Noll, J. D., 246
Norton, J. B., 157
Norton-Ford, J. D., 206
Northrop, G., 221
Nozoe, I., 15

O'Fallon, M. W., 231
Offer, D., 207, 208
Ogura, J. H., 226, 229, 230, 298, 299
Ohkubo, H., 15
Ohlsson, A. C., 108
Oldini, C., 230
Olsen, K. D., 230

Pabon, J. P. H., 29
Paesani, A., 279
Panje, W. R., 263
Pannbacker, M., 277, 278, 279, 282
Paparella, M. M., 44, 53, 141
Parker, W., 291
Partenen, T., 32
Pasternak, L., 288
Pauloski, B. R., 267
Pearl, N. B., 83, 100
Pearson, B. W., 54, 141, 230, 303
Pentz, A. L., 57
Perkell, J. S., 73
Perkins, W. H., 27, 69

Pershall, K. E., 29
Peterson-Falzone, S. J., 272, 277
Philips, B. J., 35, 126, 278, 279
Phillips, B. J., 278
Phillips, C. J., 278
Phillips, P., 278
Pignataro, O., 230
Plomp, R., 29
Portnoy, R. A., 164
Posnick, J. C., 278
Prator, R. J., 79
Prosek, R. A., 106, 180
Province, M. A., 278
Ptacek, P. H., 83
Ramig, L. A., 165, 166, 167

Randall, P., 281
Rastatter, M. P., 97, 289, 290
Ratusnik, D. L., 221
Reath, D. B., 281
Redenbaugh, M. A., 278
Redenbaugh, M. R., 74, 278
Reed, C., 175
Reich, A. R., 70, 74, 112, 113,
    161, 278
Reilly, J. S., 157
Rekart, D. M., 189
Rice, M., 21, 58, 61, 86, 87, 96, 120,
    126, 135, 139, 272
Riding, K. H., 171
Riekena, A., 233
Ringel, S. P., 166
Riski, J. E., 273, 281, 282
Robbins, J., 141, 267
Robbins, L. D., 141, 267
Rochet, A. P., 83
Rollin, W. J., 199
Rollins, A. M., 297
Rolnick, M. I., 135
Rood, S. R., 283
Rosenbek, J. C., 183
Rosenthal, P., 156
Ross, J. C., 48, 272
Ross, R. B., 48, 272
Ruben, R. J., 273
Rubin, W., 106, 107, 161, 273
Rulnick, R., 135

Rusnov, M., 158
Russell, L., 32

Sakaguchi, S., 35
Salmon, S. J., 234, 235, 239, 241, 250
Sander, E. K., 57, 83
Sataloff, R. T., 32, 48, 78, 80, 100,
    102, 132, 162, 304
Saunders, W. H., 230, 289, 299
Sawashima, M., 167
Saxman, J. H., 107
Schaefer, S. D., 304
Schattenkerk, J. K. M. E., 305
Scheer, G. E., 277
Scherer, R. C., 78, 166, 167
Schiratzki, H., 161
Schmidt, P., 85
Schneider, E., 273, 277, 279
Schramm, V. L., 283
Schuckers, G., 26
Schuller, D. E., 263
Schwartz, D. M., 106, 180
Scott, S., 166
Seaton, D. L., 274, 292
Sedory, S. E., 267
Seibert, J. J., 157
Seibert, R. W., 157
Seltzer, S., 299
Sergeant, D. C., 49, 211
Seybold, M. W., 169
Shangold, L., 79
Shanks, J. C., 268
Shapiro, A. K., 171
Shapiro, E. S., 171
Shaw, J. D., 45, 301, 304
Shearer, W. M., 84
Shelton, R. L., 272, 279
Shipp, T., 26, 27, 103, 165, 175, 246
Shprintzen, R. J., 273, 277, 278,
    279, 288
Shumrick, D. A., 44, 53, 141
Silverman, F. H., 168
Singer, M. I., 260, 263, 264
Singer, M. L., 260, 263, 264
Shin, T., 15
Skarin, B. D., 35
Skelly, M., 277

Skolnick, M. L., 9, 278, 279, 283
Smith, B. E., 221, 245, 278
Smith, F. H., 221, 245, 278
Smith, L. R., 221, 245, 278
Smitheran, J., 27, 78, 79
Snidecor, J. C., 243, 245
Solomon, N. P., 73
Sorensen, K., 134, 159
Spiegel, D., 162, 205, 206
Spiegel, H., 162, 205, 206
Spiegel, J. H., 162, 205, 206
Spitzer, J. B., 296
Stegnjajic, A., 230
Steinfatt, T. M., 75
Stevens, K. N., 2, 19, 20, 22, 36, 189,
  297, 298
Stoller, R. J., 219
Stone, R. E., Jr., 69, 85
Stout, B. M., 277
Strife, J. L., 275
Stringer, D. A., 278
Stuteville, O. H., 281
Subtelny, J., 297
Subtelny, J. D., 297
Sudderth, J. F., 126
Suen, J. Y., 54, 106, 226, 229,
  230, 261
Sundberg, J., 27, 100
Sweet, R. D., 171
Swift, R. W., 79
Syder, O., 94

Taira, T., 220
Tait, N. A., 84, 97
Tanabe, M., 220
Tange, R. A., 305
Tardy, M. E., Jr., 276, 288
Tardy, S., 276, 288
Ternstrom, S., 27
Teter, D. L., 100
Thawley, E. E., 226, 229, 230,
  298, 299
Thome, J., 112
Thompson, A. E., 157, 270, 299
Thompson, J. W., 156, 157, 299
Thorogood, P., 273
Tickle, C., 273

Titze, I. R., 17, 21, 22, 31, 32, 78,
  166, 167
Toohill, R. J., 114
Torgerson, J. K., 238
Toriumi, D., 276
Trier, W. C., 280
Trigos, I., 280
Trosset, M. W., 73
Trost-Cardamone, J. E., 270
Trudeau, M. D., 263
Tucker, H. M., 51, 54, 150, 152, 156,
  157, 158, 159, 160, 230

Unni, K. K., 228
Uppal, K., 304

Valanne, E., 32
Van Demark, D. L., 263, 284, 285
Van Demark, D. R., 284, 285
Van Riper, C., 97
Vasquez, M. C., 280
Vaughn, C., 73
Velasco, M. G., 273
Viala, P., 158
von Leden, H., 22, 52, 63, 93
Vuorenkoski, V., 32

Walden, B. E., 106, 180
Walker, E. E., 229
Walsh, M., 73
Warren, D. W., 273, 274, 278, 292
Wasz-Hocket, O., 32
Watson, P. J., 83, 100
Watterson, T. L., 48, 94, 100, 138, 161
Weinberg, B., 233, 242, 245, 246
Weiner, H. L., 168
Weismer, G. G., 106
Weiss, D. A., 179
Welborn, P., 257
Welch, G. F., 49, 211
Wenig, B. L., 230, 260
West, R., 97
Wetmore, S. J., 299
Whitehead, R. L., 75, 297
Whittingham, S., 169
Wilcox, K., 26
Williams, C. E., 157, 189, 280, 284

Williams, J. B., 157, 280, 284
Williams, W. N., 157, 278, 280, 284
Wilson, D. K., 61, 70, 81, 120, 135, 139, 211, 297
Wilson, F. B., 21, 58, 61, 81, 86, 87, 96, 120, 126, 135, 139, 272
Wilson, K. J., 81, 120, 135, 139
Winslow, 273
Witzel, M. A., 275, 278
Wolfe, S. A., 275, 280, 281
Wolfe, V. I., 75, 221, 280, 281
Wolski, W., 169
Woo, P., 79
Wood, B. G., 230
Wood, R. P., 230
Woods, J., 230
Woodson, G. E., 178
Woolff, P., 32

Wortham, D. G., 49
Wyke, B., 37

Yahr, M. D., 165
Yanagihara, N., 75, 97
Yanagisawa, E., 45
Yang, S., 188
Yorkston, K. M., 183
Youngstrom, K. A., 239, 241, 242, 250, 251, 279
Yoshioka, H., 78
Ysunza, A., 273, 280

Zagzebski, J. A., 9
Zarajczyk, D. R., 273
Zemlin, W. R., 8, 13, 15, 81, 207, 241
Zitsch, R. P., 157
Zwitman D. H., 104, 160

Subject Index

Abduction paralysis. *See* Vagus nerve lesions

Abductor spastic dysphonia, 177–178

ABR. *See* Auditory brainstem response

Acanthosis, 96

Accelerometer, 80

Adduction paralysis. *See* Vagus nerve lesions

Adductor spastic dysphonia. *See* Spastic (spasmodic) dysphonia

Adenoidectomy, 273–275

Aeromechanical instrumentation, 78–80

Aging voice, 33–35

    fundamental frequency, 34

    vocal intensity, 34

    vocal tremor, 34

    voice quality, 35

AIDS, 305

Alaryngeal phonation, 225–268

    case example, 259–260

    extrinsic sources, 232

    intrinsic sources, 231–232

    prosthetic devices (intrinsic), 232

    rehabilitation, 260

    therapy, 225–268

Alcohol. *See* Laryngeal cancer

American Joint Committee for Cancer, staging, 227–228

American Psychiatric Association classification system of mental disorders, 195–196

Amyotrophic lateral sclerosis (ALS), 166–168

    classical presentation, 166

    communication aids, 168

    phonation disorders, 167

    pitch, 167

    prognosis, 166

Anarthria, 152

Angiography, 48

Ansa cervicalis nerve, 159

Antibiotics, 50

Antihistamines, 50

Anti-inflammatory and antiedematous, 50

    drugs, 50

Aperiodicity, 75

Aphonia, 72, 194
  treatment, 203–204
Artificial larynx, 250–251
Arytenoid cartilage, 11, 14
Arytenoidectomy, 158
Assimilated nasality. See Hypernasality
Asthma, 304–305
Ataxic dysarthria, 163
Auditory brainstem response (ABR), 174
Aurex neovox electronic larynx, 237
Autonomic nervous system, 190–191

Basic metabolic rate (BMR), 190
Behavioral modification, 40, 126
Biofeedback, 145, 180–181, 206
Blepharospasm, 164
Blom-Singer Voice Prosthesis, 263
  airway resistance, 260–262
  insufflation test, 263–264
  TEP procedure, 260–262
  tracheostomal valve, 266–267
  voice restoration, 264–266
Botulinum toxin (BOTOX), 178–179
Breathiness, 73, 76, 79
Buccal speech, 235–236

Cancer
  epidemiology, 229
  etiology, 226
  symptoms, 229
  treatment, 230–232
  types, 226–229
Case history, 60–63
Central nervous system, 150
  innervation, 149
Cephalometrics. See Radiology
Cerebral palsy, 172
Cheerleader's voice, 110–111
  case study of, 110–113
Chrondromalacia (congenital), 303
Communication aids (augmentative),
  167–168
Computed tomography, 48–49
Congenital chondromalacia, 303
Consonant injection. See Esophageal
  speech
Contact ulcers, 138, 140–142
  case example, 145–148

description, 138
etiologies, 140–141
evaluation procedures, 141–142
pathogenesis, 138
therapy, 143–145
voice characteristics, 138–140
Conversion dysphonia, 204–205
CO_2 laser surgery, 53–54
Cooper-Rand Electronic Speech Aid,
  232–233
Cordectomy or hemilaryngectomy, 230
Corniculates cartilages, 14
Coup de glotte, 145
  description, 100–101
  elimination of, 145
Craniofacial anomalies. See Orofacial
  clefting
Cricoid cartilage, 11–12
Cri du chat syndrome, 303–304
Cul-de-sac resonance, 292
Cuneiforms, 14
Cyst, 305

Deafness (hearing impairment), 295–297
Deglutition, 3, 14–15
Denasality. See Hyponasality
Digital manipulation of larynx, 206
Digital Speech Spectrograph, 78. See
  also Spectrograph
Diplophonia, 76–77, 153, 179
Dysarthria, 34, 152, 163–17
Dyspnea, 154
Dysphonia, 74–77
  breathiness, 76
  diplophonia, 74, 76–77, 96
  factors, 74–77
  hoarseness, 74–76
  tension, 76
Dystonia, 164–165

Edema, 141
Electroglottograph (EEG), 22, 77–78
Electromyography (EMG), 9–10, 17, 22,
  35–37
Endoscopy, 44–45
  fiber optic, 45
  laryngoscope, 43–44
  nasopharyngolaryngoscope, 44

stroboscope, 45–48
videostroboscope, 45–46
Epiglottis, 11, 12, 14
Erythema, 141
Esophageal phonation, 238–241
  consonant injection, 240
  glossopress, 239–240
  inhalation, 240–241
  injection, 239
  methods of air intake, 238
Esophageal speech, 238
  case example, 248–250
  goals, 258–259
  mechanisms involved, 238
  methods of air intake, 238
  perceptual & acoustic characteristics,
    242–245
  phrasing, 255–256
  reduced loudness, 243
  steps in therapy, 247
Esophageal speech phrasing, 255–256
Esophageal voice production, 253–255
  burp and belch, 253
  consonant injection, 253
  glossopress or glossopharyngeal press,
    254–255
  inhalation, 254
Esophagus, 3–5
Essential tremor (organic voice tremor),
  172–173
Excessive tension, 73–74
Extrinsic laryngeal muscle, 15

Falsetto. *See* Puberphonia. *See also*
  Organic mutational falsetto
Fiber optic endoscopy, 45
Focal dystonia, 256–257
Frequency. *See* Pitch evaluation. *See*
  also Voice characteristics
Functional dysphonia, 188. *See also*
  Psychogenic voice disorder
Functional esophageal speech, 258–259

Gelfer Rating Scale, 89–90
Gilles de al Tourette's syndrome,
  171–172
Glossopress (glossopharyngeal press).
  See Esophageal speech

Granulomas. *See* Contact ulcers

Hammer and anvil action, 141
Hard glottal attack, 98, 100–101,
  141, 145
Hearing impairment, 295–297
  loudness, 297–298
  pitch, 297
  resonance, 298
  voice therapy, 297
Hierarchy analysis, 123, 125
Hoarseness, 74–76, 94
Hyoid bone, 11
Hyperfunctional voice, 71–73. *See also*
  Spasticity of voice; Adductor
  spasmodic dysphonia
Hypernasality (nasality), 270–272,
  291–293
  deafness, 289
  evaluation, 272–273
  rating scale, 272
  therapy, 284–289
  treatment, 277–280
  vs. hyponasality, 291
Hyperrhinolalia. *See* Hypernasality
Hypnosis, 205–206
Hypofunctional voice, 71–73. *See also*
  Breathiness
Hyponasality, 80, 289–294
  and nasal breathing, 292
  referral procedures, 293–294
  vs. hypernasality, 291

Idiopathic. *See* Vagus nerve lesions,
  etiologies
Inadequate breath support, 108–110
Indirect laryngoscopy, 43–44
Inhalation method. *See* Esophageal
  speech
Innervation of larynx and pharynx
  central nervous system (CNS), 150
  peripheral nervous system (PNS),
    150–152
  recurrent laryngeal nerve, 151–152
  superior laryngeal nerve, 139, 152
Intelligibility of esophageal speech,
  245–247
Intensity. *See* Loudness measurement

Interferon therapy, 300–301
Intrinsic laryngeal muscle, 15

Jako forceps, 52–53

Keratosis, 96

La belle indifference, 194
Lamina propria, 18, 20
  conus elasticus, 18
  vocal ligament, 18
Laryngeal cancer (carcinoma)
  epidimiological factors, 229
  etiology, 226
  staging, 227–228
  treatment, 230
Laryngeal paralysis, 158
Laryngeal polyps, 301
Laryngeal surgery, 51–53
  anesthesia, 51–52
  biopsy, 51–53
  forceps, 52–53
  intubation (extubation), 51–52,
    140–141
Laryngeal trauma, 60, 304
Laryngeal web, 60, 303
Laryngectomy, 230–231
Laryngology, 44, 47, 52–53
Laryngopharynx, 3, 5, 11
Laryngoscope. See Endoscopy
Laryngoscopy, indirect, 43–44
Larynx, 2, 10–21
  arytenoid cartilages, 11, 13, 93
  blood supply, 20–21
  corniculate cartilages, 11, 14
  cricoid cartilage, 11, 12
  cricothyroid muscle, 11, 16–18, 24
  cuneiform cartilages, 11, 14
  diagrams, 12–13, 16, 19
  epiglottis, 11, 12, 14
  epithelium, 20
  extrinsic muscles, 11, 15
  false vocal folds (ventricular), 11, 18, 20
  glottis, 17–18, 21–22, 24, 29, 34, 36
  hyoid bone, 11, 13, 19
  innervation, 16, 139–140
  interaytenoid muscles (transverse and
    oblique), 11, 17

intrinsic muscles, 11, 15
  lateral cricoarytenoid muscle, 11, 17
  membranes, 11, 18
  posterior cricoarytenoid muscle,
    11, 17
  sex characteristics, 13
  thyroarytenoid muscle, 11, 15, 24
  thyroid cartilage, 11–12
  ventricle, 3
  vocal folds, 2, 14–15, 18–21, 23–25,
    32–36, 38, 40, 43–44
  vocalis muscle, 11, 15, 20
Laser surgery. See CO_2 laser surgery
Leukoplakia. See Keratosis
Levator veli palatini, 5, 9–10
Limbic system, 191
Lou Gehrig's disease. See Amyotropic
  lateral sclerosis (ALS)
Loudness (intensity) measurement, 79–80

Magnetic resonance imaging (MRI), 49
Malignancy. See Laryngeal cancer
Maxillary advancement, 275
Maximum phonation duration (MPD),
  83–85
Medical referral, 56–58
Menstrual periods and the voice, 107
  speaking abusively, 107
Microsurgery. See Laryngeal surgery
Multiple sclerosis (MS), 168–169
  clinical manifestations, 168
  etiology, 168
  lesions, 168
  speech disorders, 168–169
Musical scale frequency values, 24
Mutational falsetto, 207–210
Myasthenia gravis (laryngis), 169–170
  forms of, 169
  speech, 169–170
Myoelastic-aerodynamic theory, 22
Myotomy, 264

Nasal airflow, 78–80. See also
  Aeromechanical instrumentation
Nasal cavity, 3–4
  conchea, 4
  cranial nerve, 4
  eustachian (auditory) tubes, 4

pharyngeal tonsils (adenoid tissue), 4
torus tubarius, 4, 6
Nasal consonants, 4, 10
Nasal listening devices, 293
Nasal polyps, 290
Nasality. *See* Hypernasality
Nasometer (Kay Elemetrics), 287
Nasopharyngoscopy. *See* Endoscopy
Nasopharynx, 3–5
Neolung, 241
Nerve anastomosis, 159
Neurogenic voice disorder, 179
Neurology, 41

Obturation (velopharynx), 282–283
Oral cavity, 3–5
    dentition, 4
    examination of, 11, 22, 43–50
    facial pillars, 4
    hard palate, 4
    lips, 4
    palatine tonsils, 4
    posterior pharyngeal wall, 4
    tongue, 4
    velum (soft palate), 4, 8–10
Oral panendoscopy. *See* Endoscopy
Organic mutational falsetto, 218
Organic voice tremor (essential tremor), 165
Orofacial clefting, 272–273
    audiological and otological
      considerations, 273
    communication disorder, 273
    dental orthodontic & prosthodontic
      aspects, 272
    etiological factors, 272
    maxillary advancement, 275
    surgical considerations, 272
Oromandibular dystonia, 164
Oropharynx, 3, 5
Otolaryngology: Head and Neck
    Surgery (Association), 40–41

P-E junction (pharyngoesophageal),
    241–242
PERCI-IIC instrument, 80. *See also*
    Aeromechanical instrumentation
Pachydermia, 96
Palatal lift prosthesis, 183

Palatoglossus muscle, 8
Palatopharyngeal structures, 8. *See also*
    Velopharyngeal closure
Papillomatosis (papillomas), 298–301
    description, 299
    interferon therapy, 300–301
    symptoms, 299
    treatment, 299–300
Paralysis (laryngeal),
    abduction, 158–159
    adduction, 159–163
Parkinsonism, 165–166
Partial laryngectomy. *See* Cordectomy or
    hemilaryngectomy
Pathology (medical specialty), 42–43
Patulous eustachian tubes, 291
P-E Junction, 231, 264
Peripheral nervous system (PNS), 150–152
    innervation, 150
Pharyngeal cavity, 4–6. *See also*
    Velopharyngeal closure
    diagram, 6
    inferior constrictor, 5
    middle constrictor, 5
    superior constrictor, 5, 9
Pharyngeal flap surgery, 280–282
Pharyngeal speech, 236–238
Pharyngoplasty. *See also* Pharyngeal flap
    surgery
    Teflon, 280
Phonation, phase of, 2, 22–24
Phonation theory, 22–23
    airflow and laryngeal airway, 23–24,
      27
    Bernoulli's principle, 23
    myoelastic-aerodynamic, 22
    neurochronaxic, 22
    resistance, 23
    vibrating vocal folds (glottal tone),
      23–24, 27
Phonosurgery, 51–53
Physician's Desk Reference (PDR), 50
Pitch, changing of, 25–26, 143–145,
    210–212, 242–243
Pitch evaluation, 64–67
    basal pitch, ceiling pitch, range, 68
    habitual, 67–68

jitter (perturbation), 25–27
   optimal, 67–70
Pitch pipe, 64–68
Plastic surgery, 42
Polyps, 60, 79
Progressive relaxation, 205
Pseudobulbar palsy, 163
Psychiatry (medical specialty), 41–42
Psychogenic voice disorders, 187–224
   aphonia (conversion), 194
   case examples, 192–194
   diagnosis, 188–189
   dysphonia, 194
   endocrine system affects, 190–191
   evaluation procedures, 199–201
   nature of, 188–189
   physiological changes under stress, 190
   somatoform disorders, 194
   specific disorders, 194
   therapy, 201–203
   vocal symptoms, 189–190
   vocal symptoms of dysphonia, 194, 196
Psychology, 41–42
Puberphonia (mutational falsetto),
   207–210
   adolescence, 208
   case example, 214–215
   evaluation procedures, 213–214
   factors in sexual maturation, 209
   laryngeal growth factor, 207
   management, 213–214
   nature of, 207
   organic mutational falsetto, 218
   puberty, 207
   special considerations in therapy,
      216–217
   voice characteristics, 210–212

Radiology, 42, 48
   angiography, 48
   fluroscopy, 48
   magnetic resonance imaging, 49
   roentgenography, 48
   tomography (CT scans), 48–49
   ultrasound, 50
   xeroradiography, 49
Reinforcement, 123–125
Reinke's edema, 52

Relaxation therapy. *See* Progressive
   relaxation, 181
Resonance disorder, 269–305
Resonance, evaluation of, 80. *See
   also* Nasal listening devices;
   Aeromechanical instrumentation
Respiration, evaluation of, 81–83
   chest and diaphragm movement, 83
   expiratory reserve volume (ERV), 81
   inadequate support for speech,
      108–110
   inspiratory reserve volume (IRV), 81
   magnetometers, 83
   plethysmography, 83
   tidal volume (TV), 81
   vital capacity (VC), 81
   wet spirometer (respirometer), 82
Respirometer. *See* Wet spirometer
Respitrace, 83
Reverse phonation, 115
Reye's syndrome, 156
Rhinolalia aperta. *See* Hypernasality
Roentgenography (x ray), 48

S/Z ratio, 84–85
Servox electronic larynx, 235
Singing, abusive style, 98, 100–103
Smoking, effect on voice, 63, 98,
   106–107
   cause of cancer, 226
   cause of polyps, 107
   marijuana, 107
Spastic dysarthria, 163
Spastic (spasmodic) dysphonia (adductor
   type), 164, 173–178
   abductor type, 177–178
   case example, 183–185
   description, 173
   neurogenic basis, 174
   psychogenic history, 173
   terms used, 173
   treatment, 176–177
   vocal symptoms, 175–176
Spastic torticollis, 164
Spasticity of voice, 74. *See also* Spastic
   (spasmodic) dysphonia
Speaking, abusive style, 98, 103, 105–107

Speaking rate, 245
Spectrograph, 30, 77–78
Speech appliances. *See* Obturation
Speech-language pathologist, 222–223
  psychology of voice, 222–223
Stage fright, 222
Stoma management. *See* Tracheostomy
Stoma noise, 257
Stroboscopy, 45–48
Suprabulbal palsy, 163

Teflon injection, 283–284
Teflon laryngoplasty, 51, 159–163
  contraindications for, 160–161
  documentation of change, 161–163
  indications for, 160
  voice characteristics following, 161
Tensor veli palatini, 8
Thyroarytenoid, 16
Thyroid cartilage, 11–12
Thyroid gland. *See* Vagus nerve lesions
Tokyo artificial larynx, 233–234
Tomography, 48
Tone focus, 182–183
Tonsillectomy, 273–275
Tracheoesophageal puncture (TEP),
  260–267
Tracheoesophageal voice. *See* Alaryngeal
  phonation; Tracheoesophageal puncture
  (TEP)
Tracheostoma valve, 262
Tracheostomy (tracheotomy), 231
Transsexual voice disorder, 219–222
  hormonal treatment, 219
  pitch factors, 220–222
  surgical alteration of larynx, 219–220

Ultrasound, 50
Upper respirator infection (URI),
  105–106
Uvulus, 8

Vagus nerve lesions, 153–154
  arytenoidectomy, 158–159
  etiologies, 157–158
  in infants, 157–158
  nerve-muscle pedical reinnervation,
    159

positions of vocal folds, 153–154
  recurrent laryngeal nerve, 154
  superior laryngeal nerve, 154, 156
  symptoms, 153
  treatment, 158
Velopharyngeal closure, 5, 7–10. *See
  also* Velopharyngeal structures;
  Pharyngoplasty; Pharyngeal flat
  surgery
  examination techniques, 294–295
  insufficiency, 269
  management techniques, 277–289
  movement, 5, 9
  terms pertaining to, 269–270
Velopharyngeal structures, 5–10
  diagram, 7
  innervation, 151–152
  levator veli palatini, 5, 9–10
  palatoglossus, 8
  palatopharyngeus, 8
  port, 4–6, 8–10, 88
  tensor veli palatini, 8
  uvulus, 8
  velum, 4–10
Ventricular dysphonia, 301–302
  digital pressure, 302
  pitch, 302
  relaxation training, 302
VisiPitch, 66–69, 78–79, 144
Vocal Abuse, 207. *See also* Contact
  ulcers; Vocal Nodules; Erythema; Edema
  case history form (adult), 121–123, 142
  case history form (child), 118–120, 142
  check list, 124, 142
  forms of, 93–94, 207
  hierarchy of, 123–125
  in polyps, 135
  psychogenic factor, 131
  Vocal Abuse Reduction Program
    (VARP), 135
Vocal folds, 2, 18, 21
Vocal fry, 31, 139, 142
Vocal Nodules, 94–116. *See also* Vocal
  abuse; Contact Ulcers; Erythema;
  Edema
  case example, 133–137
  etiologies, 98–99

evaluation procedures, 116–131, 137–138
group therapy, 130
pathogenesis, 94
phonosurgery, 51–53, 131–132
surgery for, 131–132
telephone therapy, 130
therapy, 116–131
voice characteristics, 96–97
Vocal quality, 27–29
aphonia, 72
breathiness, 73
evaluation instrumentation, 77
electroglottograph, 77–78
spectrograph, 77
excessive tension, 73–74
hyperfunctional voice, 71–72
hypofunctional voice, 71
spasticity, 74
whisper, 72–73
Vocal tract, 2–3, 5, 25, 29, 32–34
hypopharynx, 3–5
laryngopharynx, 3–5
nasopharynx, 3–5
oropharynx, 3–5
Vocal tremors, 37, 39–40, 165, 172–173
Voice characteristics (normal), 24–33
age & sex characteristics, 32–33
frequency (F_0) or pitch, 24
intensity or loudness, 26–27, 34
jitter (perturbation), 25–26, 75

periodicity, 31–32
quality, 27–29, 35, 243–245
registers (pulse, modal, loft), 29–32, 49
resonance, 32
shimmer, 27
Voice parameters, evaluation of, 63
pitch, 63–66
pitch range, 70
Voice evaluation, case example, 90–92
Voice fundamental frequency (F_0) or pitch, 24
Voice profile, 86–89, 96, 117
Voice screening, 58–60

Waldeyer's ring. *See* Adenoidectomy
Western Electric 5C electrolarynx, 234–235
Wet Spirometer (respirometer), 82
Wheezing. *See* Asthma
Whisper, 72–73
Wilson's disease, 170–171
Wilson and Rice voice profile, 86–89, 96, 117

Xeroradiography, 49
X ray. *See* Radiology

Yawn-sign technique, 181
Yelling, 99
etiology of vocal nodules, 98–100

About the Author

DR. JAMES L. CASE is an Associate Professor of Speech and Hearing Science at Arizona State University in Tempe, Arizona. He received his M.S. and Ph.D. degrees from the University of Utah. He is a member of the American Speech–Language–Hearing Association, the American Cleft Palate Craniofacial Association, the International Association of Orofacial Myology, the International Association of Laryngectomees, and the Arizona Speech–Language–Hearing Association. He is a Fellow in the American Speech–Language–Hearing Association. Dr. Case has been chosen as the outstanding teacher in the College of Liberal Arts at Arizona State University.